Health
COMMUNICATION

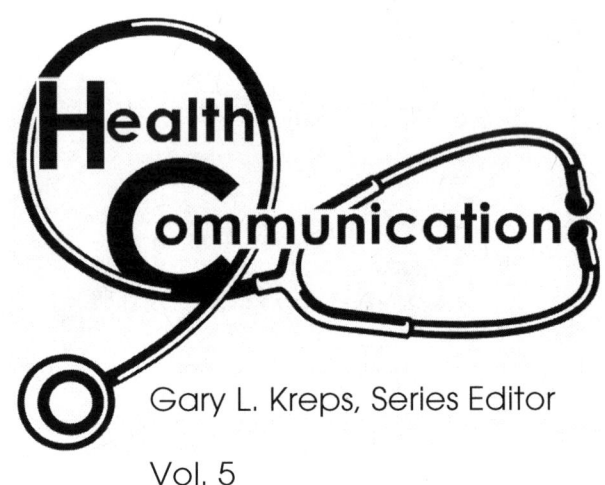

Gary L. Kreps, Series Editor

Vol. 5

The Health Communication series is part of
the Peter Lang Media and Communication list.
Every volume is peer reviewed and meets
the highest quality standards for content and production.

PETER LANG
New York • Washington, D.C./Baltimore • Bern
Frankfurt • Berlin • Brussels • Vienna • Oxford

Health
COMMUNICATION

Strategies for Developing
Global Health Programs

Edited by
Do Kyun Kim,
Arvind Singhal,
& Gary L. Kreps

PETER LANG
New York • Washington, D.C./Baltimore • Bern
Frankfurt • Berlin • Brussels • Vienna • Oxford

Library of Congress Cataloging-in-Publication Data

Strategies for developing global health programs / edited by Do Kyun Kim,
Arvind Singhal, Gary L. Kreps.
p. cm. — (Health communication; vol. 5)
Includes bibliographical references and index.
1. Health Communication—methods. 2. Health Promotion—methods.
3. International Cooperation. 4. World Health. I. Kim, Do kyun, editor of compilation.
II. Singhal, Arvind, editor of compilation. III. Kreps, Gary L., editor of compilation.
IV. Series: Health communication (New York, N.Y.); v. 5. 2153-1277
RA418 362.1—dc23 2013026977
ISBN 978-1-4331-1865-4 (hardcover)
ISBN 978-1-4331-1864-7 (paperback)
ISBN 978-1-4539-1196-9 (e-book)
ISSN 2153-1277

Bibliographic information published by **Die Deutsche Nationalbibliothek**
Die Deutsche Nationalbibliothek lists this publication in the "Deutsche
Nationalbibliografie"; detailed bibliographic data is available
on the Internet at http://dnb.d-nb.de/.

The paper in this book meets the guidelines for permanence and durability
of the Committee on Production Guidelines for Book Longevity
of the Council of Library Resources.

© 2014 Peter Lang Publishing, Inc., New York
29 Broadway, 18th floor, New York, NY 10006
www.peterlang.com

All rights reserved.
Reprint or reproduction, even partially, in all forms such as microfilm,
xerography, microfiche, microcard, and offset strictly prohibited.

Printed in the United States of America

Contents

Introduction: Design, Implementation, and Evaluation of Health Communication Strategies for Global Health Promotion   1
Do Kyun Kim, Arvind Singhal, & Gary Kreps

Leveraging Technology

Chapter 1
Strategies and Principles for Using Mass and Online/Digital Media in Health Communication Campaigns   13
Charles K. Atkin, Michigan State University
Ronald E. Rice, University of California Santa Barbara

Chapter 2
Developing and Testing Mobile Health Applications to Affect Behavior Change: Lessons from the Field   37
Andrew Isham, Bret R. Shaw, & Dave Gustafson, University of Wisconsin-Madison

Chapter 3
A Primer for Using Mobile Apps and Social Media in Healthcare   51
Carolyn Lauckner & Pamela Whitten, Michigan State University

Chapter 4
Digital Games: The SECRET of Alternative Health Realities   67
Hua Wang, University at Buffalo, The State University of New York
Arvind Singhal, University of Texas at El Paso

Performance and Narrative Power

Chapter 5
Entertainment Education Saves Lives and Improves Health: Key Steps to Developing Effective Programs   83
Caroline Jacoby, Jane Brown, Uttara Bharath Kumar, Rajiv N. Rimal, & Sanjanthi Velu, Johns Hopkins University

Chapter 6
Conversations about Cancer (CAC): A National and Global Strategy for Impacting Family and Medical Interactions   101
Wayne A. Beach, Kyle Gutzmer & David M. Dozier, San Diego State University
Mary K. Buller & David B. Buller, Klein Buendel, Inc.

Chapter 7
Narrative-based Health Communication Interventions: Using Survivor Stories to Increase Breast Cancer Knowledge and Promote Mammography   118
Tess Thompson & Matthew W. Kreuter, Washington University in St. Louis

Chapter 8
Drama as a Rhetorical Health Communication Strategy   134
Anat Gesser-Edelsburg, University of Haifa

Applied Communication Strategies

Chapter 9
Communication Network Analysis for the Diffusion of Health:
Identifying Key Individuals 153
Do Kyun Kim, *University of Louisiana at Lafayette*
James W. Dearing, *Michigan State University*

Chapter 10
The Positive Deviance Approach to Designing and Implementing
Health Communication Interventions 174
Arvind Singhal, *University of Texas at El Paso*

Chapter 11
Using Theory and Audience Research to Convey the Human
Implications of Climate Change 190
Melinda R. Weathers, *Clemson University*
Edward Maibach, *George Mason University*
Matthew Nisbet, *American University*

Chapter 12
Integrating the Diffusion of Innovations and Social Marketing for Designing
an HIV/AIDS-Prevention Strategy among a Hard-to-Reach Population 208
Do Kyun Kim, *University of Louisiana at Lafayette*

Community Participatory Design

Chapter 13
Community Participatory Design of Health Communication Interventions 227
Linda Neuhauser, *University of California, Berkeley*
Gary L. Kreps, *George Mason University*
S. Leonard Syme, *University of California, Berkeley*

Chapter 14
Faith-based Community Health Interventions: Incorporating Cultural Ecology,
the Social Ecological Framework, and Gender Analysis 244
Kari Hartwig, *Walden University*

Chapter 15
Designing Logos for Health Campaigns: Convergence of Semiotics
and the Diffusion of Innovations 262
Do Kyun Kim, *University of Louisiana at Lafayette*

Health Advocacy and Activism

Chapter 16
Strategic Communication for Health Advocacy and Social Change 281
Gary L. Kreps, *George Mason University*

Chapter 17
Health Activism as Resistance: MOSOP as a Site
of Culture-Centered Resistance in Niger Delta Region of Nigeria 297
Mohan J. Dutta, *National University of Singapore & Purdue University*

Valuing Data

Chapter 18
National Health Communication Surveillance Systems 317
Bradford W. Hesse, David E. Nelson, Richard P. Moser, Kelly D. Blake,
& Wen-ying Sylvia Chou, National Cancer Institute
Lila J Finney, Mayo Clinic
Ellen Burke Beckjord, University of Pittsburgh

Chapter 19
Cultural Beacons in Health Communication:
Leveraging Overlooked Indicators and Grassroots Wisdoms 334
Laurel J. Felt, University of Southern California
Lucía Durá & Arvind Singhal, University of Texas at El Paso

Chapter 20
Evaluating Health Communication Interventions 352
Gary L. Kreps, George Mason University

Editors and Chapter Contributors 369
Index 381

We dedicate this book to the enduring legacy
of Everett M. Rogers and Charles Atkin.

Introduction

Design, Implementation, and Evaluation of Health Communication Strategies for Global Health Promotion

Do Kyun Kim, *University of Louisiana at Lafayette*
Arvind Singhal, *University of Texas-El Paso*
Gary Kreps, *George Mason University*

The word *Ubuntu*, common to the Bantu languages of Southern Africa, represents a communicative ethic, a humanist philosophy, and a world view of interconnectedness. It essentially means "I am what I am because of what we all are." For communication scholars, *Ubuntu* finds utterance in symbolic interactionism, Kenneth Burke's dramatism, relational dialectics, and other theories that believe that an individual's identity is defined through their interactions with others. This communicative foundation provides the reason for why the health of an individual, a community, a nation state, or the world is intimately intertwined. When one person experiences suffering, they do not suffer alone. When one individual is afflicted, we are all affected.

If we pose the question, "What do people suffer from the most?" political scientists may refer to "wars." Economists may emphasize "poverty." Postmodern critical thinkers may say "power inequality." Others may say, ill-health, a condition that has been a constant companion in humankind's journey. Infant mortality may be down by millions and life expectancies up by decades; however illness and suffering are an inseparable part of our lives. Modern and traditional medicine can fix what may be physically broken, but healing comes wrapped in a relational and communicative package—a compassionate touch, social support, or life-saving information. The present book, through its collection of diverse essays, takes a communicative route to healing and well-being.

Over the past decades, the field of health communication has expanded rapidly through multiple theoretical frames, accumulated empirical research, and a plethora of lessons learned. With growing public and policy interest in meeting global development and health goals, e.g., the Millennium Development Goals (MDGs), the stock of health communication scholars and practitioners has risen sharply. Courses in health communication have mushroomed in schools of communication, public health, nursing, social work, and international development. Today, health communication scholars work hand-in-hand with practitioners of governmental agencies, public health organizations, and NGOs, both domestically and internationally, addressing complex health topics such as HIV/AIDS, infant and maternal mortality, substance abuse, obesity and diabetes, and mental and psychological illnesses.

Promotion of healthy behaviors and prevention of disease are inextricably linked to cultural understandings of health and well-being, relational and kinship structures, as also public awareness of health, health literacy, and behavior change. Health communication scholarship and practice can substantially and strategically contribute to people living, safer, healthier, and happier lives. Strategy, guided by research and deep cultural understandings, can help close the gap between knowledge and practice of healthy behaviors. The present book represents a concrete step in that direction.

In the 21st century, health communication as a field of scholarship and practice has been increasingly globalized, and the rapid interactivity and connectivity offered by the Internet, mobile platforms, and social media have greatly accelerated the diffusion and consumption of global health information and programs. Concurrently, there is a growing movement toward increased localization of health interventions, community participation, and reverence for indigenous knowledge, grassroots epistemologies, and cultural metrics of evaluation and assessment. The rise of the positive deviance approach is illustrative of this inside-out, bottom-up, community-centric view of health and well-being.

The present book establishes a strategic framework for guiding global and local health practice by describing, analyzing, and illustrating a wide range of health communication interventions in diverse cultural contexts. The book values a multi-disciplinary approach to understanding and influencing human behavior, providing readers theoretical frameworks coupled with "how-to" knowledge and applied case studies. We expect the readers of this book will not only be introduced to the foundational tenets of health communication, but will also be able to see its applications to improve global health and well-being.

Notable features of this book include a wide range of state-of-the-art strategies which can be applied to health communication interventions and provide readers with *practical guidelines about how to design, implement, and evaluate effective health communication interventions.* Few books to date have synthesized a broad range of relevant theories and strategies of health communication that are applicable globally and provide clear advice about *how to apply* such strategies based on practical guidelines and empirical evidence. Here, this book will fill the perceived gap between academic research and practical skills in health communication, simultaneously suggesting innovative future research agendas and opportunities. The contents of this book, all 20 chapters, draw upon the extensive professional experiences of the chapter contributors. The book is organized around six primary themes that characterize key perspectives on strategic health communication interventions.

Thematic section #1 on *Leveraging Technology* notes how the rapid and growing adoption of new communication technologies provides health professionals with many unprecedented opportunities to promote health. Technology must be leveraged to meet the unique needs, expectations, and competencies of different audiences to communicate relevant health information meaningfully and influentially. This section consists of 4 chapters specifically describing strategic use of e-health communication applications.

Chapter 1 entitled *"Strategies and Principles for Using Mass and Online/Digital Media in Health Communication Campaigns"* presents strategic phases and components of the use of mass, online, and mobile media in health communication campaigns. This chapter primarily focuses on campaign design frameworks, formative evaluation, types of effects, types of messages, message content and style, media channels, quantitative dissemination factors, and summative evaluation, referencing a wide array of resources and case studies. Chapter 2, *"Developing and Testing Mobile Health Applications to Affect Behavior Change: Lessons from the Field,"* deals with mobile health (mHealth) applications to be potentially powerful behavioral change tools. mHealth researchers at the Center for Health Enhancement Systems Studies at the University of Wisconsin-Madison share their experiences related to this rapidly expanding field of research and discuss what they have learned about theory-guided design, mobile platform selection, understanding user experience, social and familial implications, feature selection, clinician involvement in design, privacy concerns, keeping up with technological advancement, integrating social media, and provision of hardware to test subjects. Chapter 3, *"A Primer for Using Mobile Apps and Social Media in Healthcare,"* discusses two increasingly important models of health information and healthcare delivery: mobile apps and social media. As smartphones are increasingly adopted and with the heavy use of websites like Facebook, Twitter, and YouTube, this chapter will highlight examples of how mobile phones and social media have been used in health and will review research that has been done in this area. It will also discuss methods of implementing and evaluating these technologies in health initiatives, with a focus on creating user-centered, well-designed tools. Chapter 4, *"Digital Games: The SECRET of Alternative Health Realities,"* investigates the use of digital games for health promotion. It does so in three parts: The chapter first points out the distinct media attributes of digital games that are relevant to health communication; second, explicates, with recent cases, the major functions of health games and summarizes them in an acronym, SECRET; and finally concludes with lessons learned for intervention design and evaluation of health games, as well as future implications.

Thematic section #2 on *Performance and Narrative Power* examines the potential for using performance, narratives, and entertainment-education as unique communication tools to enhance the effectiveness of health communication programs. If used strategically, performance- and narrative-based interventions can engage audience members encouraging health education, informed health decision making, and the adoption of recommended health behaviors. There are 4 chapters in this section.

Chapter 5, *"Entertainment Education Saves Lives and Improves Health: Key Steps to Developing Effective Programs,"* reinforces that EE works and outlines a step-by-step process of how to design, implement, and evaluate quality EE programs. Each step in the process is illustrated by the award-winning Zambian TV drama, *Club Risky Business*. This chapter provides the building blocks of how to develop similarly powerful EE programs. Chapter 6, *"Conversations about Cancer (CAC): A National and Global Strategy for Impacting Family and Medical Interactions,"* reports how these basic research findings have been transformed into a parallel project entitled Conversations about Cancer (CAC). The foundation for CAC is *The Cancer Play*, a unique and professional theatrical production adapting *A Natural History of Family Cancer* to the stage. This chapter includes preliminary and compelling findings from Phase I viewings of *The Cancer Play*, and describes the methods employed to design, implement, and evaluate CAC outcomes. Chapter 7, *"Narrative-based Health Communication Interventions: Using Survivor Stories to Increase Breast Cancer Knowledge and Promote Mammography"* introduces a narrative strategy based on a project that employed a three-step biographic narrative interview process. This chapter shows important predictors of a viewer's being engaged in a story and having positive thoughts about it, comparing a narrative DVD to an informational DVD about breast cancer. Chapter 8, *"Drama as a Rhetorical Health Communication Strategy"* explain how drama can be used as an effective means of intervention on health issues while employing rhetorical elements in creating the dramatic narrative. This chapter also provides researchers and practitioners in the field of health communication with a strategy for a) building a drama that is an effective means to convey public health issues and b) conducting evaluations measuring the effectiveness of drama.

Thematic section #3 on *Applied Communication Strategies* examines how communication strategies can be informed by relevant theories and applied to create effective communication interventions for health promotion. The chapters in this section suggest how theory can inform directed change within complex social systems, taking into account the powerful influences of culture, socio-political systems, and historical precedent. This section has another 4 chapters dealing with various applied communication strategies.

Chapter 9, *"Identifying Key Individuals for the Diffusion of Health Information and Practices: A Communication Network Method"* is about how to harness the existing personal influence of certain key individuals for many health communication projects. Specifically, this chapter focuses on identification of such individuals, commonly referred to as *opinion leaders*, in the diffusion process. The identification of opinion leaders is explained in two sequential steps: a) communication network data collection and b) network analysis. This chapter briefly explains how to design an intervention that employs an opinion leader strategy. Chapter 10, *"The Positive Deviance Approach to Designing and Implementing Health Communication Interventions,"* introduces Positive Deviance (PD), highlighting the solutions to intractable health problems that lie hidden within the community. This chapter begins by describing how PD sensibilities guide the formative research process to design a family planning and maternal-child health communication intervention in India, and explains how the PD approach can be applied to global health promotion with international cases. Chapter 11, *"Using Theory and Audience Research to Convey the Human Implications of Climate Change"* describes how to use framing theory, audience segmentation, and message testing research to inform the development of communication resources. This chapter additionally offers the tips for operating training workshops for public health professionals seeking to engage their communities in climate change. Chapter 12, "*Integrating the Diffusion of Innovations and Social Marketing for Designing an HIV/AIDS-Prevention Strategy among a Hard-to-Reach Population*" presents an advanced health intervention design using a strategic amalgam of the diffusion of innovations and social marketing. This intervention is designed to maximize the effectiveness of HIV prevention in what is considered a hard-to-reach population—young African-American men who have sex with men (MSM)—in New Orleans, Louisiana. This technique can also be applicable to a diversity of health interventions targeting people with differences.

Thematic section #4 on *Community Participatory Design* emphasizes the importance of involving audiences in the design, implementation, evaluation, and maintenance of health communication interventions. The section focuses on how health communication professionals co-construct health interventions with their target populations through participatory processes that meet the needs, expectations, and goals of at-risk populations. Three chapters contribute to this section.

Chapter 13, *Community Participatory Design of Health Communication Interventions*, describes applications of the community participatory design model for developing, evaluating and extending health communication programs. The model includes strategies for identifying diverse stakeholders, defining communication issues, creating user-designed interventions, evaluating program effects, and adapting programs to other populations. Case examples of global health communication programs developed with community participatory design are described to illustrate how the model can be used to enhance global health outcomes. Chapter 14, *Faith-based Community Health Interventions: Incorporating Cultural Ecology, the Social Ecological Framework, and Gender Analysis*, deals with faith-based interventions for health promotion. This chapter specifically provides examples of how to incorporate multiple theoretical frameworks and principles to develop a culturally appropriate, gender sensitive health communication program that incorporates the local realities and expertise of the faith-based participants. For detailed information, the author provided her experience working with a faith-based institution on an HIV and AIDS training workshop in Tanzania. Chapter 15, *Designing Logos for Health Campaigns: Convergence of Semiotics and the Diffusion of Innovations*, highlights the importance of a logo as a visual representation of a health campaign. To foster a greater public understanding of a logo and enhance its effectiveness for global health campaigns dealing with culturally different target populations, this study provides theoretical and practical frames for designing a health campaign logo. To do so, the *red ribbon* logo that has been frequently used for international HIV/AIDS campaigns is analyzed from the perspectives based on *semiotics* and *the diffusion of innovations*.

Thematic section #5 describes *Health Advocacy and Activism* as critical factors for enhancing health practices, programs, and policies to meet the needs of consumers and caregivers. Since health communication is an applied social science geared toward improving the quality of health care and health promotion practices and policies, it is important to recognize the role of health advocacy in facilitating change within health care systems. Health advocacy leaders depend on strategic communication to represent the needs of consumers in the development and refinement of health care practices.

Related to the themes of section #5, Chapter 16, *Strategic Communication for Health Advocacy and Social Change*, focuses on the important communication activities that health advocates can perform to effectively represent the needs of consumers for reforming modern health care systems. Strategic health advocacy communication can have important influences on the development and refinement of health policies and practices, helping to recalibrate the balance of power in health care and health promotion efforts. Health advocates can actively represent the voices, concerns, and needs of consumers within the health care system to help make health care programs responsive and adaptive to consumer needs. However, health advocates must learn how to communicate patients' perspectives and needs in compelling ways to key audiences using a variety of different media to influence health policies and practices. The chapter also examines major communication challenges facing health advocates and suggests strategies for promoting effective health advocacy. As a case-oriented research, Chapter 17, *Health Activism as Resistance: MOSOP as a Site of Culture-Centered Resistance in Niger Delta Region of Nigeria*, offers an overview of the Ogoni resistance movement as an example of health activism originating from the global South. Attending to the adverse health outcomes that are produced by the extractive industries, this chapter documents the communicative strategies that are deployed in the articulation of the problem and in the collective framing of solutions. A variety of communicative processes are mobilized together, bringing community members in a unified voice in resistance to the State and to Shell, and creating frameworks of accountability in the community located in the global South.

The final thematic section #6 on valuing data examines the value of data in designing, implementing, evaluating, refining, and sustaining health communication interventions. Good data are instrumental in guiding strategic health communication interventions, particularly when health communication scholars are working in foreign lands and with diverse populations where good data are needed to increase understanding about the unique opportunities and constraints for health communication efforts. This section emphasizes the value of population data and careful evaluation of data for maximizing the effectiveness of health communication strategies. The last three chapters deal with this topic of valuing data.

Chapter 18, *National Health Communication Surveillance Systems*, introduces a national surveillance data system established in the United States. Surveillance data, which can come from a variety of sources, may help a community track the origins and spread of an infectious disease, document the problems associated with chronic conditions, monitor control efforts, generate hypotheses, and inform applied research. This chapter traces how the theoretical and pragmatic origins of the public health surveillance system can be expanded to monitor changes in the communication environment. This chapter additionally presents how complementary data systems may be linked within countries and internationally to inform research and policy over time. Chapter 19, *Cultural Beacons in Health Communication: Leveraging Overlooked Indicators and Grassroots Wisdoms*, argues that (1) traditional methods for gathering data do not wholly capture program-related effects, (2) non-traditional, non-textual, and participatory forms of knowledge generation can yield overlooked data; and (3) local wisdoms can enrich research and evaluation. This chapter particularly recognizes a cultural beacon (CB), an embedded indicator illuminating local conditions and illustrates different types of CBs with case studies from Uganda and India, sharing instructions for incorporating CBs within health communication projects and methods of assessing CBs.

The last chapter, Chapter 20, "*Evaluating Health Communication Interventions,*" outlines several key strategies for conducting meaningful evaluation research for guiding the development, implementation, refinement, and institutionalization of effective health communication programs. Health communication programs have developed as essential and ubiquitous tools in the delivery of care and promotion of health in the modern health care system. Yet, while the use of health communication programs has proliferated, we are not always well informed about the influences these important communication programs are having on the different key audiences they are designed to help. Too often health communication programs can evoke differential responses from diverse audiences, unintended influences, and even negative (iatrogenic) effects on health outcomes. It is critically important to conduct regular, ongoing, and strategic evaluations of health communication intervention programs to assess their effectiveness in achieving primary program goals. Evaluation data should guide program refinements and strategic planning.

The editors of this book believe this book contains a uniquely comprehensive set of health communication strategies in comparison with previous publications with similar purposes. We are certain that our collective scholarship, as represented in this volume, can contribute broadly to promoting health and well-being. Finally, our hope is that this book will spur the development of culturally sensitive, engaged, and strategic health communication intervention research programs that will effectively address important health issues both locally and globally.

Leveraging Technology

Chapter 1

Strategies and Principles for Using Mass and Online/Digital Media in Health Communication Campaigns

Charles K. Atkin, *Michigan State University*
Ronald E. Rice, *University of California Santa Barbara*

Introduction

Sophisticated public communication campaigns using mass and online media apply social science theories to strategically affect audience awareness, knowledge, attitudes and ultimately behavior across a variety of public service domains, most notably in health contexts. The following sections describe eight main strategies and principles for increasing their effectiveness: campaign design framework, formative evaluation, dual approaches, types and mix of messages, message content and style, mass media and online/digital communication channels, quantitative media dissemination factors, and summative and process evaluation.

1. Develop a Campaign Design Framework Based on Situation Analysis, Target Audiences and Behaviors, Models of Influence Pathways, Major Theories of Communication and Persuasion. These Provide the Foundation for the Nature of the Messages and Media Used in the Campaign

The initial step in campaign design is a conceptual examination of the situation to *determine opportunities and barriers* and to *identify specific outcome behaviors* of *specific subgroups of the public*. The second step is to trace backwards from the outcomes to identify their *proximate and distal determinants* (especially the role played by the mass media but also of societal and situational constraints), and then create *models* of the pathways of influence via attitudes, beliefs, knowledge, social influences, and environmental forces. The next step is to specify *goal (target) audiences* and *goal behaviors* that can be directly influenced by campaign messages and interventions.

A variety of *theoretical frameworks* is available to guide campaign design (Atkin & Rice, 2013; Glanz, Rimer, & Viswanath, 2008). The most comprehensive conceptualizations applied to campaigns are the communication-persuasion matrix and the social marketing framework. McGuire (2013) developed a classic *communication-persuasion matrix* featuring an input-output model; the five communication *input variables* include source, message, channel, and audience, and the *output process* proceeds through 13 stages from exposure through processing, learning, yielding, behavior, and integration, to encouraging others. This framework emphasizes the centrality of formative evaluation (discussed below) in selecting source messengers, designing mediated messages, and identifying the goal audience's media patterns (see Section 2).

Social marketing emphasizes an audience-centered consumer orientation and uses the media to attractively package the social product and to focus campaign strategies on attaining pragmatic goals (Kotler, Roberto, & Lee, 2002; McKenzie-Mohr, 2010). These goal responses vary in palatability associated with degree of effort, sacrifice, and monetary expense; a central strategic consideration in determining the degree of difficulty is receptiveness of the focal segment. Other key features are the multifaceted conceptions of product, costs and benefits, as well as audience segmentation, policy change, and competition. A valuable resource is the Centers for Disease Control and Prevention's online course for social marketing for nutrition, physical activity, and obesity-prevention programs, which covers problem description, formative evaluation, strategy development, intervention design, evaluation, and implementation (Detailed information available at CDC's website: http://www.cdc.gov/nccdphp/dnpa/socialmarketing/training/). The Social Marketing Institute develops social marketing campaigns based on marketing practices, and offers resources for carrying out and disseminating research, training and educating organizations, and sponsoring academic research (http://www.social-marketing.org/index.html).

Community-based prevention marketing is conducted within and guided by a social marketing perspective, emphasizing product, price, place, and promotion, competitive analysis (current risky behaviors), audience segmentation (to tailor the message and exchanges to specific groups in the community), formative evaluation (especially concerning the local audience's viewpoints), and ongoing monitoring and tracking evaluation (via surveys, measures of media exposure, website hits), that seeks satisfying exchanges (low social costs for changing behavior that fosters benefits) between promoter and audience (community members) (Bracht, 2001; Bryant et al., 2009; McKenzie-Mohr, 2010). Croft et al. (1994) described how a comprehensive community-based nutrition intervention to reduce risk of cardiovascular disease included community classes, grocery store tours, a supermarket point-of-purchase program, a restaurant labeling program, speakers' bureaus, home study courses, worksite nutrition programs, and mass media coverage (such as local radio and TV public service announcements, talk shows, and newspaper articles).

Focusing specifically on message design, the *message framing* theoretical approach (Quick & Bates, 2010) proposes message appeals with gain-frame promotion of positive behavior vs. loss-frame prevention of negative behavior (such as in fear-appeal campaigns; Yzer, Southwell, & Stephenson, 2013). Appropriate message framing (gain- versus loss-oriented) emphasizes the benefits and costs of prevention or detection/treatment, especially when matched to the goal audience's orientation (e.g., risk aversion, based on *perceptions* of and *sensitivity* to the possible outcomes of action or non-action, short-term and long-term) (Rothman, Bartels, Wlaschin, & Salovey, 2006). Very broadly, gain-framed messages are more appropriate for prevention, while loss-framed ones are more appropriate for detection/treatment, especially when goal audience members are involved with (or are encouraged to attend to) the particular issue (e.g., breast cancer screening), partially because they are more likely to engage in systematic processing. In particular, the advantages of gain-framed messages appear to accrue to promoting prevention behaviors, but not for attitudes, intentions, or detection (Gallagher & Updegraff, 2012).

Other frequent theoretical approaches include *social cognitive theory* (Bandura, 1986), the *theory of reasoned action* and the *theory of planned behavior* (Ajzen, Albarracin, & Hornik, 1997), the *diffusion of innovations* model (Rogers, 2003), and the *transtheoretical (stages of change) model of health behavior* (Prochaska & Velicer, 1997).

2. Perform Formative Evaluation by Gathering Information about Audience Predispositions, Channel Usage Patterns, Evaluation of Prospective Messengers and Appeals, and Social Structure Constraints, and Pretest Responses to Preliminary Versions of Messages

Formative evaluation research is necessary to identify and understand the goal audiences, which tend to differ in media use (channels, genres, frequency), involvement in the issue, information-retention, attitudinal orientations, at-risk behaviors, at-risk conditions, demographic and sociopsychological characteristics (for example, gender, sensation-seeking, promotion orientation), location, sources of social influence and support, temporal variations, constraints from peers, culture, and societal structures (Atkin & Freimuth, 2013; Centers for Disease Control and Prevention, 2009; National Cancer Institute, 2009; Noar, 2006; Rice & Foote, 2013).

The first stage of formative evaluation involves *pre-production information gathering* to learn more about the situation and audiences. Databases, focus groups, personal interviews and observations, and custom surveys help to provide useful understanding and insights into audience predispositions. For example, formative evaluation for a campaign to reduce HIV-associated risk behaviors among African-Americans identified three major salient messages (Romer, et al., 2009). The analysis also uncovered "counter-narratives" that might allow the audience to resist dominant arguments and myths fostering risky sex (i.e., disassociate the belief that condoms reduce pleasure, waiting to initiate sex is a sign of respect, and use condoms even with steady partners). These insights provided the basis for developing dramatic depictions of modeling these narratives (somewhat similar to entertainment-education campaigns) in campaign spots via radio and television channels popular among the goal audience, for 15 months.

The other primary area of information gathering is about patterns of usage of specific media—typically amount of time viewing television, listening to radio, and reading print publications, and exposure to specific channels such as cable networks, local radio stations, and newspapers and magazines. These include circulation audits for print circulation and readership, pass-on readers, impacts and impressions (Audit Bureau of Circulation, Mediamark Research Inc.); ratings, households, reach, share, frequency, duration, impressions, loyalty for mass and online media and ad tracking (Arbitron, Burrelle's or Nielsen; Audience Dialogue, www.audiencedialogue.net; Webster, Phalen, & Lichty, 2006); media use and consumption patterns (Claritas' PRIZM segmentation, Simmons Market Research); ad viewing and attention (e.g., Starch Readership), recognition and recall; website navigation patterns and stickiness, website postings, email prompts, and social media links, likes or retweets (Alexa Internet, Google analytics, Twitalyzer; Danaher, Boles, Akers, Gordon, & Severson, 2006).

The second stage of formative research involves *pretesting* of rough versions of specific prospective media messages to stimulate qualitative reactions in focus group or in-theater sessions and to measure quantitative ratings in message testing labs. Pretesting helps to determine whether the audience regards the message content and style positively (e.g., informative, believable, motivating, convincing, useful, on-target, enjoyable) or negatively (e.g., preachy, disturbing, confusing, irritating, dull). Pretesting can detect problematic elements that may trigger psychological reactance, which can lead to boomerang effects that reinforce counter-productive behaviors (Fishbein et al., 2002; McGuire, 2013).

3. Utilize Dual Approaches in Using Media for Attaining Impact in Order to Achieve Direct Effects on Focal Segments of Audiences and Exert Influence Indirectly via Interpersonal Influencers and Policy Makers

Mass media campaigns must diversify the pathways of impact, including purposely activating multi-step flows. Most mass media campaigns aim messages *directly* at the *goal audiences*, such as at-risk subpopulations that might benefit most from the campaign. Campaigns often seek to attain impact by using either behavior-triggering or attitude-reinforcing media messages designed for people who are already favorably predisposed (e.g., applying the transtheoretical model). Another key audience segment is composed of those who have not yet tried the undesirable behavior but whose background characteristics suggest they are prone to do so soon. Goal audience segments that are already committed to unsuitable practices are high in priority but not readily influenced by directly targeted media-based campaigns. Other ways of subdividing the overall population for purposes of targeting via mass media include demographic or socio-psychological-based subgroups (e.g., higher- vs. lower-income strata, high vs. low sensation seekers, lifestyle categories), subgroups experiencing social obstacles in accomplishing certain behaviors, and members of different cultures.

There are two basic *indirect* influence strategies used in campaigns. One approach is to initiate a multi-step flow by disseminating messages to potential *interpersonal influencers* who are in a position to personally influence goal audience individuals (Rogers, 2003). Opinion leaders tend to be receptive to media campaign messages, and they can customize messages to the unique needs and values of individuals, and the relevant social norms, in a more precise manner than mediated messages (Rice, Wu, Li, Detels, & Rotheram-Borus, 2012; Valente, 2012). A more macro-oriented indirect influence campaign approach provides messages to *societal and organizational policymakers* who are responsible for devising constraints and creating opportunities that shape focal individuals' decisions and behaviors. In the past quarter century, reformers have successfully combined community organizing and media publicity to advance healthy public policies via *media advocacy* (The Berkeley Media Studies Group, http://www.bmsg.org/; Dorfman & Wallack, 2013). This approach typically frames public health issues by emphasizing policy-related systemic and societal solutions rather than individual responsibility for good health. News coverage of the campaign and its issues can shape the public agenda, and the policy agenda pertaining to new policy initiatives and rule-making.

4. Determine the Appropriate Mix of Informational and Persuasive Messages in Campaigns Based Primarily on Audience Predispositions

There are two basic kinds of *informational* messages. *Awareness* messages typically offer relatively simple content that informs people about the prevalence and risk of the issue and what behaviors to perform, specifies which segments should do it, or provides cues about when and where it should be done (e.g., a radio spot that reminds drivers to buckle safety belts in icy conditions). These awareness messages can stimulate the audience to pursue additional, more detailed content from resources such as web pages, books, or opinion leaders. *Instructional* messages present more complex "how to do it" information in campaigns seeking knowledge gain or skills acquisition (e.g., a magazine feature story that presents recipes for healthy dinners), along with messages specifically designed to enhance personal efficacy (e.g., bolstering resistance to non-complying peers).

The other type of message is the *persuasive* appeal, which features influential reasons why the audience should adopt an advocated action or avoid a proscribed behavior. This generally involves mechanisms of attitude creation or change, usually building on knowledge gain and belief formation (e.g., smoking-cessation TV spots designed to strengthen beliefs about severity of health harms, which in turn may alter attitudes toward tobacco use). For audience segments that are already favorably inclined, the campaign has the easier persuasive task of *reinforcing* existing predispositions (e.g., motivating behavioral maintenance). Because prolonged campaigns disseminate a broad array of persuasive messages, strategists typically marshal a variety of appeals.

5. Create Qualitatively Sophisticated Messages Featuring Credible Content, Engaging Style, Relevant Portrayals, Understandable Exposition, and Persuasive Incentives

Based on the formative evaluation discussed in Section 2, message design for mass media campaigns involves the strategic selection of substantive material and creative production values that emphasize one or more of five key qualitative factors (Atkin & Rice, 2013; Cho, 2012). *Credibility* refers to the believability of message content, as conveyed by convincing evidence, the trustworthiness and competence of the source (persons, characters, organizations) appearing in the message or the media vehicle disseminating the message (Metzger, Flanagin, Eyal, Lemus, & McCann, 2003). Second, the ideas and manner of presentation should be *engaging*, by using stylistic features that are attractive and entertaining, along with substantive content that is interesting or emotionally arousing.

Third, the presentation should include elements to boost personal *relevance*, so receivers regard the subject matter as applicable to their situation and needs. Next, the *understandability* of the message contributes to recipient processing and learning, provided that the material is presented in a comprehensive and comprehensible manner that is simple, explicit, and sufficiently detailed. The fifth and final qualitative factor involves *persuasive incentives*, notably motivational appeals to influence the audience. Note that all these factors are explicitly considered in the McGuire (2013) hierarchy-of-effects model. Persuasive media messages often utilize a basic expectancy-value mechanism through which content affects beliefs regarding the subjective likelihood of each outcome occurring and the severity of its consequences. The operational formula for preventing undesirable behaviors is *vulnerability* x *severity,* which is central to many fear appeals (Yzer, Southwell, & Stephenson, 2013).

For campaigns in the health domain, the array of *incentives* includes not only physical health, but time/effort, group, moral, legal, economic, social, psychological and aspirational aspects. Rather than over-emphasizing the narrow domain of negative health threats such as death or illness, campaigners diversify by including both negative appeals (e.g., psychological regret or social rejection) and positive incentives (e.g., physical well-being or saving money) (possibly using the prevention/promotion framing approach). Regarding the number of different incentives, it is generally advantageous to use multiple persuasive appeals across a series of messages in a campaign, particularly when seeking to influence varied audiences. In conveying incentive appeals, campaign designers often provide evidence to support claims made in messages. The most effective type of evidence varies according to characteristics of the medium (e.g., short, image-oriented video, more informative audio, and interlinked multi-media online) and to audience predispositions and characteristics. For example, audiences who are knowledgeable tend to be more influenced by messages citing statistics (as in print or online media) or quoting technical experts, whereas dramatized case examples and testimonials by celebrities (as on television or online videos) work better for low-involvement audience segments (Perloff, 2003).

Message sources also convey qualitative features in media campaign messages. The *source messenger* appears in broadcast and print messages to provide information, demonstrate behavior, or present a testimonial. These messengers help enhance each qualitative factor by being *engaging* (displaying attractiveness or likability), *credible* (conveying trustworthiness or expertise; but are also affected by media credibility characteristics), and *relevant* to the audience (demonstrating that they share attributes similar to receivers). These qualities can attract audience attention and facilitate comprehension by personalizing abstract concepts, eliciting supportive cognitive responses during processing, heightening emotional arousal via identification or transfer of affect, and increasing retention and recall due to memorability and cues. The key categories of messengers appearing in mass media campaign messages are celebrities, public officials, topical expert specialists, professional performers, ordinary people, specially experienced individuals (e.g., victims or beneficiaries), unique characters (e.g., animated or costumed), and organizations (via a brand or logo).

6. Select the Mass Media and Online/Digital Communication Channels that Are Most Appropriate for Reaching and Influencing Key Audience Segments

Mass and local media

In assessing each option for channeling campaign messages, campaign designers take into account myriad advantages and disadvantages along a number of communicative dimensions. Atkin and Salmon (2010) discuss channel differences in terms of *reach* (the proportion of population exposed to the message), *specialization* (enabling basic targeting to specific subgroups or precise tailoring to individuals), *intrusiveness* (capacity for commanding attention), *personalization* (human relational nature of source-receiver interaction), *depth* (channel capacity for conveying detailed and complex content), *credibility* (believability of material conveyed), *agenda-setting* (potency of channel for raising salience priority of issues), *accessibility* (ease of placing messages in channel), and *economy* (low cost for producing and disseminating stimuli). Determining the most appropriate channels is based on budget, audience usage patterns, and the nature of the message, determined through formative evaluation (Section 2). Huge budgets for commercial spots on television and radio are no guarantee of success, however. Note, for example, the apparent failure of the extensively mass-mediated National Anti-Youth Drug campaign (Hornik, Jacobsohn, Orwin, Piesse, & Kalton, 2008), although other analyses have found specific positive results, especially for girls, high sensation seekers, and in combination with school-based prevention programs (http://www.whitehouse.gov/ondcp/Campaign-Effectiveness-and-Rigor).

Community campaigns use local media (from radio stations to social service center posters and brochures) to provide exposure to messages developed with community members (Bracht, 2001). The practice of *entertainment-education*, which involves embedding campaign topic-related material in entertaining contexts, has demonstrable potential for impact but low implementation in the US media compared to developing countries (Singhal, Cody, Rogers, & Sabido, 2004). The main problem in gaining visibility for health topics in the entertainment media is lack of access to popular vehicles, partially due to low campaign budgets and relatively dull subject matter. More subtle challenges include differing norms and goals between commercial and research professionals, as well as concerns by commercial broadcasters about advocacy and industry or sponsor critique. Thus an important potential audience for health messages is new scriptwriters for films, television, and online video, who can then apply entertainment-education resources within media programming (Beck, 2004). For example, see the evaluation of the treatment of organ donation in the primetime drama *Numb3rs*, sponsored by USC's Hollywood, Health & Society (Details available at http://hollywoodhealthandsociety.org/; Movius, Cody, Huang, Berkowitz, & Morgan, 2007). For health communication resources for entertainment writers and producers, and case examples of and storylines from entertainment-education, see the CDC's Gateway to Health Communication & Social Marketing Tools & Templates (For more information, check

CDC's website at http://www.cdc.gov/healthcommunication/ToolsTemplates/EntertainmentEd/index.html).

Campaigns may also rely on creative publicity techniques for generating magazine feature story coverage or placement in daytime TV talk shows. This strategy is most viable for certain topics in the health, safety, and environmental domain that are regarded by the public as risky, controversial, or personally salient.

Online and digital media attributes

Public communication campaigns increasingly emphasize digital/online media technologies (Lieberman, 2013; Murero & Rice, 2006; Noar & Harrington, 2012; Parker & Thorson, 2009; Strecher, 2007). Online health systems offer a variety of attributes that foster effective online interactions among users, such as interactivity, anonymity, narrowcasting, and tailoring, presence, homophily, social distance, and interaction management, which promote learning, social influence, stigma management, and coping (Walther, Pingree, Hawkins, & Buller, 2005).

Interactivity encompasses direction of communication and level of receiver control over the communication process, which shape relationships between user and source in the context of specific design features (e.g., games, email, and hyperlinks). The value of *anonymity* inherent in web information search and online discussion groups is valuable for private topics such as STD/HIV prevention and testing. *Narrowcasting* employs segmentation and targeting (key concepts in social marketing), which are especially applicable to Internet users.

Tailoring utilizes an online screening questionnaire to assess audience factors such as readiness stage, stylistic tastes, knowledge levels, current beliefs, and health condition, and then directs them to narrowly targeted and personalized messages or activities. This approach increases the likelihood of learning and persuasion while decreasing the potential boomerang effects. Lustria, Cortese, Noar, and Glueckauf (2009) reviewed 30 studies of computer-based tailoring interventions covering four general health areas: nutrition and diet, physical activity, alcoholism, and smoking cessation, most emphasizing risk prevention and health maintenance. Their Figure 2 provides a useful cross-tabulation of technical implementation strategies (extent and timing of program, online and digital media, features, and user tools) with message tailoring strategies (goal audience criteria, such as information needs and stages of change), and tailoring mechanisms (such as personalization and feedback). Because of the ability of online/digital campaigns to provide tailored messages, most online interventions reviewed by Cugelman, Thelwall, and Dawed (2011) applied strategies from the transtheoretical approach, which, along with self-efficacy and processes of change, were significantly more effective than other frameworks (Noar, Benac, & Harris (2007).

Online and digital media applications

Complementing mass media and workplace campaigns with a series of *emails* providing strategies, reminders, and links to online resources strengthens impacts, such as for a half-year worksite campaign aimed at increasing physical activity and fruit/vegetable consumption (Franklin, Rosenbaum, Carey, & Roizen, 2006). The *Internet* is a major source for online health information, support, discussion, therapy, support, prescriptions, and access to physicians (Murero & Rice, 2006; Rice, 2006). Computer-delivered intervention (including tailoring) improves knowledge, attitudes, intentions, health behaviors and general health maintenance, social support, quality of life, and self-efficacy, across a variety of health domains (Portnoy, Scott-Sheldon, Johnson, & Carey, 2008; Rains & Young, 2009). A meta-analysis of studies examining the role of the Internet in health behavior change reported an overall small but significant positive effect; stronger results were found for interventions applying health behavior theories, communication approaches, and behavior change techniques (Webb, Joseph, Yardley, & Michie, 2010). Another extensive meta-analysis of online interventions found small but consistent significant effects, though with over-time dropoff (Cugelman, Thelwall, & Dawed, 2011). Campaigns can utilize the *Internet* for low-cost message dissemination via online public service promos and spots (e.g., brief banner ad messages or solicitations to click through to a website) and long-form video messages on sites such as *YouTube*. For example, YouTube organ donation videos (and comments posted) stimulate actual organ donor registration (Tian, 2010).

Websites can provide the primary infrastructure for an integrated multimedia campaign. A meta-analysis comparing web-based to non-web-based interventions in 22 articles involving nearly 12,000 participants found improved health knowledge and/or behavioral outcomes in all but one of the studies (Wantland, Wantland, Portillo, Holzemer, Slaughter, & McGhee, 2004). The CHESS (Comprehensive Health Enhancement Support System) provides an integrated system for a wide range of health crisis campaigns. Over-time use of the CHESS site offering information, support, decision and analysis tools related to breast cancer, compared to use of Internet links to high-quality breast cancer sites, and to a control group, showed greater log-ons, use of more health resources, and greater outcomes (quality of life, health-care competence, and social support) (Detailed information available at http://chess.wisc.edu/chess/projects/about_chess.aspx; Gustafson et al., 2008; Walther, Pingree, Hawkins, & Buller, 2005). The CDC's national VERB campaign promoting exercise among pre-teens attained wide-scale engagement (based on a hierarchy-of-effects framework) in website activities (Berkowitz et al., 2008).

Texting via mobile phones is well-suited to offer tailored, wide-reaching, interactive and continuing campaign interventions (Fjeldsoe, Marshall, & Miller, 2009). It has a variety of advantages as a medium for health campaigns: interactive as well as broadcast modes, asynchronous which increased convenience, short messages are less susceptible to selective perception, tailoring, widespread accessibility, appropriate to low-income or low-educated audiences, ability to provide prompts or random reminders, etc. Meta-analysis shows significant positive effects of text messaging as a tool for health behavior change (Cole-Lewis & Kershaw, 2010). Another meta-analysis concluded that health outcomes and care processes can be improved through complementing standard care with reminders, monitoring and managing diseases, and education via mobile phone voice and text messages (Krishna, Boren, & Balas, 2009). *Podcasts* can provide relevant audio information (e.g., social support, persuasive messages, or news items) to motivated audiences at their convenience, and would be especially relevant to low-literacy or non-English-speaking audiences.

The more interactive, social, communicative, and collaborative *web 2.0* applications also enable users to participate more directly in producing, sharing, and discussing health-promotion messages (Thacheray, Neiger, Hanson, & McKenzie, 2008). *Blogs* link users with similar information needs and concerns to share their views and experiences (Rains & Keating, 2011), while *wikis* support group collaboration. *Twitter* provides updates and protocol reminders to campaign-specific followers; however, tweets (like much Internet content) may include considerable misunderstandings or misuses of health information and medicines (Scanfeld, Scanfeld, & Larson, 2010). *Social bookmarking* allows health-oriented communities to develop and share useful online resources (Thackeray, Neiger, Hanson, & McKenzie, 2008).

For guidelines on using *social media* (blogs, video-sharing, mobile applications, RSS feeds, Facebook, Twitter, buttons and badges, e-cards, text messaging, widgets) for health campaign interventions, see Centers for Disease Control and Prevention (Detailed information available at CDC's website at http://www.cdc.gov/healthcommunication/ToolsTemplates/index.html).

Voice-response systems, interactive video, DVD and CD-ROM, mobile phones and *computer games* can be effective in reaching young people. Game players can acquire skills and improve self-efficacy from role-playing, modeling, and vicarious experiences, or directly experience health benefits through physical movement as part of the game (Lieberman, 2013). More broadly, a meta-analysis of video game research findings shows a positive impact on health behaviors such as chronic disease management, exercise, and diet (Baranowski, Buday, Thompson, & Baranowski, 2008).

7. Deploy Quantitative Media Dissemination Factors that Enhance Effects by Amplifying the Volume and Repetition of Messages, the Prominence and Scheduling of Placements, and the Length of the Campaign

A major problem in mass media campaigns is simply reaching the audience and attaining attention to the messages (Hornik, 2002; Rice & Foote, 2013). The exposure problem is also due to both *selective exposure* (notably when individuals with unhealthy habits defensively avoid threatening media messages, much easier to do with media than with interpersonal influences), and simple *lack of motivation* to access health information (notably when lower-income, less-educated at-risk segments of the population ignore health messages that are encountered). Audiences may also misperceive their susceptibility to negative consequences, fail to learn many types of informational content, deny the applicability of message incentives to self, defensively counter-argue against persuasive appeals, and reject unappealing behavioral recommendations.

However, four key quantitative dissemination factors can partially overcome some of those challenges, and improve campaign effectiveness. A substantial *volume* of messages provided by the media helps attain adequate reach and frequency of exposure, as well as audience responses such as comprehension, recognition, and image formation. An appropriate level of *repetition* of specific executions facilitates message comprehension and positive affect toward the recommended behavior, although overly high repetition can produce wear-out or diminishing returns. Placement *prominence* of messages in conspicuous positions within media vehicles (e.g., front-page newspaper positioning, or high-rankings in popular search engine websites) enhances both exposure levels and perceived significance of the topic on the public agenda. Paid health promotion ads on *social media* sites have greater potential for impact because of more prominent placement and more precise targeting. Depending on campaign objectives, the *scheduling* of a fixed number of presentations may be most effectively concentrated over a short duration, dispersed thinly over a long period of time, or distributed in intermittent bursts of "flighting" (periods of no ads interspersed among periods of strategically timed ads) or "pulsing" (combining low-level continuous ads with flighting).

To maximize dissemination quantity, campaigners may gain greater media access by aggressively pursuing free public service time or space, soliciting monetary support from government and corporations to fund paid placements, skillfully using publicity techniques for generating entertainment and journalistic coverage, and exploiting low-cost channels of communication such as websites and social media. Since 1942, the Ad Council has helped create a wide range of pro-social campaigns, and provides extensive ad resources in the areas of community, education, and health/safety (http://www.adcouncil.org/default.aspx?id=15). However, effectiveness of PSAs varies extensively, and, if not designed carefully, may have negative impacts (Fishbein, Hall-Jamieson, Zimmer, von Haeften, & Nabi, 2002).

Moreover, the reach of a campaign can be widened by sensitizing audiences to appropriate content already available in the media and by stimulating subsequent information-seeking from specialty sources. The "mass" media include more than just radio, newspapers, magazines, and television; consider also films, press coverage, organizational and community public relations activities, posters and leaflets, "shopper" and free local papers, billboards and bus signs, toll-free hotlines, Internet sites and other digital and online media, school materials, work-site programs, direct marketing and coupons, merchandise with logos, music and concerts, information on the campaign resources themselves (e.g., condom packets, exercise cards), etc. (Noar, 2006). However, the primary challenge to mass media campaigns is the pervasive media environment promoting risky and unhealthy behaviors. For example, tobacco and smoking campaigns exist in a life-long environment of massive advertisements, media coverage, and entertainment media content promoting smoking (National Cancer Institute, 2008).

Regarding the *length* of a media campaign, the difficult health problems addressed by campaigners usually require exceptional persistence of effort over long periods of time. A campaign may require several months or even many years as successive phases are implemented. In many cases, perpetual campaigning is necessary because various goal audience segments are in constant need of influence, or are being regularly replaced (e.g., college students). Although lengthy campaigning can be quite expensive and probably pays diminishing returns over long periods, there are at least five types of subgroups that require lengthy time to be influenced: newcomers who move into the priority audience, backsliders who revert to prior misbehavior, evolvers who gradually adopt recommended practices, vacillators who need regular reinforcement to stay the course, and latecomers who eventually become receptive to the campaign. Further, summative evaluation and cost-effectiveness analyses can determine the relative value of such lengthy and focused media campaigns.

8. Conduct Summative and Process Evaluation Research to Measure Effects on Individuals' Knowledge, Attitudes and Behavior, and to Assess Outcomes among Policy Makers, Organizations, and Communities

Summative evaluation research is performed to quantitatively and qualitatively assess impact; cross-sectional, field experimental, and time-series designs are most widely used at this stage. *Process evaluation* assesses how well the planned implementation was accomplished (including placements of messages in media channels, using the measures in Sections 2 and 7), and how weaknesses or problems in message conduct and media exposure may have reduced the potential for the theoretical processes to actually obtain (Steckler & Linnan, 2006). Both kinds of evaluation research are conducted during and after campaigns. Evaluations also use many of the same general audience media use measures identified in Section 2.

At the individual level, evaluation researchers typically measure exposure to mediated messages and changes in awareness, knowledge, attitude and behavior. The preponderance of evaluation data suggests that campaigns exert moderate to small influences on cognitive outcomes, less influence on attitudinal outcomes, and still less influence on behavioral outcomes, and are typically more effective at prevention than cessation (Atkin & Rice, 2013; Snyder & LaCroix, 2013). Effects on behaviors depend on the dose of information carried in the media channels, duration of campaign message dissemination, integration of mass media and interpersonal communication systems, and supplementation of media stimuli by interpersonal communication (Section 4) and social-change strategies (deterrence, enforcement, education and engineering of the physical context).

Evaluation may also assess campaign impacts on policy-makers, organizations, and communities, both via exposure to campaign media and messages, but also through coverage in the media and greater prominence in the public agenda (e.g., indirect influence via media advocacy, Section 3). These outcomes usually involve alterations in environmental factors that produce improvements in societal systems and consequently individual health status (Rice & Foote, 2013).

Desired changes in individual knowledge, attitudes or behavior are typically intended evaluation outcomes. Salmon and Murray-Johnson (2013) draw distinctions among various types of campaign effectiveness, including *definitional effectiveness* (e.g., defining a social phenomenon as a significant problem or elevating the topic on the public agenda via prominence in the mass media), *cost-effectiveness* (e.g., comparing mass media campaign messages vs. interpersonal interventions), and *programmatic effectiveness* (e.g., assessing campaign outcomes associated with the media campaign relative to stated goals and objectives). Emphasizing less traditional campaign effects, Cho and Salmon (2007) identify five dimensions where *unintended effects* may occur—time (short or long term), level (individual or societal), audience (targeted or other), content (related to specific content or indirectly related to the use of the medium), and valence (desirable or undesirable).

Case Studies

There are, of course, many useful and exemplary case studies. For example, in the nearly two-year *Safer Sex* campaign using intensive television public service announcements, messages about safer sex specifically designed for sensation-seeking/impulsive-decision-making audiences in two cities achieved very high exposure and recall, which was associated with increased condom use, self-efficacy, and behavioral intentions, with no changes in the control city (Zimmerman et al., 2007). Edgar, Noar, and Freimuth (2008) present cases of the use of a wide array of communication channels (including entertainment media and Internet media) in several countries for HIV/AIDS issues.

Begun in 2000, *Truth* is the largest U.S. youth smoking campaign not directed by the tobacco industry, and integrates mass, online and social media (http://www.thetruth.com), with components targeted toward facts, music, games, and sports. Based on large nationally representative surveys, exposure to and recall of *Truth* campaign messages were associated with positive changes in attitudes, beliefs, and intentions to smoke. However, during the same time period, Philip Morris ads from their *Think. Don't Smoke* increased positive beliefs and attitudes toward the tobacco industry (Farrelly, Davis, Duke, & Messeri, 2009). California's *Anti-Tobacco Media Campaign* is one of the longest-running, most comprehensive, and best-funded anti-smoking efforts in the U.S. (More detailed information available at their website at http://www.cdph.ca.gov/programs/tobacco/Pages/CTCPMediaCampaign.aspx). The site notes the development of culturally and linguistically relevant campaign messages, and also documents difficulties in reducing smoking in adults versus kids.

The National *Youth Anti-Drug Media Campaign* produced extensive mass media exposure of rigorously designed messages (More information available at http://www.whitehouse.gov/ondcp/Campaign-Effectiveness-and-Rigor). This process first involved exploratory research involving literature reviews, expert advice, frequent studies of teens, parents, and community stakeholders, and ongoing recommendations from an advisory team. Focus groups of the goal audience in two different markets were conducted to select and improve the ad concepts. Copy-testing then sought responses from groups viewing the ad compared to control groups to verify the efficacy of the messages. Finally, regular tracking studies measured awareness and recall of the ads by goal audience members.

A campaign by the *Center for Science in the Public Interest* seeks to combat marketing of sweetened, high alcohol-concentration beverages ("alcopops") that appeal to young drinkers (Detailed information available at http://www.cspinet.org/booze/iss_alcopops.htm). The main media-based strategy was to generate news publicity, intended primarily for policy-makers in government and the alcohol industry (Freudenberg et al., 2009; one of their 12 case studies). For an analysis of a college campus risky-drinking campaign, see DeJong and Smith (2013).

The Johns Hopkins University *Center for Communication Programs* has summarized 52 lessons in 8 implementation stages from international health communication programs in 43 countries (Piotrow, Rimon, Merritt, & Saffitz, 2003). Green and Tones (2010) also provide international cases of public information campaigns.

Conclusion

Media-based health communication campaigns typically attain a low-to-modest rather than strong degree of impact. The limited effects are due to meager dissemination budgets, unsophisticated application of theory and models, poorly conceived strategic approaches, substantial resistance among key audience segments (individuals, cultural groups, and social structures), the complex or difficult nature of behaviors to be influenced (addiction, social rewards, societal systems), and the prevalence of (in some cases, massive and continuous, as in commercial advertising for unhealthy products) messages promoting the at-risk behaviors (e.g., smoking, drinking, fast foods, risky sex).

However, the evaluation research literature shows many success stories over the past several decades. For example, mass-mediated health campaigns have made significant progress in addressing important problems involving seat belt use, smoking, drunk driving, AIDS, and heart disease. The theoretical and practical literature suggests that campaign designers should give greater emphasis to relatively attainable impacts by engaging in more thorough formative evaluation, seeking more receptive focal segments, promoting more palatable positive products perceived to have a favorable benefit-cost ratio, creatively generating free publicity, and shifting campaign resources to indirect pathways that facilitate or reduce behavior of the goal audience segment via interpersonal, organizational, political and societal influences (Noar, 2006). Due to the current trends of campaigners employing sophisticated strategies, digital and online media enabling precise targeting and tailoring, and society giving increased priority to healthy and prosocial practices, it can be expected that mass-mediated health campaigns will produce stronger impacts in future years.

Recommended Readings

Bartholomew, L. K., Parcel, G. S., Kok, G., & Gottlieb, N. H. (2011). *Planning health promotion programs: An intervention mapping approach.* San Francisco: Jossey-Bass.

Burroughs, C. M., & Wood, F. B. (2000). *Measuring the difference. Guide to planning and evaluating health information outreach.* Seattle, WA: National Library of Medicine. http://nnlm.gov/evaluation/guides.html#A1

Harris, M. J. (2010). *Evaluating public and community health programs.* San Francisco, CA: Jossey-Bass.

Noar, S. M. (2006). A 10-year retrospective of research in health mass media campaigns: Where do we go from here? *Journal of Health Communication, 11*(1), 21–42.

Rice, R. E., & Atkin, C. K. (Eds.) (2013). *Public communication campaigns* (4th ed.). Sage, Thousand Oaks, CA.

Additional Resources

Centers for Disease Control and Prevention (n.d.) *CDC social media tools guidelines & best practices.* Atlanta, GA: CDC. Check its website, available at http://www.cdc.gov/Social Media/Tools/guidelines

The Community Guide, http://www.thecommunityguide.org/index.html

Crano, W. D., & Burgoon, M. (Eds.) (2002). *Mass media and drug prevention: Classic and contemporary theories and research.* Mahwah, NJ: Lawrence Erlbaum.

Health Communication Materials Network, http://www.m-mc.org/hcmn

Interactive Smart Chart, http://www.smartchart.org

McKenzie, J. F., Neiger, B. L., & Thackeray, R. (2012). National Cancer Institute's *Making health communication programs work: A planner's guide.* Check the website at http://www.cancer.gov/cancertopics/cancerlibrary/pinkbook

Noar, S. M. (2006). A 10-year retrospective of research in health mass media campaigns: Where do we go from here? *Journal of Health Communication, 11*(1), 21–42.

References

Abroms, L. C., & Maibach, E. W. (2008). The effectiveness of mass communication to change public behavior. *Annual Review of Public Health, 29,* 219–234.

Ajzen, I., Albarracin, D., & Hornik, R. C. (Eds.) (2007). *Prediction and change of health behavior: Applying the reasoned action approach.* Mahwah, NJ: Lawrence Erlbaum Associates.

Atkin, C. K., & Freimuth, V. (2013). Guidelines for formative evaluation research in campaign design. In R. E. Rice & C. K. Atkin (Eds.), *Public communication campaigns* (4th ed., pp. 53–68). Thousand Oaks, CA: Sage.

Atkin, C. K., & Rice, R. E. (2013). Theory and principles of public communication campaigns. In R. E. Rice & C. K. Atkin (Eds.), *Public communication campaigns* (4th ed., pp. 3–20). Thousand Oaks, CA: Sage.

Atkin, C. K., & Salmon, C. (2010). Communication campaigns. In C. Berger, M. Roloff & D. Roskos-Ewoldsen (Eds.), *Handbook of communication science* (2nd ed., pp. 419–435). Thousand Oaks, CA: Sage.

Bandura, A. (1986). *Social foundations of thought and action: A social cognitive theory.* Englewood Cliffs, NJ: Prentice-Hall.

Baranowski, T., Buday, R., Thompson, D. I., & Baranowski, J. (2008). Playing for real: Video games and stories for health-related behavior change. *American Journal of Preventive Medicine, 34*(1), 74–82.

Bartholomew, L. K., Parcel, G. S., Kok, G., & Gottlieb, N. H. (2011). *Planning health promotion programs: An intervention mapping approach*. San Francisco: Jossey-Bass.

Beck, V. (2004). Working with daytime and prime-time television shows in the United States to promote health. In Singhal, A., Cody, M. J., Rogers, E. M., & Sabido, M. (Eds.), *Entertainment-education and social change: History, research, and practice* (pp. 207–224). Mahwah, NJ: Lawrence Erlbaum Associates.

Berkowitz, J., Huhman, M., Heitzler, C., Potter, L., Nolin, M., & Banspach, S. (2008). Overview of formative, process, and outcome evaluation methods used in the VERB™ campaign. *American Journal of Preventive Medicine, 34*(6), S222–S229.

Bracht, N. (2001). Community partnership strategies in health campaigns. In R. E. Rice & C. K. Atkin (Eds.), *Public communication campaigns* (3rd ed., pp. 323–342). Thousand Oaks, CA: Sage.

Bryant, C. A., McCormack Brown, K., McDermott, R. J., Debate, R. D., Alfonso, M. A., Baldwin, J. L., Monaghan, P., & Phillips, L. M. (2009). Community-based prevention marketing: A new framework for health promotion interventions. In R. DiClemente, R. A. Crosby, & M. C. Kegler (Eds.), *Emerging theories in health promotion practice and research: Strategies for improving public health* (2nd ed., pp. 331–356). San Francisco, CA: Jossey-Bass.

Burroughs, C. M., & Wood, F. B. (2000). *Measuring the difference. Guide to planning and evaluating health information outreach*. Seattle, WA: National Library of Medicine. http://nnlm.gov/evaluation/guides.html#A1

Centers for Disease Control and Prevention (2009). *Health marketing*. http://www.cdc.gov/healthmarketing/entertainment_education/healthstyles_survey.htm

Centers for Disease Control and Prevention (n.d.) *CDC social media tools guidelines & best practices*. Atlanta, GA: CDC. Website information available at http://www.cdc.gov/SocialMedia/Tools/guidelines

Cho, H. (Ed.) (2012). *Health communication message design: Theory and practice*. Thousand Oaks, CA: Sage.

Cho, H., & Salmon, C. T. (2007). Unintended effects of health communication campaigns. *Journal of Communication, 57*(2), 293–317.

Cole-Lewis, H., & Kershaw, T. (2010). Text messaging as a tool for behavior change in disease prevention and management. *Epidemiologic Reviews, 32*(1), 56–69.

Crano, W. D., & Burgoon, M. (Eds.) (2002). *Mass media and drug prevention: Classic and contemporary theories and research*. Mahwah, NJ: Lawrence Erlbaum.

Croft, J. B., Temple, S. P., Lankenau, B., Heath, G. W., Macera, C. A., Eaker, E. D., et al. (1994). Community intervention and trends in dietary fat consumption among black and white adults. *Journal of the American Dietetic Association, 94* (11), 1284–1290.

Cugelman, B., Thelwall, M., & Dawed, P. (2011). Online interventions for social marketing health behavior change campaigns: A meta-analysis of psychological architectures and adherence factors. *Journal of Medical Internet Research, 13*(1), e17.

Danaher, B. G., Boles, S. M., Akers, L., Gordon, J. S., & Severson, H. H. (2006). Defining participant exposure measures in web-based health behavior change programs. *Journal of Medical Internet Research, 8*(3):e15 http://www.jmir.org/2006/3/e15/

DeJong, W., & Smith, S. W. (2013). Truth in advertising: Social norms marketing campaigns to reduce college student drinking. In R. E. Rice & C. K. Atkin (Eds.), *Public communication campaigns* (4th ed., pp. 177–189). Thousand Oaks, CA: Sage.

Dorfman, L., & Wallack, L. (2013). Putting policy into health communication: The role of media advocacy. In R. E. Rice & C. K. Atkin (Eds.), *Public communication campaigns* (4th ed., pp. 335–348). Thousand Oaks, CA: Sage.

Edgar, T. M., Noar, S. M., & Freimuth, V. S. (Eds.) (2008). *Communication perspectives on HIV/AIDS for the 21st century*. New York: Lawrence Erlbaum.

Farrelly, M. C., Davis, K. C., Duke, J., & Messeri, P. (2009). Sustaining 'truth': Changes in youth tobacco attitudes and smoking intentions after 3 years of a national antismoking campaign. *Health Education Research, 24*(1), 42–48.

Fishbein, M., Hall-Jamieson, K., Zimmer, E., von Haeften, I., & Nabi, R. (2002). Avoiding the boomerang: Testing the relative effectiveness of antidrug public service announcements before a national campaign. *American Journal of Public Health, 92*(2), 238–245.

Fjeldsoe, B. S., Marshall, A. L., & Miller, Y. D. (2009). Behavior change interventions delivered by mobile telephone short-message service. *American Journal of Preventive Medicine, 36*(2), 165–173.

Franklin, P. D., Rosenbaum, P. F., Carey, M. P., & Roizen, M. F. (2006). Using sequential email messages to promote health behaviors: Evidence of feasibility and reach in a worksite sample. *Journal of Medical Internet Research,* 8(1):e3 http://www.jmir.org/2006/1/e3/

Freudenberg, N., Bradley, S. P., & Serrano, M. (2009). Public health campaigns to change industry practices that damage health: An analysis of 12 case studies. *Health Education and Behavior, 36*, 230–245.

Gallagher, K. M., & Updegraff, J. A. (2012). Health message framing effects on attitudes, intentions, and behavior: A meta-analytic review. *Annals of Behavioral Medicine, 43*(1), 101–116.

Glanz, K., Rimer, B. K., & Viswanath, K. (Eds.) (2008). *Health behavior and health education: Theory, research, and practice* (4th ed.). San Francisco, CA: Jossey-Bass.

Green, G., & Tones, K. (2010). *Health promotion: Planning and strategies* (2nd ed.). London: Sage.

Gustafson, D. H., Hawkins, R., McTavish, F., Pingree, S., Chen, W. C., Volrathongchai, K., Stengle, W., Stewart, J. A., & Serlin, R. C. (2008). Internet-based interactive support for cancer patients: Are integrated systems better? *Journal of Communication, 58*, 238–257.

Harris, M. J. (2010). *Evaluating public and community health programs*. San Francisco: Jossey-Bass.

Hornik, R. (Ed.) (2002). *Public health communication: Evidence for behavior change*. Mahwah, NJ: Lawrence Erlbaum Associates.

Hornik, R., Jacobsohn, L., Orwin, R., Piesse, A., & Kalton, G. (2008). Effects of the national youth anti-drug media campaign on youths. *American Journal of Public Health, 98*(12), 2229–2236.

Kotler, P., Roberto, N., & Lee, N. (2002). *Social marketing: Improving the quality of life*. Thousand Oaks, CA: Sage.

Krishna, S., Boren, S. A., & Balas, E. A. (2009). Healthcare via cell phones: A systematic review. *Telemedicine and e-Health, 15*(3), 231–240.

Lieberman, D. (2013). Using interactive media in communication campaigns for children and adolescents. In R. E. Rice & C. K. Atkin (Eds.), *Public communication campaigns* (4th ed., pp. 273–287). Thousand Oaks, CA: Sage.

Lustria, M. L. A., Cortese, J., Noar, S. M., & Glueckauf, R. L. (2009). Computer-tailored health interventions delivered over the web: Review and analysis of key components. *Patient Education and Counseling, 74*(2), 156–173.

McGuire, W. J. (2013). McGuire's classic input-output framework for constructing persuasive messages. In R. E. Rice & C. K. Atkin (Eds.), *Public communication campaigns* (4th ed., pp. 133–145). Thousand Oaks, CA: Sage.

McKenzie, J. F., Neiger, B. L., & Thackeray, R. (2012). *Planning, implementing, and evaluating health promotion programs: A primer* (6th ed.). San Francisco: Benjamin Cummings.

McKenzie-Mohr, D. (2010). *Fostering sustainable behavior: An introduction to community-based social marketing* (4th ed.). Gabriola Island, British Columbia: New Society Publishers.

Metzger, M., Flanagin, A., Eyal, K., Lemus, D., & McCann, R. (2003). Credibility for the 21st century: Integrating perspectives on source, message, and media credibility in the contemporary media environment. In P. Kalbfleisch (Ed.), *Communication yearbook 27* (pp. 293–335). Mahwah, NJ: Lawrence Erlbaum.

Movius, L., Cody, M., Huang, G., Berkowitz, M., & Morgan, S. (2007). Motivating television viewers to become organ donors. *Cases in Public Health Communication & Marketing*. June. For instant access, check http://www.casesjournal.org/volume1/peer-reviewed/cases_1_08.cfm

Murero, M., & Rice, R. E. (Eds.) (2006). *The Internet and health care: Theory, research and practice*. Mahwah, NJ: Lawrence Erlbaum Associates.

National Cancer Institute. (2008). *The role of the media in promoting and reducing tobacco use*. Tobacco Control Monograph 19. Bethesda, MD: U.S. Department of Health and Human Services, National Institutes of Health, National Cancer Institute. NIH Pub. No. 07-6242.

National Cancer Institute. (2009). *Health information national trends survey*. http://www.hints.cancer.gov/dataset.jsp

Noar, S. M. (2006). A 10-year retrospective of research in health mass media campaigns: Where do we go from here? *Journal of Health Communication, 11*(1), 21–42.

Noar, S. M., Benac, C. N., & Harris, M. S. (2007). Does tailoring matter? Meta-analytic review of tailored print health behavior change interventions. *Psychological Bulletin, 133*(4), 673–693. doi: 10.1037/0033-2909.133.4.673

Noar, S. M., & Harrington, N. G. (Eds.) (2012). *eHealth applications: Promising strategies for behavior change*. New York: Routledge.

Parker, J. C., & Thorson, E. (2009). *Health communication in the new media landscape*. New York: Springer Publishing Co.

Perloff, R. M. (2003). *The dynamics of persuasion: Communication and attitudes in the 21st century* (2nd ed.). Mahwah, NJ: Lawrence Erlbaum Associates.

Piotrow, P. T., Rimon J. G. II, Merritt, A. P., & Saffitz, G. (2003). *Advancing health communication: The PCS experience in the field*. Center Publication 103. Baltimore: Johns Hopkins University, Bloomberg School of Public Health, Center for Communication Programs. For more information, check http://pdf.usaid.gov/pdf_docs/Pnact765.pdf

Portnoy, D. B., Scott-Sheldon, L. A. J., Johnson, B. T., & Carey, M. P. (2008). Computer-delivered interventions for health promotion and behavioral risk reduction: A meta-analysis of 75 randomized controlled trials, 1988–2007. *Preventive Medicine, 47*(1), 3–16.

Prochaska, J., & Velicer, W. (1997). The Transtheoretical Model of health behavior change. *American Journal of Health Promotion, 12*(1), 38–48.

Rains, S. A., & Keating, D. M. (2011). The social dimension of blogging about health: Health blogging, social support, and well-being. *Communication Monographs, 78*(4), 511–534.

Rains, S. A., & Young, V. (2009). A meta-analysis of research on formal computer-mediated support groups: Examining group characteristics and health outcomes. *Human Communication Research, 35*, 309–336.

Rice, R. E. (2006). Influences, usage, and outcomes of Internet health information searching: Multivariate results from the Pew surveys. *International Journal of Medical Informatics, 75*(1), 8–28.

Rice, R. E., & Atkin, C. K. (Eds.) (2013). *Public communication campaigns* (4th ed.). Thousand Oaks, CA: Sage.

Rice, R. E., & Foote, D. (2013). A systems-based evaluation planning model for health communication campaigns in developing countries. In R. E. Rice & C. K. Atkin (Eds.), *Public communication campaigns* (4th ed., pp. 69–81). Thousand Oaks, CA: Sage.

Rice, R. E., Wu, Z., Li, L., Detels, R., & Rotheram-Borus, M. J. (2012). Reducing STD/HIV stigmatizing attitudes through community popular opinion leaders in Chinese markets. *Human Communication Research, 38*, 379–405.

Rogers, E. M. (2003). *Diffusion of innovations* (5th ed.). New York: Free Press.

Romer, D., Sznitman, S., DiClemente, R., Salazar, L. F., Vanable, P. A., Carey, M. P., Hennessy, M., Brown, L. K., Valois, R. F., Stanton, B. F., Fortune, T., & Juzang, I. (2009). Mass media as an HIV-prevention strategy: Using culturally sensitive messages to reduce HIV-associated sexual behavior of at-risk African American Youth. *American Journal of Public Health, 99*(12), 2150–2159.

Rothman, A. J., Bartels, R. D., Wlaschin, J., & Salovey, P. (2006). The strategic use of gain- and loss-framed messages to promote healthy behavior: How theory can inform practice. *Journal of Communication, 56*, S202–S220.

Salmon, C. T., & Murray-Johnson, L. (2013). Communication campaign effectiveness and effects: Some critical distinctions. In R. E. Rice & C. K. Atkin (Eds.), *Public communication campaigns* (4th ed., pp. 99–112). Thousand Oaks, CA: Sage.

Scanfeld, D., Scanfeld, V., & Larson, E. L. (2010). Dissemination of health information through social networks: Twitter and antibiotics. *American Journal of Infection Control, 38*(3), 182–188.

Singhal, A., Cody, M., Rogers, E., & Sabido, M. (2004). *Entertainment-education and social change: History, research, and practice*. Mahwah, NJ: Lawrence Erlbaum Associates.

Snyder, L. B., & LaCroix, J. M. (2013). How effective are mediated health campaigns? A synthesis of meta-analyses. In R. E. Rice & C. K. Atkin (Eds.), *Public communication campaigns* (4th ed., pp. 113–129). Thousand Oaks, CA: Sage.

Steckler, A., & Linnan, L. (Eds.) (2006). *Process evaluation for public health interventions and research.* New York: John Wiley and Sons.

Strecher, V. (2007). Internet methods for delivering behavioral and health-related interventions (eHealth). *Annual Review of Clinical Psychology, 3,* 53–76.

Thackeray, R., Neiger, B. L., Hanson, C. L., & McKenzie, J. F. (2008). Enhancing promotional strategies within social marketing programs: Use of Web 2.0 social media. *Health Promotion Practice, 9*(4), 338–343.

Tian, Y. (2010). Organ donation on Web 2.0: Content and audience analysis of organ donation videos on YouTube. *Health Communication, 25*(3), 238–246.

Valente, T. W. (2012). Network interventions. *Science, 337*(6 July), 49–53.

Walther, J. B., Pingree, S., Hawkins, R. P., & Buller, D. B. (2005). Attributes of interactive online health information systems. *Journal of Medical Internet Research, 7*(3):e33 http://www.jmir.org/2005/3/e33/

Wantland, D. J., Portillo, C. J., Holzemer, W. L., Slaughter, R., & McGhee, E. M. (2004). The effectiveness of web-based vs. non-web-based interventions: A meta-analysis of behavioral change outcomes. *Journal of Medical Internet Research, 6*(4):e40 http://www.jmir.org/2004/4/e40/

Webb, T. L., Joseph, J., Yardley, L., & Michie, S. (2010). Using the Internet to promote health behavior change: A systematic review and meta-analysis of the impact of theoretical basis, use of behavior change techniques, and mode of delivery on efficacy. *Journal of Medical Internet Research, 12*(1):e4. http://www.jmir.org/2010/1/e4

Webster, J. G., Phalen, P. F., & Lichty, L. W. (2006). *Ratings analysis: The theory and practice of audience research* (3rd ed.). Mahwah, NJ: Lawrence Erlbaum.

Witte, K., Meyer, G., & Martell, D. P. (2001). *Effective health risk messages: A step-by-step guide.* Thousand Oaks, CA: Sage.

Yzer, M. C., Southwell, B .G., & Stephenson, M. T. (2013). Inducing fear as a public communication campaign strategy. In R. E. Rice & C. K. Atkin (Eds.), *Public communication campaigns* (4th ed., pp. 163–176). Thousand Oaks, CA: Sage.

Zimmerman, R. S., Palmgreen, P. M., Noar, S. M., Lustria, M. L. A., Lu, H-Y., & Horosewski, M. L. (2007). Effects of a televised two-city safer sex mass media campaign targeting high-sensation-seeking and impulsive-decision-making young adults. *Health Education & Behavior, 34,* 810–826.

Chapter 2

Developing and Testing Mobile Health Applications to Affect Behavior Change: Lessons from the Field

Andrew Isham, Bret R. Shaw, & Dave Gustafson,
University of Wisconsin-Madison

Introduction

Today, mobile communication technologies are being adopted faster than any information technology in human history (Waegemann, 2010). Mobile health (mHealth) applications are advantageous because they can be used 24 hours a day, 7 days a week, anywhere there is cellular coverage (Evans, Abroms, Poropatich, Nielsen & Wallace, 2012). Additionally, many people carry their mobile devices with them everywhere, making them a potentially powerful behavioral change tool. Promisingly, early studies indicate that mHealth applications can be efficacious across a variety of behavioral domains (e.g., Burke et al., 2012; Cole-Lewis & Kershaw, 2010; Dowshen, Kuhns, Johnson, Holoyda, & Garofalo, 2012; Fjeldsoe, Marshall, & Miller, 2009; Stockwell et al., 2012; Whittaker et al., 2009). Not surprisingly, there is a great deal of interest in mHealth solutions among both consumers and clinicians (Dolan, 2009). Others have observed there are few areas in the field of health communication that have generated as many enthusiasts in such a short time as has mHealth (Sherry & Ratzan, 2012). Clearly, mHealth opportunities abound.

At the Center for Health Enhancement Systems Studies at the University of Wisconsin—Madison, we have developed and tested several mobile health applications designed to manage chronic conditions via behavioral change. This is an attempt to collate and synthesize the learning that has taken place in order to provide practical guidelines to developers and researchers about how to design, implement, and evaluate successful mobile health communication interventions.

Examples of mHealth Applications

CHESS (Comprehensive Health Enhancement Support System) is the umbrella name for a variety of computer- and smartphone-based eHealth programs (e.g., Baker et al., 2011; DeBenske, Gustafson, Shaw & Cleary, 2010; Gustafson et al., 2002; Gustafson, Boyle, Shaw et al., 2011; Gustafson, Shaw, Isham et al., 2011; Shaw, Gustafson, Hawkins et al., 2006). The CHESS development process utilizes an interdisciplinary team of researchers, administrators, clinicians and programmers working in close collaboration with patients and their families. This process can serve as an example for other teams developing smartphone-based health interventions. Prior to sharing our lessons learned in designing, implementing and evaluating mHealth applications, we briefly describe three mHealth interventions we have developed to provide context for our recommendations.

Addiction Comprehensive Health Enhancement Support System (A-CHESS)

A-CHESS is a smartphone application for people leaving residential treatment designed to prevent relapse and build support for long-term recovery. Development of all A-CHESS features took into account the smaller screens available with content, interfaces, and when/how they were delivered optimized for a handheld device. Some key features of A-CHESS include the following: *Discussion Groups* let patients exchange emotional support and information with other A-CHESS users via online support groups. *Ask an Expert* allows users to receive responses within 24 hours (weekdays) from addiction experts to request information and advice. *Personal Stories* are audio narratives based on interviews of patients and family members focused on recovery experiences and strategies to avoid relapse. *Recovery Info* offers answers to common questions, articles on addiction management, and links to recovery-related web resources. *Easing Distress* is a computerized cognitive behavioral therapy program. *Healthy Events Newsletter* offers information about local healthy, recovery-friendly events and includes the capability to automatically link users to other individuals in recovery who share similar interests, which helps facilitate companionship and enhance feelings of relatedness while participating in activities likely to contribute to a lasting recovery. *Electronic Care Manager* connects the user to a case manager who has access to data about the patient so the person in recovery can access one-on-one support and receive tailored recommendations about educational content available on A-CHESS. The *High-Risk Patient Locator* uses Global Positioning System (GPS) technology to track when somebody in recovery is approaching an area where he or she has traditionally obtained alcohol so they can be contacted to receive support to work through what might be a high-risk situation for relapse. *Weekly Check-ins* are short surveys to gauge environmental, social, physical and psychological factors that may contribute to relapse so users can receive additional support if needed for their recovery. *Panic Button* provides the patient the means to immediately seek support from others (e.g., counselor, sponsor, friend, family member) if they feel the need for immediate support to avoid an imminent relapse (e.g., if urges and cravings become severe and they want assistance). *My Profile* allows users to share pictures and interests, expanding/enhancing their support networks. Users can receive alerts that notify them when there is new content to access.

Mobile CHESS (M-CHESS) for Adolescents with Asthma

Mobile CHESS is an application to help underserved teens with asthma improve their medication compliance and reduce symptoms. The M-CHESS intervention was designed to test whether an asthma care management system delivered via a smartphone could support low-income teenagers to improve symptom control and reduce asthma-related emergency or urgent care visits and hospitalizations. The secondary aims included whether M-CHESS could increase adherence to asthma control medication and reduce absenteeism from school or work. The interface was intended to provide easy-to-access, immediate information about asthma and disease care management and to facilitate communication between the participants, the asthma case manager, their health care providers and families. To do this, intervention participants were provided a smartphone with Internet and text messaging capabilities along with access to M-CHESS. Key features of M-CHESS include the following: *Medications* offers reminders to take medications to control asthma and instruction on when and how to take rescue medications. *Asthma Action Plan* provides customized guidance on when to contact health care providers or go to the emergency room. *Asthma Info* includes answers to common questions and brief animated instructional videos. *My Team* allows users to share pictures and interests with other M-CHESS users. Individuals earn points for taking their medication and accessing different M-CHESS features. These points contribute to the teams' score, incentivizing participation and adherence. M-CHESS users can communicate with both other users and case managers using *My Messages*.

Survivorship CHESS (S-CHESS) for People Leaving Colon Cancer Treatment

A third mobile program has been developed to help colon cancer patients leaving treatment improve daily activity. It differs in two ways from the alcohol and asthma programs. First, it uses an avatar (virtual guide) to help users navigate the system and second, its approach involves goal setting, progress monitoring and feedback. While it also offers many other features provided by the asthma and alcohol programs, such as discussion group and ask an expert, its focus is on guided behavior change (exercise) rather than on improved coping strategies (relapse prevention). And while the typical users of asthma (M-CHESS) tend to be much younger and A-CHESS users tend to be young to middle age, S-CHESS tends to serve people in later stages of life.

Mobile Health Application Design Opportunities and Challenges

Based on our Center's experience developing and evaluating smartphone-based mHealth applications, we highlight key lessons about opportunities and challenges below.

1. Use theory to guide design and evaluation

mHealth interventions tend to be complex, potentially involving interactions between patients, their families, clinicians, and the healthcare system. Such complexity challenges designers to select useful features from the large array of what might work. Behavioral models can be used to inform which features to include, and when and how they might be most useful. However, mHealth studies to date typically fail to explicitly test theoretical assumptions (Evans, Abroms, Poropatich, Nielsen & Wallace, 2012). During evaluation, specifying the 'innards' of one's theory offers the potential to track more explanatory, proximate outcomes, which serve as valuable initial measures informing and complementing more distal outcomes.

We've used Self Determination Theory (SDT) to guide the design and evaluation of the mHealth interventions we have brought to trial. SDT posits that three fundamental needs contribute to adaptive functioning; i.e., perceived competence, a feeling of relatedness, and autonomous motivation

(Ryan & Deci, 2006). Many studies have verified the importance of these three domains (Pingree, Hawkins, Baker et al., 2010). A generalizable behavioral change model such as SDT can be used in conjunction with condition-specific models; for example, we've used SDT in conjunction with Marlatt's Relapse Prevention model to develop A-CHESS (Gustafson, Shaw, Isham et al., 2010).

However, design does not need to be limited to addressing only elements of specific model(s), as many existing models were developed and tested prior to the introduction of mobile applications and the anywhere/anytime monitoring and intervention they potentially facilitate. Rather, a model should be used to identify novel, high-value opportunities for intervention presented by the new data-rich and more dynamic platform. The framework provided by such models provides a starting point for design, but, again, it is important to not limit your thinking to address only the components of the model, as the technology may open new opportunities for theory-building and behavioral interventions that are not included in traditional models. For example, the A-CHESS *High Risk Locator* responds to a potential high-risk situation by automatically engaging supportive others via text message, potentially overcoming the potential for relapse. Marlatt's relapse prevention model suggests self-monitoring to identify high-risk situations, but the smartphone GPS technology presents the opportunity for the application to take some of the burden of self-monitoring off of the user, as well as serve as a vehicle for supportive response from peers, family members or clinicians.

2. Pick platform based on target audience's needs

An mHealth intervention can be developed for a smartphone, a basic cellphone, a tablet, or any combination of the above. The first question a developer should ask is "Given the array of monitoring and support features that we want to provide, what is the most suitable platform(s) to develop for?" For example, if there aren't time and location-based features and the content presented is text-intensive, developing primarily for the web may be more effective than developing for a mobile device (Cartman, 2009). It is a mistake to conceive of an mHealth application as a smaller version of a website. Doing so not only neglects the strengths of the mobile platform (e.g., time and location sensitivity, anywhere access, push capabilities, etc.), it also makes it likely that user experience will overwhelm and quickly frustrate because it can be difficult to sift through as much content on a mobile device as can be done with ease on a larger screen.

For users with special needs, the universal access features offered by a technology platform must be considered. For example, when designing a mobile application for the hard of hearing, a device that is highly compatible with hearing aids should be used. For users who cannot read, screen readers are available for most major smart phones. Users with motor control issues may benefit from intelligent keyboards with predictive text entry, which is an option on current Android and iOS devices. As voice navigation, voice to text and text to voice becomes progressively more effective, its availability will certainly increase the accessibility of these systems to those with low literacy. These are just a few examples of the wide range of accessibility features available. Some of these accessibility features are built into operating systems, and some will need to be added to an application sometimes for free, sometimes for purchase.

3. Understand context in which application will be used

The mobile platform allows developers to present information using text, pictures, audio, video, and even tactile cues (e.g., touchscreen with haptic feedback, custom vibration ringtones). There are a couple of considerations that may be unique to mHealth user populations—for example: (1) Some target users might have cognitive impairments that involve low literacy (as mentioned earlier) and low attention span, so the duration and complexity of the user experience designed must be kept to a minimum; (2) The mHealth application will likely be used in public and any audio/visual indicators of private health information might betray the user's desire for confidentiality. Convenience and privacy are sometimes in conflict with each other. We've successfully overcome such privacy concerns by training participants to use the security features on the phone (screen lock, password, etc.) as well as demonstrating enough potential value of the applications during training to make it worth the minimal risk of privacy breach.

4. Understand social and familial implications

A clinician is simply a visitor in a patient's life, not a central part of it as the family usually is. There may be key clinically relevant communication with family members that could be aided or facilitated by mHealth solutions. Family members or caregivers may benefit from portals into a system that are customized according to their needs. For example, if a teenager with asthma has reported (via a reminder/survey application) that they have not been taking their asthma control medication, a report to the clinician may prove useful in the longer term, but a text message or email to a parent may be a more immediate (and therefore, effective) means of encouraging positive behavioral change. Social context may be monitored to inform the delivery of behavioral change features, for example, a person in addiction recovery may benefit from avoiding certain bars, which can be monitored using GPS. In such a case, a response could be generated and sent to the individual's phone, a counselor, a peer, a sponsor, a relative or all of the above, depending on the preferences of those involved. Broadly, once important information has been captured, there may be many ways to make it actionable, both immediately and in the long term, to a number of people. Designers should carefully consider those people who have the most access and impact in the life of a user, not just clinicians. It may well be that the influence of a patient's family and friends eclipses that of even the most engaged health care providers.

Another contextual issue is thoroughly understanding the needs and environment within which users exist. For instance, in a new program we are developing for elderly people and their family caregivers (not mentioned prior), our programmers and technical development team are volunteering at an elderly day care center so as to better understand what the lives of their system's users are like. And by visiting elders in their homes in a rural county of Wisconsin, they personally experienced how the hills and valleys affect reception of cellular signals. This helped them rethink the design of the system, leading them in some cases to see the next-door neighbor and family member as key users of the mobile system being developed to support the intended target users. And by better understanding the near paranoia the elderly have of being scammed, they appreciated the challenge of employing some of the social media sites that exist.

Broadly speaking, the patient and their supportive others (family, friends) should be a part of each stage of the design and development processes, not just the implementation and evaluation phases. Without this input and involvement, researchers and developers make themselves susceptible to misconceptions, false assumptions and lost opportunities that can undermine the effectiveness of their interventions.

Focus groups, pilot testing, surveys, and nominal group process are all methods that we have employed to gather input and feedback from patients and their families. In the initial version of A-CHESS, we only generated notifications for the user if it was time to take a weekly survey. We thought that notifications for other events and activities within A-CHESS would pile up quickly and become a burden to users. After demonstrating these features to a focus group of potential users, they let us know that they would much prefer to receive notifications for any new posting in A-CHESS (messages, healthy events, discussion group activity, etc.), and they did not think it would be a burden at all, so we made such changes. As a result, some users ended up rapidly responding to discussion group posts asking for support—something that could not have happened had we not used the focus group feedback. Our initial assumption was wrong, the change was easy, and the result of the change was more engaged, connected users.

5. More functionality is not always better

To most effectively take advantage of opportunities presented by mHealth, a developer must carefully consider which features to include and which to leave out—based on what is well suited to the mobile platform, as opposed to what could be developed, but is not well suited to the platform (in other words, determine the difference between what should be done vs. what could be done). The challenge is to identify which services would likely provide enough value (benefit) to justify the use of crucial screen/attentional real estate (cost). Generally, compact screen size requires a minimal feature set optimized for common use cases. Researchers are often equipped with limited development resources, requiring them to be selective about which features of an application are most important and ensure they are created with a mind for both usability and usefulness to maximize the potential effectiveness of their mHealth application.

6. Reconceptualize existing clinical approaches

In addition to the patients and their families and friends, clinicians (e.g., physician, specialist, nurse, counselor) should be a part of each step in the design and development process, in order to (1) make sure that they are aware of all of the input/output capabilities of the smartphone or other mobile device, so that they do not limit their thinking to the confines of traditional interventions and data collection procedures; (2) if the clinician will be accessing patient data gathered via the application, it is important to identify what is useful to them, and when, and how (platform could be mobile, web, etc.) the information is delivered. For example, if a typical practice is to have a patient learn about and remember key side effects associated with a new medication in order to self monitor, an mHealth application may circumvent or reduce such a burden on the patient by generating symptom-monitoring assessment surveys. In such a case, limited patient/clinician time need not be used to educate patients about what to watch out for, as the survey remembers for them. At follow up appointments, the clinician would have access to data collected along the way and need not rely on patients' recall. Further, this data could be used to alert clinicians of adverse events in real time between appointments.

7. Privacy concerns may limit design options

Much of the attraction of non-mHealth applications may be attributable to social media—indeed, social media features are some of the most frequently used features of the applications we've developed—this allure can and ideally should be harnessed by mHealth developers. However, if an application is designed to work with protected personal health information, Institutional Review Boards (IRBs) may require mHealth researchers to restrict interaction between test participants, for example, our IRB prevented us from allowing men to interact with women via A-CHESS because of the risk of predatory behavior, so we traded the potential power of the broader pool of supportive others, which may have limited the benefit of integrated social media for added safety. Additionally, IRB may require that all personal health information be stored on encrypted servers (as opposed to on a device or 3rd-party servers). This presents two challenges to developers and researchers: (1) applications that require personal health information may not be able to run in areas with poor cell coverage and may not respond as quickly as they would if such data were stored locally on the mobile device, (2) developers may be prevented from integrating with 3rd-party features that may otherwise provide value—for example, using Facebook to manage support groups, Google Calendar to coordinate events, etc.

In some cases, these concerns can be addressed by explaining the security features on the device (screen lock, passwords, etc.) to study participants as a part of the consenting process, allowing them a range of security options to protect their personal information. Development teams should work closely with IRBs to negotiate and determine an appropriate application of the guidelines so as not to hamstring the key features of the intervention.

Most research groups will be subject to an IRB that presents its own security requirements. Researchers should seek to develop relationships with their IRB that foster greater understanding of the nature and potential benefits (as well as the risks) of the social media being developed.

8. The technology evolves faster than it can be tested

The traditional clinical trial testing model is not well suited to test mHealth interventions. Many trials will take at least a couple of years to complete. As a result, the best available mobile devices at the beginning of the trial period are outmoded or obsolete by the end. Methods for evaluating mHealth need to include not only randomized clinical trials but also other complementary, alternative methodologies to ensure research studies can provide timely information within a rapidly evolving field (Nilsen et al., 2012). As it relates to evaluating mHealth applications, research should be designed to test an intervention approach rather than an instantiation tied to a specific device or interface. For example, we developed a meeting locator for 12-step programs, for A-CHESS that initially existed exclusively on our servers, with the database maintained by us. As the hardware and Google Maps improved, we decided to query Google from within our application to expand the reach of the meetings that could be found using the meeting locator feature. This made analysis of the usefulness of this feature more complex, because we wanted to compare the effect of the first version of the meeting locator with the effect of the second version in addition to evaluating them as one feature, albeit one that evolved over time. In this way, evaluating many mHealth features may be more difficult because they are 'moving targets.' Researchers should be prepared to analyze the use and usefulness of evolving features from multiple angles, including comparing before/after significant changes to allow room for developmental advancement within the trial period. In summary, since the clinical trial model was created to test more static interventions, researchers using the model to test mHealth interventions will have to be flexible as they update applications and analyze data. Other more efficient designs (such as fractional factorials and stepped wedge) should be considered, along with ways to speed recruitment of subjects.

9. Interventions that feature social media require critical mass

Social media may require a minimum number of users to provide value. Since the number of participants using an mHealth application during a testing period is usually determined by power calculations and logistical/financial limitations for recruitment, there may be patient-to-patient interactive features that, even though they have potential to work in a scaled-up context, do not show effects in a testing context. It may be necessary for researchers to simulate social interaction in the early stages of a trial to create the communicative momentum necessary to stimulate ongoing supportive interactions. We ended up seeding discussion groups to provide initial impetus within the social media of our applications. Additionally, we created a tool for A-CHESS users to share information about recovery-oriented meetings (time, place, rating, etc.) with each other. Fully scaled up, there would presumably be a sufficient number of A-CHESS contributors to keep the feature populated with meetings. Since we were testing with numbers much smaller than full-scale, we had the counselors at the test sites enter meetings to ensure there were options for those who sought them out.

10. Consider using test subjects' primary telephone for intervention

Our Center has been developing and evaluating technology-based information and support systems to help people facing health challenges now for almost 25 years. When we first began this work, owning a computer was a rarity, and therefore we would provide hardware to subjects who participated in our studies. However, the technology landscape has changed substantially over this time period, and now we've found a significant majority of our subjects already own computers and many own smart phones. As a result, we have found that where provisioning technology such as computers or smart phones to patients was once a necessity for conducting our studies, it may now actually be a liability in some cases for a successful implementation.

Despite concerns about the 'digital divide,' other research supports our observation that the traditionally underserved often have access to mobile devices. For example, one recent study found that 92% of low-income families had mobile phones. Of these, 96% could receive text messages and 81% had unlimited data plans (Ahlers-Schmidt, Chesser, Hart, Paschal, Nguyen & Wittler, 2010). Another report by the Pew Internet and American Life Project found that African Americans and Latinos had higher than average levels of smartphone adoption and—even among those with a household income of $30,000 or less—smartphone ownership rates for people ages 18–29 was equal to the national average (Smith, 2011). Dowshen et al. (2012) also conducted a study in which they demonstrated the feasibility of implementing an mHealth intervention for a difficult-to-reach population using their own mobile phones.

In addition to the cost of providing all test subjects with smart phones, there are a few obstacles to be aware of: (1) If the mHealth application is not on a participant's primary phone, they are less likely to have it with them at all/most times and places, so the power of pushing time/location sensitive interventions may be diminished; (2) The participant may have to learn how to navigate the phone and the operating system before benefiting from the mHealth application. For these reasons, it is important to train new users on the phone (not just the mHealth applications), and leverage the devices that people are already using to the extent possible.

Conclusion

mHealth researchers face a unique set of challenges and opportunities. Mobile technology may hold the potential to extend the reach of behavioral monitoring and intervention well beyond its present-day limitations. In terms of diagnosis and treatment, barriers between the clinic and the real world may effectively begin to blur. Additionally, family and friends can be included as integral partners in mHealth interventions designed to influence behavior change and adherence, as they are often already connected to the patient via mobile devices or could be if they are not. To make the most of these opportunities, research teams seeking to design, implement, and evaluate such systems should be ready to address the potential barriers outlined here. We invite readers to determine which of the recommendations that we've made here apply to their circumstance. You may not use them all at once. And there may be exceptions—these strategies might not always apply—but we find the promise of these strategies has generally been made evident in our pilot studies, our trial results, and our synthesis of the mobile app design literature (for more on mobile app design, we recommend *Strategic Mobile Design: Creating Engaging Experiences* by Cartman and Ting and *Usability of Mobile Websites & Applications: 237 Design Guidelines for Improving User Experience of Mobile Sites and Apps* by Nielsen Norman Group). Researchers should stay mindful of the strengths and weaknesses of the mobile platform, so as to keep themselves open to prospective shifts in clinical and psychosocial paradigms that can usher in true, useful innovation (for more on behavior change mobile interventions, we recommend Fjeldsoe et al., 2009 and Gustafson et al., 2011). We've learned a lot—often via trial and error—but mHealth is an interdiscipline in its infancy. Hopefully, our lessons learned thus far will be helpful.

Recommended Readings

Cartman, J., Ting, R. (2008). *Strategic Mobile Design: Creating Engaging Experiences.* Berkeley, CA: New Riders.

Budiu, R., Nielsen, J. (2010). *Usability of Mobile Websites & Applications: 237 Design Guidelines for Improving User Experience of Mobile Sites and Apps.* Fremont, CA: Nielsen Norman Group.

Fjeldsoe, B. S., Marshall, A. L., & Miller, Y. D. (2009). Behavior change interventions delivered by mobile telephone short-message service. *American Journal of Preventive Medicine, 36,* 165–173.

Gustafson, D.H., Shaw, B.R., Isham, A., Baker, T., Boyle, M.G., & Levy, M. (2011). Explicating an evidence-based, theoretically informed, mobile technology-based system to improve outcomes for people in recovery for alcohol dependence. *Substance Use and Misuse, 46(1),* 96–111.

References

Ahlers-Schmidt, C.R., Chesser, A., Hart, T., Paschal, A., Nguyen, T., & Wittler, B.R (2010). Text messaging immunization reminders: feasibility of implementation with low-income parents. *Preventive Medicine,* 50, 306–307.

Baker, T.B., Hawkins, R., Pingree, S., Roberts, L.J., McDowell, H.E., Shaw, B.R., Serlin, R., Dillenburg, L., Swoboda, C.M., Han, J.Y., Stewart, J.A., Carmack-Taylor, C.L., Salner, A., Schlam, T.R., McTavish, F., & Gustafson, D.H. (2011). Optimizing eHealth breast cancer interventions: Which types of eHealth services are effective? *Translational Behavioral Medicine: Practice, Policy, Research, 1*(1), 134–145.

Burke, L.E., Styn, M.A., Sereika, S.M., Conroy, M.B., Ye, L., Glanz, K., Sevick, M.A., & Ewing, L.J. (2012). Using mHealth technology to enhance self-monitoring for weight loss: A randomized trial. *American Journal of Preventive Medicine,* 43, 20–26.

Cole-Lewis, H., & Kershaw, T. (2010). Text messaging as a tool for behavior change in disease prevention and management. *Epidemiologic Reviews, 32*(1), 56–69.

Dowshen, N., Kuhns, L.M., Johnson, A., Holoyda, B.J., Garofalo, R. (2012). Improving adherence to antiretroviral therapy for youth living with HIV/AIDS: A pilot study using personalized, interactive, daily text message reminders. *Journal of Medical Internet Research,* 14, e51.

DuBenske, L.L., Gustafson, D.H., Shaw, B.R., & Cleary, J.F. (2010). Web-based cancer communication and decision making systems: Connecting patients, caregivers, and clinicians for improved health outcomes. *Medical Decision Making,* 30(6), 732–744.

Evans, D.W., Abroms, L.C., Poropatich, R., Nielsen, P.E., & Wallace, J.L. (2012). Mobile health evaluation methods: The Text4baby case study. *Journal of Health Communication,* 17, 22–29.

Fjeldsoe, B. S., Marshall, A. L., & Miller, Y. D. (2009). Behavior change interventions delivered by mobile telephone short-message service. *American Journal of Preventive Medicine, 36,* 165–173.

Gustafson, D.H., Boyle, M.G., Shaw, B.R., Isham, A., McTavish, F., Richards, S., Schubert, C., Levy, M., & Johnson, K. (2011). An e-Health solution for people with alcohol problems. *Alcohol Research & Health,* 33(4), 327–337.

Gustafson, D.H., Shaw, B.R., Isham, A., Baker, T., Boyle, M.G., & Levy, M. (2011). Explicating an evidence-based, theoretically informed, mobile technology-based system to improve outcomes for people in recovery for alcohol dependence. *Substance Use and Misuse,* 46(1), 96–111.

Nilsen, W., Kumar, S., Shar, A., Varoquiers, C., Wiley, T., Riley, W.T., Pavel, M., & Atienza, A.A. (2012). Advancing the science of mHealth, *Journal of Health Communication,* 17, 5–10.

Shaw, B., Gustafson, D., Hawkins, R., McTavish, F., McDowell, H., Pingree, S. & Ballard, D. (2006). How underserved breast cancer patients use and benefit from eHealth programs: Implications for closing the digital divide. *American Behavioral Scientist,* 49, 1–12.

Sherry, J.M., & Ratzan, S.C. (2012): Measurement and evaluation outcomes for mHealth communication: Don't we have an app for that? *Journal of Health Communication*: International Perspectives, 17:sup1, 1–3.

Smith, A. (2011). Smartphone adoption and usage. *Pew Internet and American Life Project.* Retrieved on June 27, 2012: http://pewinternet.org/Reports/2011/Smartphones/Summary.aspx

Stockwell, M.S., Kharbanda, E.O., Martinez, R.A., Vargas, C.Y., Vawdrey, D.K., Camargo, S. (2012). Effect of a text messaging intervention on influenza vaccination in an urban, low-income pediatric and adolescent population: A randomized controlled trial. *Journal of the American Medical Association* (JAMA), 307, 1702–1708.

Whittaker, R., Borland, R., Bullen, C., Lin, R. B., McRobbie, H., & Rodgers, A. (2009). Mobile phone-based interventions for smoking cessation. *Cochrane Database of Systematic Reviews, 4.* Art. No.: CD006611.

Chapter 3

A Primer for Using Mobile Apps and Social Media in Healthcare

Carolyn Lauckner & Pamela Whitten,
Michigan State University

Introduction

Consider this scenario: a diabetic patient, after a visit with her doctor, logs on to a web portal to see how thousands of similar patients have reacted to the treatment her physician has just recommended. She can see their ratings of the treatment's effectiveness and the severity of side effects experienced, along with personal tips for taking the medication. Armed with the knowledge of these many other patients, she contemplates the pros and cons of beginning the treatment. While on this website, she also logs into her personal profile and enters in her blood glucose levels for the past few days. To get this information, she opens the app on her phone that receives data on her blood sugar wirelessly via Bluetooth from her glucometer. With these two technologies, she can view how her health has changed over time and look for patterns in her glucose levels to aid in better self-management of her condition.

Such a scenario would have been impossible in the recent past. One patient could not easily access the opinions of thousands of similar others, and keeping track of glucose levels required manual recording and charting. New technologies, including social media sites and smartphones, have evolved rapidly and are becoming increasingly useful for patients, as well as healthcare providers, health educators, and individuals wanting to make healthy changes. The wide proliferation of these technologies and their integration into daily routines is helping to increase their utility for healthcare: recent statistics show that 44% of American adults, including 58% of 18–29 year olds, have smartphones. Worldwide, there are seven countries in which more than half of the population have smartphones: Singapore (62%), United Arab Emirates (61%), Saudi Arabia (60%), Norway (54%), Australia (52%), Sweden (51%), and the United Kingdom (51%) (Think Insights with Google, 2012). Recently, there has also been a significant increase in the use of social media technologies. Market research has found that, worldwide, 65% of individuals use social networking sites. In Brazil, China, Russia, the U. S., and India, more than 65% of Internet users actively manage social media profiles. Globally, 88% of people have watched video clips online, 63.2% have read blogs, and 42.9% have used a microblogging service (e.g., Twitter) (Universal Media, 2012).

Importantly, research has suggested that individuals are already using smartphones and social media for health-related purposes, although there is much room for growth. Findings from Pew Internet have shown that 17% of cell phone owners have used their phone to look up health information and 9% have used mobile apps for tracking their health. Among Internet users, 34% have read others' online commentary on health issues (Fox, 2011). Although these percentages are not high, they do represent a significant amount of individuals who are, of their own volition, using these technologies for health. With targeted public health initiatives and health providers' recommendations, it is likely that the usage of these tools for health could be increased.

This chapter will discuss how smartphones, specifically mobile apps, and social media have been and can be used in healthcare initiatives. Because these two technologies are discussed together, it is important to consider their similarities and differences. Both mobile apps and social media represent emerging and customizable technology platforms that have gained widespread use. Additionally, using apps and social media are activities that are increasingly a part of individuals' daily routines, making them effective methods of reaching populations. In many cases, social media and apps actually overlap, such as with the popular Facebook and Twitter apps. There are important distinctions between the two technologies, however. Social media sites are, as their name implies, tools for connecting individuals. Their primary goal is facilitating interactions between people who have existing connections. Apps, conversely, are not always social. Many are used in isolation on an individual's smartphone for personal purposes. As a consequence, the purposes associated with mobile apps are much more varied than those found in social media. Still, in spite of these differences, the principles applied to using these technologies in healthcare are similar, as will be demonstrated in this chapter.

The uses of social media and mobile apps discussed here cover a broad spectrum of health-related contexts, including clinical care, health promotion, and personal health uses. Specific projects will be highlighted as exemplars of use and to provide models for implementation across several areas of healthcare. Additionally, the authors will put forth recommendations for using these technologies in health promotion efforts by describing steps required in creation, implementation, and evaluation. Issues that are important to address in using these platforms will also be highlighted.

Mobile Apps in Health: The State of Research and Examples of Use

Mobile apps, due to their customizability, open development systems, and relative inexpensiveness, can be powerful tools for health. The following sections highlight some of the research that has been done on mobile apps, as well as examples of current applications, with the goal of providing insight as to the varied uses of these tools.

Research on Mobile Apps: Feasibility Studies and Interventions

Due to the new nature of apps, most of the articles that have been published concern the development of apps and efforts to establish their reliability or usability. Baerlocher, Tamanow, and Baerlocher (2010), for example, describe the development and potential benefits of an app they created to track an individuals' long-term exposure to radiation from medical procedures. Such articles merely introduce an app and provide insight as to its creation. Bergman, Spellman, Hall, and Bergman (2012) went one step further and tested the validity of an existing app: a free pedometer for iPhones. Their results showed that, for a treadmill, the app did not accurately measure steps—demonstrating that apps are not always of the highest quality. Other researchers have assessed usability, such as Morris et al. (2010), who created an app for delivering cognitive behavioral therapy. In their article, the authors describe the experiences of participants and the different ways they used the app in daily life. Qualitative studies such as these, although they tell us little about the effectiveness of apps, help to determine if more rigorous studies are worth pursuing and can inform future development.

Interventions and experiments represent the next step in research on mobile apps. To date, studies published tend to focus on short-term outcomes, with few researchers examining long-term effects. Rizvi et al. (2011) created an app, *DBT Coach*, for delivering therapy to individuals with substance abuse or borderline personality disorder. Participants used the app for 10–14 days as needed, and results indicated that it had positive effects on emotion intensity and urges to use substances. Another app addressing mental health was tested among a group of adolescents as a means of monitoring several indicators, including stress, coping strategies, exercise, and alcohol and drug use. Results indicated that use of the app significantly increased emotional self-awareness, and post-hoc analyses indicated that it led to better mental health care from providers (Reid, et al., 2011). Other studies, however, have not found such support for the use of apps. Turner-McGrievy and Tate (2011) found that the use of a monitoring app as a supplement to podcasts for a weight-loss intervention did not add to outcomes after six months. Thus, there is a definite need for further research to examine how to best use mobile apps for health.

Exemplars of Current Mobile Apps for Health

Kaiser Permanente, a managed care consortium providing health plans to individuals in eight United States regions, has been a pioneer in the use of mobile apps. Their free *KP app* contains a secure patient medical record, which individuals can reference to keep track of their health and view lab results, immunizations, and prescriptions. Patients can also refill prescriptions, schedule appointments, and securely message their providers. Lastly, a location finder shows individuals the nearest medical facilities that are covered by their insurance. Overall, this demonstrates the true power of mobile apps, as it facilities virtually every step of the healthcare process in a straightforward, easy-to-use manner (for more information, visit https://itunes.apple.com/us/app/kaiser-permanente/id493390354?mt=8).

The U.S. Department of Defense, alternatively, demonstrates the ability of mobile apps to *deliver* therapeutic care. Their award-winning app, *PTSD coach*, helps individuals cope with PTSD symptoms. It enables self-assessment and symptom tracking, and provides systematic relaxation and self-help techniques. It also contains educational materials about PTSD to help patients understand their condition. Additionally, the Department of Defense has two other apps to walk individuals through breathing exercises: *Breathe 2 Relax*, which aids in stress management and guides the user through diaphragmatic breathing, and *Tactical Breather*, which was developed for soldiers in intense combat situations (for more information on these apps, visit http://t2health.org/mobile-apps). Together, these examples demonstrate the usefulness of mobile apps for managing mental health symptoms by drawing upon psychotherapeutic techniques and interactive, feedback-based systems.

The American Red Cross has created a primarily educational *First Aid* app, which provides expert advice on delivering first aid in everyday scenarios and is also integrated with 911 for emergency situations. It includes safety tips to help prepare for emergencies and contains pre-loaded content so that it may be used in situations without an Internet connection. Users can watch videos, animations, and view step-by-step guides to performing first aid.

Altogether, the organizations' apps discussed here demonstrate the variety of purposes that may be served by these tools, such as providing information or education, using GPS capabilities to help individuals find healthcare facilities, delivering therapeutic interventions, tracking health metrics, and aiding in managing healthcare-related tasks.

Social Media and Health: The State of the Research and Examples of Use

As social media have grown in popularity, health organizations and businesses have drawn upon these technologies. Often, organizations use existing popular social media, such as Facebook or YouTube, while other developers have designed social media tools specifically for health purposes. The next section will review some of the research that has examined the intersection of social media and health, with articles chosen that represent the variety of ways in which these tools can be used for this domain.

Research on Social Media and Health: Content Analyses, Interventions, and Experiments

Most research on social media and health falls within three categories: content analyses, applications within health education, and interventions or experiments assessing effects. Because this chapter emphasizes health promotion, studies related to education will not be discussed. Content analyses have examined various social media platforms for health-related posts, including YouTube, social networking sites, and microblogs. A recent study by Briones, Nan, Madden, and Waks (2011) examined portrayals of the human papillomavirus vaccine within YouTube videos. Overall, their findings indicated that most of the videos negatively portrayed the vaccine, providing a snapshot of public opinion that could potentially inform health campaigns. Another content analysis examined breast cancer groups on Facebook, finding that fundraising groups were most popular, and that groups were associated with a low amount of wall posts (Bender, Jimenez-Marroquin, & Jadad, 2011). This suggests that Facebook may not be ideal for use in health behavior interventions, as engagement appears to be low. In a Twitter analysis, Chew and Eysenbach (2010) collected over two million tweets related to H1N1 flu, finding that mentions coincided with major news stories about the epidemic, as well as with incidence data. This Twitter study, along with other similar anlayses, demonstrate the utility of this tool for performing illness surveillance.

Many systematic tests of the effectiveness of social media tools in health are related to health education. However, a few studies have tested the usefulness of these technologies among lay audiences through interventions or experiments. Adam et al. (2011) developed an intervention to reduce stigma associated with HIV-positive gay men, which included a website and blog-based discussions. Outcome evaluations indicated statistically significant changes in individuals' stigma-related attitudes and behaviors, as well as in recognition of the effects of stigma. However, because multiple technologies were used in this intervention, it is difficult to argue for the effectiveness of blogs in bringing about change. In an experiment, Hu and Sundar (2010) tested the effects of different online sources and media on behavioral intention related to health information. Results indicated that individuals had stronger behavioral intention when reading information on a website vs. a blog or personal homepage, but that this was mediated by perceived gatekeeping and information completeness. Such results suggest that blogs may not be the most persuasive sources for health information, which could have an impact on their use in interventions.

The research on social media and health is still in its infancy, and there is a clear need for more studies that systematically test the effectiveness of these technologies. However, studies to date have allowed us to better understand the content produced in social media and the potential of such technologies for health.

Health Initiatives in Popular Social Media Sites:
Facebook, YouTube, and Twitter

One of the forerunners in health-related social media is Mayo Clinic (MC), which has developed a Center for Social Media and maintains accounts on YouTube, Facebook, and Twitter. The MC YouTube channel contains interviews with physicians, medical news updates, patient stories, and informational videos. Their Facebook and Twitter accounts are populated with recent updates in medical news, links to patient stories, information about the clinic, and interactions with stakeholders. They also host informational Facebook chat sessions, in which individuals can speak with medical professionals. Lastly, they host a Sharing Mayo Clinic blog, in which patients and employees share their stories about their clinic experience. Overall, their approach is commendable because it casts such a wide net and also remains dynamic, with new content added frequently (for more information, visit http://socialmedia.mayoclinic.org/).

Another organization that draws upon popular social media sites is the U.S. Centers for Disease Control (CDC). Like MC, the CDC uses YouTube, Twitter, and Facebook, but, due to the size of the organization, has multiple accounts for each social media service. There are approximately 50 affiliated Twitter accounts, many from doctors associated with the CDC. They also have 17 Facebook pages and promote 13 blogs related to various topics, such as increasing health literacy and preventing chronic disease (see http://www.cdc.gov/socialmedia/ for more information). This approach of segmenting their social media accounts helps individuals to subscribe to content or "like" pages that are most relevant to them. Altogether, the CDC is a good example of how a large organization can draw upon social media tools to distribute a variety of messages to more narrow, focused audiences.

Besides these two organizations, many others including the World Health Organization, LiveStrong, and the American Heart Association are beginning to draw upon popular social media tools. These efforts, if executed well, can generate awareness and distribute messages in a way that was not possible before the rise of social media. However, these tools are not always robust enough to serve healthcare needs. The next section details examples of social media tools created specifically for healthcare purposes.

Social Media Tools Created for Health Purposes

One popular health site is *PatientsLikeMe*, a social networking site designed to bring together patients with similar health conditions so they can learn from one another by sharing health data and experiences. Members maintain individual profiles containing information about illnesses, treatments, and other relevant medical information. They can also track their symptoms in order to see treatment effects and view others' data in aggregate form. Additionally, PatientsLikeMe makes data available to researchers; for example,

Wicks, Vaughan, Massagli, and Heywood (2011) studied the effects of an ALS treatment approach using self-reported data from the site. Thus, Patients LikeMe is not only helpful for connecting patients, but also provides a rich data source for studying health conditions.

Another site, *HealthTap*, brings together patients and health professionals by allowing anyone to sign up and ask a short health question for free. Then, licensed physicians respond quickly, sometimes "agreeing" with each other's responses to point the patient toward the best answers. Although physicians are not compensated for providing their expertise, they participate to build up their reputations, attract patients, and give existing patients more access to their knowledge. Although HealthTap provides a simple service, it is powerful in that it lowers the barriers to acquiring reliable health knowledge.

Altogether, the examples of social media use in healthcare point to the flexibility of these technologies. To help health professionals and educators draw upon these tools, the following section provides a guide for incorporating both social media and mobile apps into health promotion projects.

A Step-by-Step Guide: Using Mobile Apps and Social Media in Health

This section contains suggestions for using mobile apps or social media as part of health initiatives, with suggested resources provided at the end of this chapter for more information. It will cover three project phases: designing mobile app or social media tools, implementing and distributing them, and evaluating their effectiveness. Importantly, the suggestions here apply to both mobile apps and social media sites unless otherwise specified. For reference, a list of the recommended steps put forth in this chapter is included in Table 1.

Table 1. Steps for completing mobile app or social media projects

Creating, Implementing, and Evaluating a Mobile App or Social Media Project	

Creating	1. Determine your goal
	  - Try to address an existing gap
	  - Keep the goal focused

	2. Choose and research your audience
	  - Determine what tools they already have
	  - Assess their level of access

	3. Determine what and how often tasks will be completed

	4. Develop strategies to encourage use and engagement
	  - Incentives
	  - Reminders

	5. Determine the unique contribution of your tool
	6. Decide on costs for users
	7. Test mock-ups with focus groups
	8. Develop beta version and conduct usability testing - Iterate design as needed
Implementing	9. Dedicate a technical support team
	10. Recruit users - Consider external incentives for continued use
	11. Listen and respond to feedback
	12. Ensure content on social media sites stays fresh - If necessary, designate a "core" group of users
	13. For mobile apps, *avoid* too many updates
	14. Examine automated activity logs - Downloads, IP addresses, mouse clicks, pages visited

	15. Distribute surveys assessing satisfaction, attitudes, and use of tools
	  - If possible, at several different times
	  - Consider integrating surveys into the tools themselves

	16. Assess clinical outcomes - Self-reports, sensors, or in-person measures
	17. Analyze user-generated content
Issues to Consider	18. Consider HIPAA and privacy issues - Obtain consent, if necessary
	19. If physicians are involved, check on medical licensing rules in your state
	20. Address reimbursement issues

Creating Mobile Apps or Social Media-Based Projects

The first step to take when considering using mobile apps or social media for a health promotion project is determining what goal the project aims to achieve. A good place to start is figuring out where a "gap" exists—such as an area where there is a lack of communication or support, or a health issue about which people are poorly educated. Consider the previously discussed *PTSD Coach* app—this was created to provide in-time therapy to individuals as they need it. Previously, such patients would have to wait for an appointment to speak with a therapist. Working to address such a gap will help the tool to be based on an actual need, which should increase usage.

Once a goal is set, choose and research the potential audience. Find out what tools they are already using—examine their social media behaviors or their mobile app usage. Also, determine their level of access; if the population doesn't have smartphones or broadband Internet access, then the technologies discussed here may not be ideal. For a social media intervention, this is the step where developers must decide whether to create a new site or use existing platforms. If the target population is already active on social media sites, and these can be used effectively to achieve the project's goal, then that is likely the best option. Consider following the example of Mayo Clinic, which uses several popular social media services that are effective in meeting their main goals of outreach and education. This helps them to reach wider audiences and establish a "brand" across the different sites. Remember, however, that existing social media sites are not easily customized, so the types of behaviors that can be facilitated are limited.

Once a basic goal and audience is determined, then the design process can begin. First, ask, "What tasks will users be completing?" This requires breaking down the overarching goal into smaller, concrete behaviors. For example, with Kaiser Permanente's *KP App,* their overarching goal is to facilitate healthcare, and the smaller tasks include filling prescriptions, scheduling appointments, etc. Also, consider how often people will be engaging in those tasks—will individuals use the tool several times a day on a set schedule, or on an as-needed basis? If it will be used often, make sure the tool is accessible and not time-consuming. The *HealthTap* website, for example, is intended to be a resource for everyday health questions. The format of the website suits this goal, as asking questions is easy, responses come quickly, and joining the website is completely free.

The next step in the design process is to answer the question "What will encourage people to use this?" Is the tool intrinsically rewarding, in that people get satisfaction just from using it? This is the case for tools like *Patients LikeMe*, which are empowering for individuals by helping them take control of their health. Or, will the tool provide extrinsic rewards, such as giveaways or recognition? Giveaways are common techniques for engaging users in a discussion on Facebook. Typically, administrators ask for comments related to a health topic, and anyone who responds will be entered into a drawing. Other options to consider are automated reminders to encourage participation or the involvement of external parties, such as health providers or family. The study by Reid et al. (2011), for example, automatically transmitted data from an app to adolescents' doctors, motivating them to be more consistent in their self-monitoring.

Next, it is important to ask what makes the tool unique. If it performs the same functions as an existing app or site, then individuals will be less likely to use it. Thus, it is essential to not only figure out what the competitive advantage of the tool is, but to make sure that users are aware of it. *Zombies, Run!*, an immersive mobile game in which people try to escape zombies by running in real life, could easily get lost in the sea of running and pedometer-based apps. However, the novelty of the idea, in addition to the game-based components, has made the app a success.

A final important question to ask is if individuals will be charged for using your tool. If there is a charge, the design should be sophisticated, the tool should be unique, and technical support should be available. For example, one of the top paid iPhone apps is the *Sleep Cycle Alarm Clock*. This app analyzes sleep patterns using the phone's accelerometer and wakes users when they are sleeping lightly. Not only is the contribution of this app unique, but the design is also easy to use and there is a dedicated support page. Thus, many are willing to pay for it.

After concrete design ideas are in place, test several mock-ups with focus groups. Be sure to include individuals from your target audience, have a non-judgmental moderator, and conduct several groups over time. For each group, edit the design until finding one that tests well. Then, develop a beta version of the app or site and conduct usability testing. Observe individuals as they use the tool and ask them to talk through any problems they encounter. Fix bugs and issues as they arise until usability tests run smoothly. For further information on conducting focus groups and usability tests, see the resources listed at the end of this chapter.

There are several pitfalls to avoid during the design process. The first is being too ambitious and seeking to achieve several goals with one tool. Keep the goal focused and simple—it is better to do one thing really well than to do many things poorly. Another pitfall is making an app or site that already exists or failing to advertise what makes the tool unique. For apps, it is especially important to make them stand out in the crowd, as app stores grow every day. Put some time into creating a catchy title, app icon, and app description. Last, releasing a tool without any testing is likely to be disastrous, as individuals on the design team are often so invested in the project that they miss its flaws. Even if funding is short and compensation for participants is unavailable, ask colleagues, friends, and family to provide feedback.

Implementing the Project

After the design process is complete, there are a few steps to take before releasing the tool. First, identify an individual or a group of people to serve as primary technical support and troubleshoot problems as they arise. Next, recruit users by advertising at health facilities, on health websites, or through health organizations. If conducting a study, consider using established research panels, student participant pools, or traditional cold-calling recruitment procedures. If possible, provide external incentives, such as financial compensation or prize drawings, to make sure research participants use the tool.

The first days after releasing the tool are crucial. Designate one or more people to listen to feedback and respond to users' comments or questions. Staying engaged with users demonstrates investment in the project and care about their experience, which will likely increase participation. Additionally, make sure that the content in the tool stays fresh. Social media users now expect new content every time they visit so, if necessary, designate a core group of users to post frequently. These can be actual users who are recruited for this purpose or project team members that try to stimulate discussion. If releasing a mobile app or game, however, try to *avoid* too many updates. If the app keeps changing and users have to download several updates, they will get frustrated. Last, encourage continued participation by using incentives on a regular basis, as discussed in the design section.

Once the tool is released, a major pitfall would be "checking out," as many project teams have done. Personnel should remain engaged with users, making updates as needs arise and contributing new content. Additionally, do not stop recruiting. Users get bored with apps and social media sites quickly, so constantly drawing in new users is a necessity for maintaining participation. If a study is being completed that requires users to stay active over a longer period of time, then provide good incentives for doing so.

Evaluating the Project

One of the easiest ways of assessing a tool involves automated logs of users' activity. For mobile apps, the number of downloads can demonstrate its popularity. For social media sites hosted by project developers, logs of IP addresses, incoming links, pages visited, and time spent on the site can be examined, among other metrics. On externally hosted social media sites, potential metrics include the number of "fans" or comments, number of YouTube video views, and the locations of users.

For more detailed feedback, use surveys to assess satisfaction, attitudes, and uses of the tool. If possible, conduct surveys at several points in time in order to assess changes. In many cases, they can be integrated into the tool itself as part of the user's experience. For example, on a social media site, a poll can be embedded within a post. For assessing a mobile app, users could be asked to provide ratings in the Android or iPhone app stores. At the least, these ratings can provide a numeric average of people's opinions, as well as some text-based feedback. During evaluation, especially for participants who are volunteers, a big mistake is to make surveys long and cumbersome. Try to keep them simple; the easier the questionnaires are to complete, the more likely it is that people will respond. In formal research studies, there is more freedom in terms of survey length, as participants typically expect to complete thorough measures.

In order to make a strong argument for the benefits of a tool, demonstrating a positive change in individuals' health by measuring clinical outcomes is key. At the most basic level, self-reports can be used to assess health status, such as quality-of-life or reported weight. Sensors can also be used, such as accelerometers within smartphones or external sensors that automatically transmit data to phones. These are common in diabetes research for transmitting blood glucose levels. Another method is to have study personnel measure the health indicators. For smaller pilot studies, this approach is ideal, as it does not rely on the abilities or willingness of participants and is thus likely to produce more usable data. When measuring clinical outcomes, it is important to conduct at least a pre- and post-test so that changes can be assessed.

A final form of evaluation involves analyses of user-generated content to see how individuals are using the tool. Mobile apps will not generate much content, but posts or profiles on social media sites can be examined. Quantitative content analysis approaches with coding schemes and inter-coder reliability can be used to assess frequencies of certain types of content. Alternatively, qualitative approaches can be used to report on general themes. Often, these content analyses can increase understanding of acquired results.

Important Issues to Consider for Future Work

Overall, this chapter has discussed the value of using mobile apps and social media as a part of healthcare initiatives while also providing basic guidance for projects using these technologies. However, there are a few final issues to address when developing a project of this nature. First, there are legal issues, including privacy and, if in the U.S., security requirements related to the Health Insurance Portability and Accountability Act (HIPAA). If asking patients to transmit health data over the Internet, they must be completely aware of the potential dangers of doing so and, in some cases, they should sign a consent form. If there is uncertainty regarding privacy standards and their applicability, speak with the local Institutional Review Board (IRB) for guidance. For apps, this area is especially murky due to the rapid pace of technological developments and potential insecurity of mobile networks. To address privacy concerns, the U.S. National Telecommunications and Information Administration has called meetings to discuss this issue and develop a code of conduct. Such guidelines may be helpful for future projects.

Another potential problem is that most physicians are only licensed to provide healthcare in one state or region, which keeps them from seeing distant patients. Some states in the U.S., such as Arizona, California, and Texas, have adopted special licenses for telemedicine, but this is still not a widespread practice. Before working with physicians, be sure to check on the laws governing telemedicine in all areas that will be involved in the project. Also, be sure to consider reimbursement issues if involving physicians that want to be compensated for their services. In many areas, there are restrictions on the type of telemedicine that can be reimbursed such that only real-time or synchronous telemedicine is covered. Thus, it is unlikely that physicians will be reimbursed for services provided via social media or mobile apps. For more information on legal issues related to telemedicine, see the suggested resources at the end of this chapter.

Yet, in spite of these potential barriers associated with the use of mobile apps and social media for health, they represent promising tools for this area of work. Never before have there been technologies that are so easily customized while also being deeply ingrained into people's lives. Health practitioners, public health professionals, and researchers should be taking advantage of these opportunities in order to bring about healthy changes in individuals' lives. Future work should look beyond content analyses and seek to develop tools that encourage long-term use, strengthen individuals' confidence in health behaviors, and result in real clinical outcomes.

Recommended Readings

Chou, W. S., Hunt, Y. M., Beckiord, E. B., Moser, R. P., & Hesse, B. W. (2009). Social media use in the United States: Implications for health communication. *Journal of Medical Internet Research, 11,* e48. doi: 10.2196/jmir.1249

Rubin, J., & Chisnell, D. (2008). *Handbook of usability testing: How to plan, design and conduct effective tests*: Wiley-India.

Stewart, D. W., Shamdasani, P. N., & Rook, D. W. (2007). *Focus groups: Theory and practice* (Vol. 2.0): Sage Publications, Inc.

Additional Resources

Directions for designing and coding apps

General tips for app development: http://www.businessinsider.com/how-to-make-an-iphone-app-tips-and-tricks-2011-7?op=1

Step-by-step guide for creating iPhone apps: http://www.businessinsider.com/how-to-make-iphone-apps-2011-6#

Guide to developing your first Android app:
http://developer.android.com/training/basics/firstapp/index.html

Other Resources

Social Media toolkit from the CDC:
http://www.cdc.gov/socialmedia/Tools/guidelines/pdf/SocialMediaToolkit_BM.pdf

Legal issues in telemedicine: http://www.telehealthresourcecenter.org/legal-regulatory

References

Adam, B. D., Murray, J., Ross, S., Oliver, J., Lincoln, S. G., & Rynard, V. (2011). hivstigma.com, an innovative web-supported stigma reduction intervention for gay and bisexual men. *Health Education Research, 26,* 795–807. doi: 10.1093/her/cyq078

Baerlocher, M. O., Talanow, R., & Baerlocher, A. F. (2010). Radiation passport: An iPhone and iPod touch application to track radiation dose and estimate associated cancer risks. *Journal of the American College of Radiology, 7*, 277–280. doi: 10.1016/j.jacr.2009.09.016

Bender, J., Jimenez-Marroquin, M., & Jadad, A. (2011). Seeking support on Facebook: A content analysis of breast cancer groups. *Journal of Medical Internet Research, 13*, e16. doi: 10.2196/jmir.1560

Bergman, R. J., Spellman, J. W., Hall, M. E., & Bergman, S. M. (2012). Is there a valid app for that? Validity of a free pedometer iPhone application. *Journal of Physical Activity & Health, 9*, 670–676.

Briones, R., Nan, X., Madden, K., & Waks, L. (2012). When vaccines go viral: An analysis of HPV vaccine coverage on YouTube. *Health Communication, 27*, 478–485. doi: 10.1080/10410236.2011.610258

Chew, C., & Eysenbach, G. (2010). Pandemics in the age of Twitter: Content analysis of tweets during the 2009 H1N1 outbreak. *PLoS ONE, 5*, e14118. doi: 10.1371/journal.pone.0014118

Fox, S. (2011). *The social life of health information.* Retrieved from http://www.pewinternet.org/Reports/2011/Social-Life-of-Health-Info.aspx

Hu, Y. F., & Sundar, S. S. (2010). Effects of online health sources on credibility and behavioral intentions. *Communication Research, 37*, 105–132. 10.1177/0093650209351512

Reid, S., Kauer, S., Hearps, S., Crooke, A., Khor, A., Sanci, L., & Patton, G. (2011). A mobile phone application for the assessment and management of youth mental health problems in primary care: A randomised controlled trial. *BMC Family Practice, 12*, 131. doi:10.1186/1471-2296-12-131

Rizvi, S. L., Dimeff, L. A., Skutch, J., Carroll, D., & Linehan, M. M. (2011). A pilot study of the DBT Coach: An interactive mobile phone application for individuals with Borderline Personality Disorder and Substance Use Disorder. *Behavior Therapy, 42*, 589–600. doi: 10.1016/j.beth.2011.01.003

Think Insights with Google (2012). Our mobile planet. Retrieved from http://www.thinkwithgoogle.com/mobileplanet/en/

Turner-McGrievy, G., & Tate, D. (2011). Tweets, apps, and pods: Results of the 6-month mobile pounds off digitally (mobile POD) randomized weight-loss intervention among adults. *Journal of Medical Internet Research, 13*, e120. doi:10.2196/jmir.1841

Universal Media (2012). *The business of social: Social media tracker 2012.* Retrieved from http://universalmedia.rs/sr/knWave6.html

Wicks, P., Vaughan, T. E., Massagli, M. P., & Heywood, J. (2011). Accelerated clinical discovery using self-reported patient data collected online and a patient-matching algorithm. *Nature Biotechnology, 29*, 411–414. doi: 10.1038/nbt.1837

Chapter 4

Digital Games: The SECRET of Alternative Health Realities

Hua Wang, *University at Buffalo, The State University of New York*
Arvind Singhal, *The University of Texas at El Paso*

Introduction

Digital games are video games, computer games, online games, mobile games, simulations, and virtual worlds played on arcade units, console systems, handheld devices, personal computers, or the Web. Can they help manage pain, reduce infections, cope with post-traumatic stress disorder, and boost efficacy to practice healthy behaviors? We seek to answer such questions in this chapter.

In 40 years, digital games have become one of the largest and most profitable global media industries and play an important role in the everyday life of millions of people all over the world, cutting across age, gender, and socio-economic status. Although games are often seen as frivolous or harmful, more people have started to value their potential for making positive changes. Game designers have been collaborating with content experts to foster learning and promote health since the mid-1990s (Lieberman, 2009). As design strategies and evidence of effectiveness are fast accumulating in the "Games for Health" literature in recent years, health game projects are attracting more public attention, substantial funding resources, and enthusiastic research efforts (Ferguson, 2012). Annual conferences have been held in North America since 2004 and in Europe since 2011. A peer-reviewed journal *Games for Health: Research, Development, and Clinical Applications* was launched in 2012.

In this chapter, we first briefly point out the distinct media attributes of digital games relevant to health communication. We then explicate, with recent cases, the major functions of health games summarizing them in an acronym SECRET (see Figure 1). Finally, we conclude with lessons learned for intervention design and evaluation as well as implications for future projects.

Why "Digital Games" for Health?

At least five media attributes of digital games can be strategically positioned for health promotion and behavior change: two on the "game" aspect (i.e., fun nature and experiential play), two on the "digital" aspect (i.e., multimodality and interactivity), and another turbocharging feature (i.e., narrative engagement). 1. Games are *fun*; at least they are supposed to be. Player participation is voluntary. So by nature, games are intrinsically motivating and rewarding as players overcome challenges and complete missions (McGonigal, 2011). 2. Games involve *experiential play*, allowing players to self-direct their explorations and discoveries; therefore, they offer a more powerful form of user engagement than the vicarious experience offered by radio and television programs (Wang & Singhal, 2009). 3. Digital games are *multimodal*, converging multiple sensory stimuli ranging from 3D modeling to body sensors to create immersive virtual environments (Lieberman, 2013). Multimodality also makes digital games easily scalable to more people through multiple platforms with large amounts of information compressed and transmitted in short time periods. 4. Digital games are *interactive* between the player and the virtual environment, artificial intelligence-based agents, avatars controlled by human actors, and other players. Successful games can easily reach a global community of tens of millions of players, a massive human resource that can be strategically leveraged for public good (McGonigal, 2011). 5. *Narrative engagement* is the turbocharged sauce of digital games. Although characters and storylines may not be found in all games, and the role of narrative in digital games has been debated, when they are included it enhances the play experience, making it more compelling and memorable (Wang, Shen, & Ritterfeld, 2009).

Taken together, these attributes of digital games allow players to explore new horizons, experiment with different actions, and experience their consequences in a safe space. Games offer a wide-ranging variety of stimulation, interaction, challenge, and choice, providing countless opportunities for players to contemplate alternative perspectives and realities. These possibilities have significant implications for health promotion and behavioral change.

How Can Digital Games Help with Health Promotion?

Past scholarship has included comprehensive literature reviews and game applications for specific health issues. Building on the previous efforts, an extended overview is provided in this section on the major functions of health games, summarized in the acronym SECRET. Recent examples of each function, backed by empirical research, are provided when possible.

Figure 1. Specification of the Acronym SECRET

> **S**ocial connectivity and support
> **E**xercise of the body and mind
> **C**rowdsourcing for problem-solving
> **R**ehearsal of real life scenarios in a safe space
> **E**ducation of medicine and public health
> **T**reatment of illness and diseases

Social Connectivity and Support

The stereotypical loner image of gamers has relegated the social aspect of game play to the back burner. Although games were mostly perceived as a threat to individual well-being in their early days, health game research more recently has demonstrated their potential in enhancing communication about illness and engendering social support (Lieberman, 1997). For instance, *Wellness Partners* is a social game designed by an interdisciplinary team at the University of Southern California to promote physical activity among middle-aged adults and their family and friends. A Facebook-like web interface allows users to share with their alters both public updates and private messages about their physical activities as well as setbacks. Players accumulate points as rewards for such reporting which can be redeemed to collect virtual gifts and engage a virtual character in animated wellness activities. The physical activities reported by the players are presented in tag clouds. A larger-sized font in the tag clouds represents more frequently reported physical activities. Preliminary findings suggest that participants were enthusiastic about this type of health game application that marries personal social networking with fun gaming elements for healthy lifestyles (Gotsis, Wang, Spruijt-Metz, Jordan-Marsh, & Valente, 2013). During casual game play, participants gained new insights about their family members and friends, allowing them to offer timely social support, while improving their own exercise habits in conjunction with others. A significant increase in self-reported exercise frequency was found among all participants, especially those who were alters, in groups with larger age variation, and started with the game version as opposed to the control version. A significant decrease in BMI was found among the primary participants.

SuperBetter (http://superbetter.com) is a social game invented by Jane McGonigal to engage individuals on an epic journey to improve their physical, mental, emotional, and social well-being. Collaborating with experts in neuroscience, positive psychology, and medicine, the SuperBetter design team incorporated gaming elements to build compelling quests, provoke positive emotions, strengthen social connections, and improve personal resilience. Players can invite family, friends or people with similar experiences ("Allies") to help them define their personal goals ("Quests"), barriers ("Bad Guys"), motivators ("Power-ups"), and rewards ("Achievements"). *SuperBetter* thus serves as a self-management tool and a structured social support platform for family and friends to help a loved one during a time of crises. Several clinical trials are currently underway to evaluate its effectiveness in recovery from traumatic brain injury, to enhance weight loss and fitness, and to fight clinical depression.

Exercise of the Body and Mind

A big concern about excessive game play centers on sedentary habits as players tend to sit in front of a computer or a game console for hours at a time. To counter that, games have been developed to promote physical activity and cognitive functionality. Such digital games are called exergames (Lieberman, 2006). If *Dance Dance Revolution* started the first wave of exergames, the more recent sports and fitness series on Nintendo Wii, Microsoft Xbox 360 Kinect, and PlayStation Move have revolutionized the genre of exergames. Companies like Gamercize (http://gamercize.net) are developing new exergames to target specific population groups such as schoolers and office workers. Exergames invariably require the players to engage in a certain degree of body movements in a certain time period in order to progress. With the technological development and market penetration of intuitive controllers, sensors, and tracking devices, the literature on exergames is rapidly growing. A recently published meta-analysis notes that playing exergames promotes light-to-moderate intensity physical activity and can significantly increase heart rate, oxygen consumption, and energy expenditure compared to sitting on a couch (Peng, Lin, & Crouse, 2011).

Digital games are also targeted to sharpening the mind. As populations in many countries age, games are tackling the physical and psychological well-beings of senior citizens. *ElderGames*, an initiative funded by the European Union, employs digital games to help seniors in Europe improve their physical and mental health. Gaming environments are incorporated into real-life technology and senior recreational centers, and serve as a preventive and therapeutic tool for early health diagnosis, facilitating social interactions, and improving the quality of life for the elderly. Game customization guidelines have been developed based on prior research as well as specific aging challenges in the participating European countries (Gamberini et al., 2006). Digital games can help the elderly to maintain cognitive acuity, participate in social activities, and fulfill personal recreational needs. Further, a number of game applications in recent years use brain wave sensors to engage players of all ages in game play. *Mindflex* (http://mindflexgames.com) by Mattel is a fine example. Players wear an EEG headset with sensors embedded in the headband that enables them to use their mind to control a blue styrofoam ball as it hovers over multiple obstacles. Players can control the pace of the game and compete with themselves or with one other player.

Crowdsourcing for Problem-Solving

Some of the greatest games are puzzle games. Digital games are more than mere digital versions of traditional puzzle games. They take problem-solving up several notches with the possibility of engaging a global community and leveraging vast human creativity and collective intelligence. For example, *Foldit* (http://fold.it) is a multiplayer online game that invites players, including amateur non-scientist gamers, to solve puzzles related to the scientific research of protein structure (Cooper, Khatib, Treuille, Barbero, Lee, Beenen, et al., 2010). Biochemists and computer scientists at the University of Washington created this game, hoping the massive online game players could help them discover scientific breakthroughs by experimenting with the gazillion possible folding structures of protein. For over a decade, scientists could not decipher the structure of *retroviral protease* (an enzyme critical in HIV multiplication patterns), so they posed this intractable challenge to the 60,000 players in the game. Players worldwide competed to solve the puzzle and in a matter of 10 days they were able to generate new models of sufficient quality that may help biochemists develop antiretroviral drugs for HIV/AIDS.

What is most intriguing about *Foldit* is that many of the players who made this discovery did not have any background in biochemistry. Seth Cooper, the lead designer of *Foldit* noted: "People have spatial reasoning skills—something computers are not yet good at. Games provide a framework for bringing together the strengths of computers and humans" (quoted in Moore, 2011). Following the success of *Foldit*, scientists at Carnegie Mellon University and Stanford University developed *EteRNA* (Check for more details: http://eterna.cmu.edu/content/EteRNA) to capitalize on the powerful crowdsourcing capacity of digital games to uncover new ways of folding life's fundamental building blocks RNA molecules.

In addition to finding solutions directly related to health promotion and sciences, digital games can also elicit innovative ideas for solving social problems. *EVOKE* (http://urgentevoke.com) was developed by Jane McGonigal and the World Bank Institute as a 10-week crash course in changing the world. The game uses a graphic novel (as a textbook) to broach a weekly global crisis and teach players essential skills such as creativity, collaboration, entrepreneurship, and sustainability to tackle intractable world problems such as hunger, poverty, and access to clean water. The game attracted 8,000 players in 120 countries within the first week of its launch in March 2010. Players are encouraged to propose innovative solutions to urgent problems, report on their activities through blogs and videos, and take actions in the real world. *EVOKE* was the winner of the Games for Change Festival's 2011 Direct Impact Award.

Rehearsal of Real Life Scenarios in a Safe Space

Avatars often appear in digital games as the user's digital self-representation. Alternations of self-avatars in virtual reality can transform human behaviors—a phenomenon called the *"Proteus Effect"* (Yee & Bailenson, 2007). Lab experiments found that female participants who experienced a high level of presence in their self-avatars were more likely than those who experienced a low level of presence to imitate the self-avatar and suppress unhealthy eating behavior (Fox, Bailenson, & Binney, 2009). In addition, when participants could see their self-avatars lose weight through exercise in the virtual environment, they voluntarily performed significantly more physical activity in real life (Fox & Bailenson, 2009). The *Proteus Effect* research suggests that intentionally alternating certain attributes of a self-avatar's appearance can change the player's health perceptions and behaviors.

Digital games are also increasingly being adopted to address sensitive health topics such as safe sex and HIV/AIDS because they can provide people at risk opportunities to rehearse the decision-making processes through realistic scenarios in the game. *Nightlife* is a downloadable single-player adventure game targeting heterosexual, young African-American men to promote condom use, HIV/STI testing, and to reduce risk through oral sex and mutual masturbation (Snyder, Farrar, Biocca, & Bohil, 2010). The game allows the player to customize his self-avatar and make safer or riskier choices in exotic scenarios. The player is also given the option to visit a virtual clinic and the scripts are designed to be engaging and non-preachy. Preliminary results from a national randomized controlled trial suggest that within two days of download, *Nightlife* players rated higher on behavioral intentions to get tested for HIV than those in the control condition. In the follow-up post-test three to four months later, *Nightlife* players who voluntarily played *Nightlife* more often than others were more likely to have been tested (Snyder & Farrar, 2012).

Another approach to changing risky sexual behavior is called Socially Optimized Learning in Virtual Environments or SOLVE (Miller, Christensen, Godoy, Appleby, Corsbie-Massay, & Read, 2009). The premise is that effective learning takes place in social situations and decision-making processes are mediated by emotional responses to environmental triggers that mark them as "good" or "bad" situations. These triggers create affective biases to guide future decision making. Applied to HIV-prevention scenarios related to men having sex with men, research on SOLVE suggests that the use of interactive technologies in virtual gaming environments to rehearse choices in potentially risky scenarios is far more effective than traditional approaches, and has significantly higher predictive power of future risk-taking behavior (Read, Miller, Appleby, Nwosu, Raynaldo, Lauren, et al., 2006).

Education of Medicine and Public Health

Almost from the advent of commercially available digital games, applications have been developed to foster learning (Lieberman, 2009). The Entertainment Software Rating Board even has a separate rating category for *edutaiment* games. The initial round of health games was designed to educate pediatric and adolescent patients about disease and coping (Lieberman, 1997). In the past decade, with immersive virtual environments and mobile applications coming of age, health educators have grasped the true potential of gaming technologies for teaching, training, and interacting with medical students and health workers. Once *Second Life,* one of the best-known virtual worlds with 3D modeling tools, was launched in 2003, health organizations began developing simulated environments for medical, health, and patient education and skills training (Beard, Wilson, Morra, & Keelan, 2009). Medical doctors and health professionals can also organize virtual meetings and discuss patient cases in *Second Life*.

New applications similar to *Second Life* have been burgeoning. *Visualand* is a medical virtual reality based in Hungary that allows users to upload and share visual and audio files for free (Meskó, 2011). *Pharmatopia* (http://pharm.monash.edu.au/education/epharm/pharmatopia.html) is a virtual classroom created by the Faculty of Pharmacy and Pharmaceutical Sciences at Monash University in Australia to provide an immersive environment for problem-based pharmacy training. *Webicina* (http://webicina.com) is a web-based social media platform that aggregates resources on more than 80 topics for patients and medical professionals with free services in 17 languages. *Prognosis* is a free mobile game that uses an interactive cartoon-based narrative to engage players to investigate, deduce, and diagnose complex clinical cases. *Prognosis* is specifically designed to help doctors, nurses, and medical students prepare for standard exams and recall key clinical insights.

Increasingly, medical program directors and medical students are acknowledging the value of digital health games. A survey of family medicine and internal medicine residency program directors (N = 434) found 92% of the respondents supporting the use of games as an educational strategy; 80% reported already using games in their programs (Akl, Gunukula, et al., 2010), indicating great future potential in this area. Another study of medical students at the University of Michigan and University of Wisconsin-Madison (N = 217) found that 80% of the respondents believed that video games can have educational values and 77% would readily employ a multiplayer online healthcare simulation to develop health workers' skills in interacting with patients (Kron, Gjerde, Sen, & Fetters, 2010).

Treatment of Illness and Diseases

Digital games have been employed as tools for medical treatment, pain/discomfort distraction during treatment, treatment compliance, and self-care management. For example, a major barrier to traditional clinical treatment of PTSD is the patient's unwillingness or inability to recall or imagine the trauma-relevant event. A PTSD virtual reality exposure therapy system *Virtual Iraq/Afghanistan* was developed to overcome this problem. Using a head-mounted display along with a set of multisensory tracking devices, a PTSD patient can be immersed in a digitally constructed virtual environment that resembles a combat-related trauma scenario with realistic visual, auditory, olfactory, and tactile stimuli (Rizzo, Difede, Rothbaum, & Reger, 2010). During a treatment session, the therapist can use a separate clinical interface to monitor the patient's physiological and psychological parameters and adjust the emotional intensity of the scene as per the patient's directions. A number of randomized controlled trials are underway for *Virtual Iraq/Afghanistan*, and initial clinical assessments have found statistically significant reductions in PTSD symptom severity measures (Reger, Holloway, Candy, Rothbaum, Difede, Rizzo, et al., 2011).

Digital games have also been used as a therapeutic tool. Therapists have used *Guitar Hero* and Nintendo Wii series to engage patients in otherwise repetitive and tedious practices. Other programs have used games for physiotherapy such as movement recovery and muscular dystrophy, and occupational therapy such as repetitive strain injuries (Jung, Yeh, McLaughlin, Rizzo, & Winstein, 2009). Health games seem to be especially useful in pain management. Numerous studies have documented how game use can distract from the sensation of pain, particularly for children and youth (Griffiths, 2005). Handheld video games also have proven effective to modulate pain of pediatric and adolescent patients from burns and alleviate them from the discomfort of cancer treatment. *Re-Mission* (http://re-mission.net) is a third-person shooter game that allows young cancer patients to role-play a nanobot named Roxxi, and navigate through a 3D simulated human body to destroy cancer cells, battle bacterial infections, and learn to manage treatment-engendered adverse effects. Multi-site, randomized clinical trials of *Re-Mission* have been conducted with 375 cancer patients aged 13–29. Cancer-related knowledge, self-efficacy to communicate about cancer, treatment adherence behavior, and self-management of side effects increased significantly for *Re-Mission* players (Cole, Kato, Marin-Bowling, Dahl, & Pollock, 2006; Kato, Cole, Bradlyn, & Pollock, 2008). A more recent study of *Re-Mission* revealed that the interactivity experienced during gameplay helped activate players' brain circuits associated with incentive motivation, contributing to positive self-perceptions (Cole, Kato, Marin-Bowling, Dahl, & Pollock, 2012).

What Are the Lessons Learned in Health Games Research?

Clarify Purposes

Any health game project is an interdisciplinary endeavor requiring teamwork. Game designers and developers need to work closely with health professionals and researchers from start to finish. Clear purposes need to be established every step of the way including an iterative process to test out design ideas, game prototypes, and research instruments. Aligning these purposes with intended experiences and outcomes would help improve the effectiveness of game interventions.

Refine the Application

Digital games are based on advanced digital technologies and technical difficulties can hinder play and learning experience. This means all digital game projects should be extensively pretested and closely monitored during implementation for technical errors and abnormal behavioral modifications. Game refinements or adjustments should not be limited to player access or loading time, but also features associated with player's privacy protection and database security.

Base on Theories

The design and evaluation of health games must be guided by coherent theories and established principles. For example, uses and gratifications theory can be used to help game designers and researchers understand players' motivations; elaboration likelihood model and framing theory can help tailor the health messages to the target gamer characteristics; the notion of "presence" can reveal players' psychological state during game play. Theories can also guide subsequent scientific inquiries and hypothesis testing during summative research.

Develop Rigorous Research Design

Systematic reviews on health game research have found that most published evaluation studies are lacking rigor and vigor in research design. In order to make a quality causal argument about game effects on health outcomes, researchers need to conduct randomized controlled trials (when possible), include adequate control groups, recruit sufficient numbers of participants based on a priori power analysis, conduct baseline assessment to compare with post-intervention outcomes, and use valid, reliable, and objective measures. When evaluating a game intervention against other options, the control condition should ideally have similar attributes except the delivery method (i.e., the game).

Report in Details

Past game research has not sufficiently provided detailed descriptions of the game intervention or research procedures, exacerbating the challenge to conduct meta-analysis and develop systematic understanding of the field. In order to develop a body of high quality literature, researchers need to report concrete information about the game, the players, the standard procedural elements, and intended as well as unintended outcomes including negative effective and unexpected events and challenges.

Recommended Readings

Kato, P. M. (2012). Evaluating efficacy and validating games for health. *Games for Health Journal: Research, Development, and Clinical Applications, 1*(1), 74–76. doi:10.1089/g4h.2012.1017

Lieberman, D. A. (2013). Designing digital games, social media, and mobile technologies to motivate and support health behavior change. In R. E. Rice & C. K. Atkin (Eds.), *Public communication campaigns* (4th ed., pp. 273–288). Los Angeles, CA: Sage.

McGonigal, J. (2011). *Reality is broken: Why games make us better and how they can change the world.* New York: The Penguin Press.

Peng, W., & Liu, M. (2008). An overview of using electronic games for health purposes. In R. Ferdig (Ed.), *Handbook of research on effective electronic gaming in education* (pp. 388–401). Hershey, PA: IGI Global.

References

Akl, E. A., Gunukula, S., Mustafa, R., Wilson, M. C., Symons, A., Moheet, A., & Schünemann, H. J. (2010). Support for and aspects of use of educational games in family medicine and internal medicine residency programs in the U.S.: A survey. *BMC Medical Education, 10,* 26. Available at http://www.biomedcentral.com/1472-6920/10/26

Beard, L., Wilson, K., Morra, D., & Keelan, J. (2009). A survey of health-related activities on Second Life. *Journal of Medical Internet Research, 11*(2), e17. Available at http://www.jmir.org/2009/2/e17/

Cole, S. W., Kato, P. M., Marin-Bowling, V. M., Dahl, G. V., & Pollock, B. H. (2006). Clinical trial of Re-Mission: A video game for young people with cancer. *CyberPsychology & Behavior, 9,* 665–666.

Cole, S. W., Yoo, D. J., & Knutson, B. (2012). Interactivity and reward-related neural activation during a serious videogame. *PLoS ONE*, *7*(3), e33909. doi:10.1371/journal.pone.0033909

Cooper, S., Khatib, F., Treuille, A., Barbero, J., Lee, J., Beenen, M., Leaver-Fay, A., Baker, D., & Popovic, Z. Foldit players. (2010). Predicting protein structures with a multiplayer online game. *Nature*, *466*(7307), 756–760. doi:10.1038/nature09304

Ferguson, B. (2012). The emergence of games for health. *Games for Health Journal: Research, Development, and Clinical Applications*, *1*(1), 1–2.

Fox, J., & Bailenson, J. (2009). Virtual self-modeling: The effects of vicarious reinforcement and identification on exercise behaviors. *Media Psychology*, *12*(1), 1–25. doi:10.1080/15213260802669474

Fox, J., Bailenson, J., & Binney, J. (2009). Virtual experiences, physical behaviors: The effect of presence on imitation of an eating avatar. *Presence: Teleoperators & Virtual Environments*, *18*(4), 294–303.

Gamberini, L., Alcaniz, M., Barresi, G., Fabregat, M., Ibanez, F., & Prontu, L. (2006). Cognition, technology and games for the elderly: An introduction to ELDERGAMES project. *PsychNology Journal*, *4*(3), 285–308.

Gotsis, M., Wang, H., Spruijt-Metz, D., Jordan-Marsh, M., & Valente, T. (2013). Wellness partners: Design and evaluation of a web-based physical activity diary with social gaming features for adults. *JMIR Research Protocols*, *2*(1), e10. Available at http://www.researchprotocols.org/2013/1/e10/

Griffiths, M. (2005). Video games and health: Video gaming is safe for most players and can be useful in health care. *British Medical Journal*, *331*(7509), 122–123.

Jung, Y., Yeh, S., McLaughlin, M., Rizzo, A., & Winstein, C. (2009). Three-dimensional game environments for recovery from stroke. In U. Ritterfeld, M. J. Cody, & P. Vorderer (Eds.), *Serious games: Mechanism and effects* (pp. 413–428). New York: Routledge.

Kato, P. M., Cole, S. W., Bradlyn, A. S., & Pollock, B. H. (2008). A video game improves behavioral outcomes in adolescents and young adults with cancer: A randomized trial. *Pediatrics*, *122*(2), e305–e317.

Kron, F. W., Gjerde, C. L., Sen, A., & Fetters, M. D. (2010). Medical student attitudes toward video games and related new media technologies in medical education. *BMC Medical Education*, *10*, 50. Available at http://www.biomedcentral.com/1472-6920/10/50

Lieberman, D. A. (1997). Interactive video games for health promotion: Effects on knowledge, self-efficacy, social support, and health. In R. L. Street, W. R. Gold & T. Manning (Eds.), *Health promotion and interactive technology* (pp. 103–120). Mahwah, NJ: Erlbaum.

Lieberman, D. A. (2006). *Dance games and other exergames: What the research says*. Retrieved on September 27, 2007 from http://www.comm.ucsb.edu/faculty/lieberman/exergames.htm

Lieberman, D. A. (2009). Designing serious games for learning and health in informal and formal settings. In U. Ritterfeld, M. J. Cody, & P. Vorderer (Eds.), *Serious games: Mechanism and effects* (pp. 117–130). New York: Routledge.

Lieberman, D. A. (2013). Designing digital games, social media, and mobile technologies to motivate and support health behavior change. In R. E. Rice & C. K. Atkin (Eds.), *Public communication campaigns* (4th ed., pp. 273–288). Los Angeles, CA: Sage.

McGonigal, J. (2011). *Reality is broken: Why games make us better and how they can change the world.* New York: The Penguin Press.

Meskó, B. (2011). *Health games, social media and virtual education.* Keynote speech at Games for Health Europe conference, Amsterdam, the Netherlands. Retrieved on February 16, 2012 from http://www.youtube.com/watch?feature=playerembedded&v=fLgPV_vOGEE&noredirect=1

Miller, L. C., Christensen, J. L., Godoy, C. G., Appleby, P. R., Corsbie-Massay, C., & Read, S. J. (2009). Reducing risky sexual decision-making in the virtual and in the real world: Serious games, intelligent agents, and a SOLVE approach. In U. Ritterfeld, M. J. Cody, & P. Vorderer (Eds.), *Serious games: Mechanism and effects* (pp. 429–447). New York: Routledge.

Peng, W., Lin, J.-H., & Crouse, J. (2011). Is playing exergames really exercising? A meta-analysis of energy expenditure in active video games. *Cyberpsychology, Behavior, and Social Networking, 14*(11), 681–688.

Read, S. J., Miller, L. C., Appleby, P. R., Nwosu, M. E., Raynaldo, S., Lauren, A., & Putcha, A. (2006). Socially optimized learning in a virtual environment: Reducing risky sexual behavior among men who have sex with men. *Human Communication Research, 32*(1), 1–34.

Reger, G. M., Holloway, K. M., Candy, C., Rothbaum, B. O., Difede, J., Rizzo, A. A., Gahm, G. A. (2011). Effectiveness of virtual reality exposure therapy for active duty soldiers in a military mental health clinic. *Journal of Traumatic Stress, 24*(1), 93–96.

Rizzo, A., Difede, J., Rothbaum, B. O., & Reger, G. (2010). Virtual Iraq / Afghanistan: Development and early evaluation of a virtual reality exposure therapy system for combat-related PTSD. *Annals of the New York Academy of Sciences* (NYAS), *1208*, 114–125.

Snyder, L., & Farrar, D. (2012, July). *Promoting HIV testing behaviors among African-American heterosexual men using a safer sex video game.* Paper presented at the XIX International AIDS Conference, Washington, D.C.

Snyder, L., Farrar, D., Biocca, F., & Bohil, C. (2010, August). *Developing and testing the effectiveness of a safer sex video game for young adult urban African-American heterosexual men in the U.S.* Paper presented at the National Conference on Health Communication, Marketing, and Media, Atlanta, GA.

Wang, H., Shen, C., & Ritterfeld, U. (2009). Enjoyment of digital games: What makes them seriously fun? In U. Ritterfeld, M. J. Cody, & P. Vorderer (Eds.), *Serious games: Mechanism and effects* (pp. 25–47). New York: Routledge.

Wang, H., & Singhal, A. (2009). Entertainment-education through digital games. In U. Ritterfeld, M. J. Cody, & P. Vorderer (Eds.), *Serious games: Mechanisms and effects* (pp. 271–292). New York: Routledge.

Yee, N., & Bailenson, J. (2007). The Proteus effect: The effect of transformed self-representation on behavior. *Human Communication Research, 33*(3), 271–290.

Performance and Narrative Power

Chapter 5

Entertainment Education Saves Lives and Improves Health: Key Steps to Developing Effective Programs

Caroline Jacoby, Jane Brown, Uttara Bharath Kumar,
& Sanjanthi Velu, *Johns Hopkins Bloomberg School of Public Health Center for Communication Programs*
Rajiv N. Rimal, *George Washington University*

JESSICA
How could you do this to me?

SACHI
I'm sorry, I'm really sorry. Please understand that I love you. She gave me a choice between you and her tonight. And I chose you, I chose you Jessie, because I love you.

JESSICA
I thought you chose me the day you married me. And what do you mean she gave you a choice—you couldn't give yourself that choice?

SACHI
It's not like that.

JESSICA
It's not only that you cheated on me, but do you know the risks? You obviously didn't use condoms, is she alright? We have to get tested.

SACHI
No honey, I'm sure it's alright. I'm really sure it's okay.

JESSICA
(Shaking her head)
Sachi, wake up! How sure can any of us be these days? I was "sure" you weren't sleeping with anyone else, and just see how that turned out! Even people that have been tested for HIV can't be sure. Have you ever heard of the "window period?"
(Sachi looks blank and slowly shakes his head.)

JESSICA (cont'd)
Sachi, the window period is the time when an HIV-positive person is most infectious, or most likely to pass on HIV, in the first few weeks after he or she has been infected. The body has not yet started to fight the new virus, so HIV uses that chance

to start making more copies of itself. During this time, the amount of virus or "the viral load" in the newly infected person's body increases rapidly. The likelihood of transmitting HIV by having unprotected sex during this period is extremely high; about half of all HIV infections occur during the window period.

(In the next scene, Sachi explains to his friends what Jessica has told him.)

In the example above, from the award-winning Zambian TV drama, *Club Risky Business* (2009), Jessica, a nurse, reacts angrily when her husband Sachi confesses that he has a son by another woman. Not only has Sachi been unfaithful, but he has put them all at risk of contracting HIV. Developed under the auspices of the Zambian National AIDS Council and technical support from Johns Hopkins Bloomberg School of Public Health Center for Communication Programs (JHU·CCP), the drama addresses the difficult issue of multiple concurrent partners and HIV in a realistic and emotional manner so that audiences are able to relate to the story and reflect on their own behaviors. *Club Risky Business* is one of many powerful Entertainment Education (EE) productions that have shown considerable success in positively impacting people's relationships and lives. This chapter will share some recent effective EE programs and outline the key steps to developing successful EE programs.

Most conventional entertainment programs are not educational. Also, many programs with an educational intent are too didactic and do not engage audiences. The conscious aim of Entertainment Education is to grab and hold the attention of audiences and to purposely increase audience members' knowledge about an issue, create favorable attitudes, shift social norms, and change behavior (de Fossard, 2004; Singhal & Rogers, 1999; Singhal, Cody, Rogers, & Sabido 2004) by using a creative story-telling approach. The Entertainment Education approach can have significant influence on motivating people to change health behaviors (Kincaid & Figueroa, 2012; Storey, Karki, Heckert, Karmacharya, & Boulay, 1999). An important Health Communication approach, EE has been used to address a myriad of public health issues, such as family planning, gender equality, cancer, and HIV prevention and stigma reduction, among others (Beale, Kato, Marin-Bowling, Guthrie, & Cole, 2007; Storey et al., 1999).

EE is not a new concept. For millennia, people have been telling parables or stories to teach lessons. What is more recent is the blend of art and science of EE. The art is the creation of wonderful stories and characters that touch audience members' emotions and help them feel empathy for the characters and their situations. The science is the application of analysis and theory to shape a compelling story that moves audience members to examine a given issue in their own lives and, once they are thinking about making changes, provides concrete ideas on how to do that. EE shows consequences of actions and models conversations, enabling people to experience things vicariously before they test them out in real life. The science is also the measurement of an EE program's impact.

In the last 10 years, EE has evolved from the foundations of traditional TV and radio dramas to embrace new technologies and formats. Programs are becoming even more creative—some more "Hollywood-like" and yet others tapping into reality programming—in the increasingly competitive media environments. Some channels used are:

- Mass media: television, film, radio, comic books;
- Traditional media: storytelling, drama, puppetry, music;
- Internet-based: gaming, social networking, mobile phones (Storey & Sood, 2013).

Examples of effective and innovative EE approaches were recently demonstrated at the 5th International Entertainment Education conference (http://www.ee5.org/). Highlights included EE programs from Africa and Asia that had a positive effect on people and government-level policies (see Case Studies 1–3).

CASE STUDY 1: Do you know your lover's lover? *Intersexions*: Exploring sexual networks in South Africa

Intersexions (2012), an award-winning 26-episode TV drama series in South Africa, explores the lives of those infected and affected by HIV, the circumstances of their contracting the virus, and the relationships in their lives. Each stand-alone episode takes viewers closer to understanding the interconnectedness of sexual networks. The program also addresses audience self-efficacy to resist multiple concurrent partnerships, use condoms, and get tested for HIV.

A 2012 survey revealed that 9 million South Africans watched *Intersexions*—28% of men and 38% of women (Kincaid & Figueroa, 2012). Of those who watched the series, almost 50%, or 4.5 million South Africans, watched at least 13 episodes. According to the survey, *Intersexions* increased audience self-efficacy to resist multiple concurrent sexual partnerships (MCP). The series increased positive attitudes towards condom use and self-efficacy to use them. It also reinforced the perceived norm that more people are getting an HIV test and increased discussion about testing (Kinkaid & Figueroa, 2012).

For more information about *Intersexions*, see the official *Intersexions* website at http://www.intersexions-tv.co.za and "*Intersexions* wins Peabody

Award" at http://www.jhuccp.org/news/intersexions-wins-peabody-award-accolades-keep-coming-south-african-serial-drama.

CASE STUDY 2:
Award-Winning Film Influences Pakistani Health Policy

Bol ("Speak Up"), a full-length Entertainment Education feature film that addresses social realities and advocates women's rights, opened in Pakistan on June 24, 2011, and has earned more box office revenue than any other film in the nation's history. The film revolves around Zainub Khan, who has been found guilty by Pakistan's Courts and is to be hanged. Her last wish is to speak out about her father Hakim, and the lengths he went to in order to have a son instead of his seven daughters. While the film has received critical and widespread acclaim, its critical message was aimed specifically at opinion leaders and policymakers and has had an influence on national health policy. In January 2012, Pakistan's National Assembly and Senate unanimously passed bills that prohibit forced marriage (one of Bol's central issues).

For more information, see "Pakistan women hope to gather gains as bill moves forward to Senate," on the Women News Network at http://womennewsnetwork.net/2012/01/29/pakistan-women-gather-gains/ and "The Making of *Bol*," in *The Vigilant* at http://www.thevigilantinternational.com/component/content/article/34/67-November2012.html.

CASE STUDY 3: Get H2O:
Using games to promote peace among young people in urban East Africa

Get H2O is a serious game that provides young people skills to deal with themes that lead to violent conflict. Get H2O simulates the complexity of life in an informal settlement, focusing on the scarcity of resources, especially water and housing. Players learn how to manage resources, invest in the community, and prevent escalation of conflict. The mobile version of the game at www.geth2ogame.com garnered more than 85,000 downloads, including 5,000 downloads from East Africa.

Before playing the game, a majority of youth noted "friendship" and "helping people in need" as key community contributions. After playing, participants noted "building public toilets and community houses," "protecting the resources like water," and "working together and cease revenge" as other possible ways that can contribute to improve the well-being of the community (Beamer, 2012).

EE has many possibilities for application. Three additional case studies (Annex 1) showcase using comic books to prevent diabetes among Native American youth, radio reality programming in Malawi, and a short mobile film that reached Indian migrant laborers with HIV-prevention and testing information.

The EE Development Process

Although each EE program is unique, quality EE programs follow a systematic development process (Noar, 2006). EE requires dedicated, professional experts from different fields to work together. Social scientists and communication personnel research, design, implement, and monitor impact in a systematic and thoughtful way; scriptwriters, graphic designers, filmmakers, and others bring the imagination and creativity to attract the audiences (Bouman, 2002). Having a systematic process enables everyone to work together efficiently and effectively.

Below, using an illustrative example of the *Club Risky Business* case study, we describe the basic steps required in formulating and implementing EE programs.

Part 1: Design—Audience Assessment, Theory, and Technical Brief

The first and arguably most important step is to analyze and come to understand the intended audience members' social context and psychosocial profile so the program can addresses their specific needs and appeal to them in a meaningful, engaging way. Some key data that is gathered at this stage include the audience members' age and gender profile, locale, socioeconomic status, cultural beliefs, interests, media habits, and key behaviors for change, along with the facilitators and barriers the audience will encounter and information about existing policies or programs. While some audience information can be gleaned from existing demographic, epidemiological, sociological or economic studies, many programs conduct further research.

A critical part of the EE process is to determine which behavior change theory or theories will be most effective for influencing change with a given audience on a particular topic. Two widely adopted theoretical perspectives of how EE affects change are presented in this chapter.

Social cognitive theory (SCT) (Bandura, 1977, 1986) explains that individuals learn by observing the behavior of others and evaluating the apparent consequences in order to make behavioral decisions of their own. Individuals can learn from behavior modeled in the real life around them or the behavior of characters depicted in the media. The theory asserts that people will replicate behaviors they are exposed to if they perceive the behaviors to be beneficial. Similarly, negative behaviors are more likely to be emulated if those exhibiting the behaviors are shown not to suffer negative consequences. People interpret the consequences of actions, assess their own ability to enact similar behaviors, and then act (or choose not to act) accordingly.

Self-efficacy is the belief that one has the ability to exert personal control over outcomes. EE programs focus on strengthening self-efficacy through characters modeling the key positive behaviors and achieving their desired goals.

The extended parallel process model (EPPM) (Witte, 1992) suggests that, in order to promote behavior change, individuals must perceive a significant amount of threat associated with their current behavior. For example, those who do not use condoms must first perceive that this behavior puts them at risk of negative consequences. Second, individuals must perceive that they have the self-efficacy to bring about change.

Thus, EPPM proposes that behavior change occurs when both perceived threat and efficacy, or the ability to do something about it, are high. In EE programming, this is often accomplished by showing the negative consequences of high-risk behaviors (which may include an unwanted pregnancy or the realization that one is HIV-positive) and modeling the correct or desired behaviors.

Technical brief

Every successful EE program—be it a street drama, film, radio program, or video game—has a technical brief, which outlines the "education" that goes into an EE program before making any decisions about the creative aspects or the "entertainment." An effective brief is developed with participation from key stakeholders—researchers, content experts, communication professionals, social scientists, artists, writers, producers, stakeholders, and audience members, as relevant to the program. Based on the audience and theory considerations described above, the technical brief becomes the guiding document for the creative people to develop storylines, script, characters, etc. The technical brief is also the foundation for script and program review, monitoring, implementation, and evaluation.

Technical briefs are done in varying styles. For example, a long-running drama serial may have a more comprehensive document (de Fossard, 2004). Shorter programs may only have a one-page brief highlighting key points. That said, the following are the essential elements for any EE technical brief:

- Intended Audience: Determine primary audience (individuals whom the program is to reach directly) and secondary audiences (those who influence the primary audience). For both audiences, at a minimum, gender, age, income, where they live, and marital status should be included.
- Behavioral Objectives: Clarify what the program wants audience members to know, what attitude they should hold, or what they should do after they see or hear the EE program. Ensure that the objectives are SMART—Specific, Measurable, Appropriate, Realistic, and Time-bound. These objectives will serve to guide the program as well as to provide the foundation for evaluating whether the program is successful.
- Communication Objectives: Determine the two or three key messages to get across to the primary intended audience.
- Positioning Statement: Consider competition (barriers and facilitators), key promise, or main benefit of doing the behavior.
- Call to Action: Clarify what individuals can do after seeing or hearing the program.
- Creative Considerations: Consider tone, brand personality, format, color schemes, clothing to be worn, and any underlying social issues of which to be aware or to address.
- Technical Program Specifications: Identify geographical placement, media plan, languages, promotional materials, pretesting needs, and program-related issues.

The amount of detail covered in the technical brief depends on program need, but the key idea is to keep it as concise as possible.

Illustrative Example: Club Risky Business *Part 1: Design—Audience Assessment, Theory, and Technical Brief*

Zambia's HIV prevalence was high at 14.3% among 15–49 year-olds (Central Statistical Office (CSO) [Zambia] & Macro International Inc, 2007). Multiple and concurrent sexual partnerships was identified as a key driver (Halperin & Epstein, 2009). Urban residents were twice as likely to be living with HIV compared with their rural counterparts, and prevalence increased with age. While the general perception was that marriage and long-term relationships provided a safe haven from HIV, in fact, over 20% of new infections occurred among people who reported having only one sex partner (NAC, 2009). Men were not aware of the "window period" and its relation to HIV transmission.

Table 1. Club Risky Business *chapter study: Technical brief*

Intended Audience	1. Phase 1 primary target: men Age: 25–50 Income: medium to high Education: medium to high Where they live: urban/peri-urban Marital Status: married	2. Phase 1 secondary targets: women (wives and girlfriends) Age: 20–45 Income: low to medium Education: low to medium Where they live: urban/peri-urban Marital status: wives or unmarried girlfriends
Behavioral Objective	This mass media campaign will be a "wake-up call" or "epiphany" for target groups. After seeing the campaign, people engaged in multiple concurrent sexual partnerships (MCP) will do the following: (a) Realize the risks posed by MCP; (b) Have one partner at a time who has no concurrent sexual partners, or simply reduce their number of concurrent sexual partners; (c) Realize that sexual partners have mutual rights and responsibilities to know and disclose their HIV status to each other; (d) Go for Voluntary Counseling and Testing (VCT) (preferably with partners) and disclose their status to partner(s); (e) Improve relationship with primary partner (better communication and sex); (f) Use condoms correctly and consistently with all sexual partners, including regular/long-term/trusted partners.	
Communication Objective	1. Increase personal risk perception for acquiring HIV through better understanding of "window period" and sexual networks (role of concurrency); 2. Increase understanding of protective behaviors (partner reduction, condom use); 3. Increase sense of responsibility to not infect others.	
Positioning Statement	**Partner Reduction:** Having one partner at a time can greatly reduce your risk of HIV infection and can reduce the stress/strain on your resources (time and money). **VCT:** You and your partner(s) have mutual rights and responsibilities to know and disclose your HIV status to each other. **Condoms:** Condoms are not just for those who are unfaithful or infected/worried about being infected with STIs (including HIV); they are a sign of love/care for your partner.	
Call to Action	Get yourself tested.	
Creative Considerations	Concept of "risk" needs to be expanded from focusing on the individual to raising awareness that HIV risk depends on sexual patterns of both partners (and partners' partners, etc.) • Capture ideas that resonate with Zambian culture and specific target groups, as portrayed by people, clothing, phraseology, sayings; • Concept of monogamous relationships such as marriage should be re-defined and spiced up; • Challenge gender norms (e.g., having more partners does not make you more of a man); • Challenge people to take responsibility and not use cultural/social "norms" as excuses for their actions; • Model positive, healthy relationships.	
Technical/Program Specifications	Geographical placement: Nationwide Other languages: 7 local languages Materials to be used for promotion: Facebook, launch, newspaper insert, bus stop and mini-bus billboards, radio talk show, adverts on radio and TV, bumper stickers, T-shirts, caps and pens	

Urban and peri-urban men (ages 25–45 years) with some disposable income and aspirational lifestyles were identified as those most likely to engage in multiple concurrent partnerships. Many men did not know if they were in a sexual network or that being in a sexual network would put one at increased risk of HIV.

As the goal of the program was to increase self-efficacy and risk perception among Zambian men, the main theoretical framework was a combination of social cognitive theory (SCT) and extended parallel process model (EPPM). The design team decided that the main characters should be people who are just like everyone else, so that the audience would relate to them. The design team determined to use SCT by being sure to demonstrate the consequences of actions and also to model characters changing their own behaviors based on consideration of these consequences. The design team utilized EPPM by showing how characters' risk perception increased along with their self-efficacy to engage in risk-reduction behaviors. All critical partners developed the technical brief. (see Table 1).

Part 2: Artistry and Pretesting

The key to successful Entertainment Education is a good story. The creative process starts after the team completes the technical brief. Artists develop character profiles and stories. Next, a designated review team ensures that the characters and story will resonate with the audience described in the formative research and that they will demonstrate the desired behavior change outlined in the technical brief. The creative team then develops the stories into scripts, followed by storyboards (if using a visual medium like TV or gaming). Note that EE reality programming follows a different creative process where the "stories" and "characters" are based on who is interviewed, but the principles of ensuring that "characters" resonate with the audience and having an emotionally appealing story are the same.

Characters are important. Characters must be people with whom the intended audience can relate and identify (Kincaid, 2002). By representing certain characters or processes in particular ways, audience members come to adopt similar approaches in their own thinking, or integrate such thinking within their own practices (Parker, Ntlabati, & Hajiyiannis, 2005). In a South African TV Drama *Tsha Tsha* (http://www.cadre.org.za/about-tsha-tsha), viewers identified with characters to the point that particular values and problem-solving strategies were internalized and audience members "wanted to be like" the depicted characters (Parker et al., 2005). Some key characteristics of developing good characters are:

- Each character should have a unique personality, shown by the way they walk, talk, move, and react.
- Characters should be believable and someone the audience can relate to.
- Characters must have quirks or flaws.

   The main quirk or flaw of the character should drive the plot. For example, in a successful American detective drama (not an EE program), the main detective Monk is obsessive compulsive—which makes things difficult for him. But he solves crime *because* he is obsessive compulsive.
- Effective EE programs demonstrate key characters going through their own behavior-change processes in realistic ways. Rather than being perfect role models, they must be human by making mistakes, by being gullible, or by having to try something a few times before they get it right.

Elements of a good EE story

An EE story must touch the emotions of the audience (e.g., a love story, a competition, a quest). It should be exciting with lots of action or twists in the plot that catch and hold the audience's attention. A good EE story's main conflict is about something more than the health or social topic, because the depiction of only a health issue is immensely difficult to present in an engaging manner.

Pretesting

Technical program experts, and drama experts provide critical review at key points in the production process to ensure that characters, storys, scripts, storyboards, etc., are in line with the technical brief and appeal to the audience.

Despite the rigor with which the program has been developed up to this point, all EE must be pretested with the audience. This generally involves focus group discussions with audience members to pretest scripts, storyboards, and entire episodes or program segments. Pre-testing secures audience feedback on attractiveness and identification with characters, appeal of episodes or storylines, credibility and originality, cultural, religious and social authenticity and acceptability, gender sensitivity, message comprehension, take-away points, and avoidance of stereotyping.

Illustrative Example: Club Risky Business *Part 2: Artistry and Implementation*

The artists of *Club Risky Business* created characters with whom the main intended audience, Zambian men, would relate, and they made sure to include an interesting story.

Sachi, in his late 30s, is a middle-income civil servant with an infertile wife and a girlfriend who is the mother of his one-year-old son. He loves both women but has to figure out which one to be with. Formative research showed that condoms signify mistrust and disease and are rarely used in long-term relationships. Sachi does not use condoms with his wife and long-term girlfriend because he trusts them. The "window period" of acute HIV infection is not well understood.

David is a rich businessman in his early 40s with a wife and three children. He cannot communicate his sexual dissatisfaction to his wife and so seeks comfort and distraction with three other women, including a co-worker and a college student.

Charlie Lucky is a "player" in his late 20s. He is single and has many girlfriends but always uses a condom. He has to figure out what to do when the love of his life shows up.

These three friends meet at the neighborhood bar, Club Risky Business, and exchange stories about their relationships and lives. The drama intensifies as the stories illustrate each man's sexual network. The audience is surprised to find out who is HIV positive at the end of the story.

Watch the show at http://www.youtube.com/watch?v=XY00mts_uZ8.

Part 3: Implementation

An EE program is more effective when a "buzz" is created and people are talking about it with their families, friends, partners, and communities. EE programs increasingly seek to open up dialogue because audience involvement appears to be a precursor for increasing self-efficacy and collective efficacy and in promoting interpersonal communication among individuals in the audience (Sood, 2002).

Program promotion is key. With the saturated media environments that are the norm in most countries, programs must be increasingly aggressive and creative to get the audience's attention. Promotion can include TV or radio spots posters, wristbands, hats, T-shirts, competitions, launch events, public parades, mobile 'blasts,' flash mobs, among other ideas.

Media planning is a critical aspect of implementation, which, regretfully, is often left until the last minute. Media planning involves determining where and when the EE program will be broadcast or performed. Determining a media plan requires getting input from listeners about their preferred times and days for listening to and watching the programs, balanced with the high broadcast costs, as is the case in many countries.

Program implementation refers to community engagement activities, feedback and monitoring while the EE is 'on air.' Some ideas are:

- In facilitated discussion groups, audience members can see or hear the program and then talk about the issues raised in terms of their own lives in order to take action.
- Supplemental materials such as discussion guides, story books, informational brochures, and pictorial flip charts can reinforce the main motivational or educational issues.
- Social media is an emerging powerful tool through Facebook, Twitter, and mobile technology. Social media can be used to promote a program, hold discussions, gain feedback, or monitor interest in the program. Many EE programs will have their own Facebook and Twitter pages and post provocative questions after broadcast each week. This opens the space for dialogue between the program and the audience but also between audience members themselves.
- Mobile phones are becoming increasingly useful in an EE approach. For some time, texting through mobile phones has been utilized for feedback or promotional activities. In some countries mobile phones are now functioning as the radio or video screen to hear/see the EE program and as the means for audience members to engage in discussions about their experience on social media sites.

Illustrative Example: Club Risky Business *Part 3: Implementation*

The *Club Risky Business* program kicked off with a showy red-carpet launch, attended by partners, media, and senior government officials, so it grabbed attention right away. View the trailer for *Club Risky Business* at http://www.youtube.com/watch?v=NJ_ILKHs0VE&feature=related.

The series was then aired weekly on national and private TV channels. A new episode was broadcast every week with repetitions at different times that same week to maximize viewership. These were supplemented by animated commercials.

See a reinforcement spot on Saachi's network at: http://www.youtube.com/watch?v=e6Rmd8-Kg3E&list=UUgi-2Zi8Xtl05SA2XKWEwHg&index=1&feature=plcp.

Club Risky Business's Facebook page named for the campaign tag line One Love Kwasila was very popular. Facebook fans more than doubled, from 2,000 at the beginning of the campaign in 2009 to over 5,000 in August 2010. As of 2012, people were still active on the Facebook page two years after the broadcast ended. View the program's Facebook page at: http://www.facebook.com/#!/OneLoveKwasila.

Part 4: Evaluation

It is not enough just to design a program and put in on the air. The overarching evaluation question for funders, program designers, and partners is: Did the program have an impact that can be documented? They may also ask more nuanced questions, such as:

- Which segment of the population appears to have gained the most from the program and which segment appears to have been least affected? What are the reasons for this disparity?
- How did exposure to the program result in the desired outcomes? Did the program, affect perceived risk or self-efficacy, which may have affected the desired outcome?
- Which actor appears to have had the highest level of identification from audience members and did this translate into desired behavior change?

Because EE programs often use mass media, it becomes a challenge to conduct randomized trials to assess program effectiveness. One cannot, for example, randomly assign people not to watch a particular program when it is aired on mass media. Therefore, researchers use other methods to attribute outcomes to particular programs. One such technique is conducting a dose-response analysis (Piotrow et al., 1992; Storey et al., 1999)—with the idea that those who were exposed to the program more extensively would change more rapidly or drastically, in comparison with those who were exposed in only small doses. Another technique is running a propensity score analysis (Mai & Kincaid, 2006), which matches people on key variables and assesses whether exposure to the program differentiates the exposed group from the unexposed group on key behavioral outcomes.

Evaluators have also found that indirect exposure to EE programs can have significant impact on behavior. Indirect exposure refers to people who have not watched or heard the EE program directly but discussed the program with family, friends or neighbors who were exposed. Program evaluations that ignore indirect exposure underestimate the impact of a mass media program on behavior (Boulay, Storey, & Sood, 2002).

Qualitative methods can serve as a mechanism for audience members to share how they or their community were impacted by the EE program. Potential methods include in-depth interviews, focus groups, audience feedback analysis (i.e., blog posts, texts, letters, and Facebook updates, among others) (Sood, 2002).

Illustrative Example: Club Risky Business *Part 4: Evaluation*

Club Risky Business won a national award for "Best Drama Series" in Zambia (2009) and the AfriComNet 2010 award for the "Best HIV/AIDS Multichannel Campaign in Africa."

The program achieved impressive results. For example, 32% of Zambians had heard of *Club Risky Business* (Kumkum & Clark, 2010). The campaign call-in radio program reached 3 million listeners in a country of 11 million, and during the text messaging competition, over 17,000 text entries were received in response to questions posed at the end of the episodes.

The program used primarily qualitative data for the evaluation. Indications of how audience members perceived the program and the impact it made on their lives was evidenced through comments on Facebook as well as other means. One Zambian health professional shared how the program affected her community: "The series woke Zambia up and broke a huge silence around MCP. Furthermore, the wake-up happened on primetime television and went into homes, directly to families and couples."

Lessons Learned about Entertainment Education

Our experience in Entertainment Education has taught us several important lessons:

- **Plan for evaluation from the beginning.** Many EE programs are not evaluated because of cost and time issues. There is no doubt that national programs are expensive to evaluate. But if planned and budgeted for at the start, impact assessments can be done, and the findings can then feed back into the program to strengthen it. Our experience has been that, although some funders are reluctant to spend a lot of resources on conducting the campaign evaluation, they often do want to see results. Hence, an evaluation component is needed.

- **Utilize a participatory, theory-based design process.** Getting technical input from experts, audience members, and stakeholders on the program's design, theoretical foundations, objectives and content from the beginning makes the program more likely to be effective.
- **Hire the best creative minds and actors possible.** It is an art form to develop a story that is entertaining and one that weaves in educational messages in a subtle and yet effective way. When working with the best production team and talented actors, it is easier and more cost effective to develop a great product that will attract a wider audience.
- **Provide EE training for writers and/or producers.** In many cases, writers or producers may be at the top of their field but not experienced in integrating educational messages into their programs. This requires specific training.
- **Link with other resources,** such as health or social services, peer educators, community or religious leaders, talk shows, online discussion groups, Facebook, Twitter, and mobile technology.
- **Form partnerships** with TV or radio media houses, DVD, video CD (VCD), or comic book distributors, schools, implementing partners, drama groups, puppet teams, Internet service providers, mobile phone service providers, and others.
- **Work with the private sector.** Contact media houses and companies that could sponsor ads or airtime or make in-kind contributions. In South Africa, partnership with the South Africa Broadcasting Corporation facilitated free national broadcast for the *Intersexions* TV drama.

Entertainment Education is a powerful and versatile approach that can enhance the impact of communication strategies and programs. As discussed in this chapter, if implemented correctly and systematically, it works on a wide variety of health and social issues and through a number of channels: mass media, traditional media, or with the new information technologies such as social networking sites. EE has the promise to make the world a healthier, safer, and happier place for the millions of audience members who tune in every day to their TV, radio, community activities, and social networking sites.

APPENDIX

CASE STUDY: "Reaching Young Native Americans Through Comic Books"

Type 2 diabetes is an emerging problem among young Native Americans. In response, a comic book series was developed for Native children in grades K–4. Diabetes prevention messages are integrated into a mystery-adventure plot, in which the child characters foil a ring of fossil poachers with the help of three animal heroes that embody the cultural values of their tribe. Due to high demand, approximately 500,000 comic book sets have been distributed, and the program has expanded. The books were developed by Westat with support from the U.S. Centers for Disease Control and Prevention (CDC). For more information, see http://www.cdc.gov/diabetes/pubs/eagle/index.html.

CASE STUDY: "Reality Radio in Malawi—A Fresh Approach"

In rural Malawi, the rates of HIV infection hover around 10%. Programmers developed *Chenicheni Nchiti?* ("What is Real?"), a weekly 30-minute radio program broadcasting real individuals, community leaders, and action groups telling their stories. Stories were gathered by trained community reporters and then edited before broadcast. Listener demand for the show, which was produced by StoryWorkshop with support from the Johns Hopkins Bloomberg School of Public Health · Center for Communication Programs, has risen exponentially. Initially broadcast three times each week on the national local-language radio station, the show expanded to broadcasts on nine radio stations up to 15 times each week. For more information, see http://www.jhuccp.org/whatwedo/regions/africa/malawi.

CASE STUDY: "Reaching Migrant Laborers Through a Short Film in India"

In India, migrant workers are at higher risk of HIV than the general population because the loneliness and isolation combined with negative peer influence makes them vulnerable to engaging in high-risk behaviors, such as unprotected sex or drug abuse. Part of a larger "Safe Migrant Package," the short film *Jeelo Zindagi* ("Embrace Life"), produced by JHU/CCP, tells the tale of a shy, young man who is new in the city and encounters temptations. The film presents choices that either protect or make a migrant worker vulnerable to the risk of HIV infection. The short film touched a chord with the audience. More migrants went for HIV testing where the film was shown than elsewhere. One audience member explained, "All these characters are among us. We have more people like Raju and Shambhu (risk takers in the film) and less like Mohan (one who behaves responsibly). We liked Mohan."

Recommended Readings

de Fossard, E. (2004). *Communication for behavior change, volume 1: Writing and producing radio dramas.* India: Sage Publications Pvt Ltd. Provides a detailed step-by-step process of developing a long-running radio drama using the design document process.

de Fossard, E. (2005). *Communication for behavior change, volume 2: Writing and producing for television and film.* India: Sage Publications Pvt Ltd. Describes the step-by-step process of developing a long-running TV drama using the design document process.

McKee, R. (1997). *Story substance, structure, style and the principles of screenwriting.* Regan Books. Explains the fundamentals of character and story development.

References

Bandura, A. (1977). *Social learning theory.* Englewood Cliffs, NJ: Prentice Hall.

Bandura, A. (1986). *Social foundations of thought and action.* Englewood Cliffs, NJ: Prentice-Hall.

Beale, I.L., Kato, P.M., Marin-Bowling, V.M, Guthrie, N., & Cole, S. (2007). Improvement in cancer-related knowledge following use of a psychoeducational video game for adolescents and young adults with cancer. *Journal of Adolescent Health, 41,* 263–270.

Beamer, E. (2012). Get H2O Game from the website address at http://www.butterflyworks.org/content/13802/geth2o_serious_games.

Boulay, M., Storey, J.D., Sood, S. (2002) Indirect exposure to a family planning mass media campaign in Nepal. *Journal of Health Communication, 7,* 379–399.

Bouman, M. (2002). Turtles and peacocks: Collaboration in entertainment-education television. *Communication Theory, 12,* 225–244. doi: 10.1111/j.1468-2885.2002.tb00268.x

Central Statistical Office (CSO) [Zambia] & Macro International Inc. (2009). *Zambia Demographic and Health Survey 2007: Key findings.* Calverton, MD: CSO and Macro International Inc.

de Fossard, E. (2004). *Communication for behavior change, volume 1: Writing and producing radio dramas.* New Delhi, India: Sage.

Halperin, D., & Epstein, H. (2009). *Strategic communication for communications on multiple and concurrent partnerships.* Handout for Participants in the Expert Multiple Concurrent Partnership Meeting, Gabarone, Botswana.

Kincaid, D.L. (2002). Drama, emotion, and cultural convergence. *Communication Theory, 12*(2), 136–152.

Kincaid, D. L., & Figueroa, M. (2012). *The impact of* Intersexions *TV drama on prevention behavior: National communication survey, 2012 preliminary results.* Presented at South Africa Broadcasting Corporation, Johannesburg, South Africa.

Kumkum, A., & Clark, M. (2010). *'Club Risky Business': A Zambian television series challenges multiple and concurrent sexual partnerships.* Case Study Series. Arlington, VA: USAID.

Mah, T.L., & Halperin, D.T. (2010). Concurrent sexual partnerships and the HIV epidemic in sub-Saharan Africa: The evidence to move forward. *AIDS and Behavior, 14,* 11–16.

Mai, P., & Kincaid, L. (2006). Impact of an entertainment education television drama on health knowledge and behavior: An application of propensity score matching. *Journal of Health Communication, 11*, 301–325.

National AIDS Council (NAC). (2009). *National Strategy for the Prevention of HIV and STIs*. April 2009. Lusaka, Zambia: Government of Zambia and National HIV/AIDS/STI/TB Council.

Noar, S. (2006). A 10-year retrospective of research in health mass media campaigns: Where do we go from here? *Journal of Health Communication, 11*(1), 21–42.

Parker, W., Ntlabati, P., & Hajiyiannis, H. (2005, June). *Television drama and audience identification: Experiences from Tsha Tsha*. Presented at the 2nd South African AIDS Conference, Durban, South Africa.

Piotrow, P.T., Kincaid, D.L., Hindin, M.J., Lettenmaier, C.L., Kuseka, I., Silberman, T., & Mbizvo, M.T. (1992). Changing men's attitudes and behavior: The Zimbabwe male motivation project. *Studies in Family Planning, 23*, 365–375.

Singhal, A., Cody, M.J., Rogers, E.M., & Sabido, M. (2004). *Entertainment-education and social change: History, research, and practice*. Mahwah, NJ: Lawrence Erlbaum Associates.

Singhal, A., & Rogers, E.M. (1999). Entertainment-education: A communication strategy for social change. Mahway, NH: Lawrence Erlbaum.

Sood, S. (2002). Audience involvement in entertainment education. *Communication Theory, 12*, 153–172.

Storey, D., Karki, Y., Heckert, K., Karmacharya, D.M., & Boulay, M. (1999). Impact of the integrated Radio Communication Project in Nepal, 1994–1997. *Journal of Health Communication, 4*, 271–294.

Storey. D., & Sood, S. (2013). Increasing equity, affirming the power of narrative and expanding dialogue: The evolution of entertainment education over two decades. *Critical Arts: South-North Cultural and Media Studies, 27*(1), 9–35.

Witte, K. (1992). Putting the fear back in fear appeals: The extended parallel process model. *Communication Monographs, 59*, 225–249.

Chapter 6

Conversations about Cancer (CAC): A National and Global Strategy for Impacting Family and Medical Interactions

Wayne A. Beach, Kyle Gutzmer, & David M. Dozier,
San Diego State University
Mary K. Buller & David B. Buller, *Klein Buendel, Inc.*

Introduction

Cancer is a highly insidious and uncertain disease involving ambiguous diagnostic and treatment outcomes, changes in lifestyle and appearance, altered relationships, increased stress, and frequent financial hardships. Throughout cancer journeys cancer (the 'C' word) is understandably feared more than any other medical condition by Americans and one of the primary causes of health anxiety worldwide. When managing the trials and tribulations of cancer, from diagnosis through possible death of loved ones, the communication challenges faced by cancer patients, family members, and medical experts are considerable: For example, updating and making sense of both good and bad news, managing inherently uncertain futures, adjusting to changes in lifestyles and relationships (e.g., caregiving burdens), describing and assessing what doctors have reported and the overall quality of medical care being delivered (Beach, 2009). These and considerably more activities can create ongoing difficulties, but also unique opportunities exist to remain hopeful in the midst of fearful and uncertain events. Being hopeful exemplifies primal survival responses to managing diseases that cannot be fully controlled, events occurring over time that threaten quality and length of living.

While research in the social and medical sciences acknowledges these diverse challenges, and hopeful opportunities, little has been revealed about actual family communication when making sense of and coping with ordinary cancer circumstances. Direct access to interactions comprising family interactions has been constrained by a predominant focus on individuals' perceptions of, and reportings about, cancer experiences. Recently, however, a detailed and longitudinal analysis of a naturally occurring family cancer journey (Beach, 2009) has examined how a cancer patient and family members talk about and through cancer on the telephone. The basis of *A Natural History of Family Cancer* is a close analysis of 61 phone calls over a period of 13 months.[1] Many enduring and endearing moments occur in these calls, including how family members commiserate with each other, tell stories about everyday life experiences, and utilize humor to de-trigger cancer's impacts in the face of a loved one's gradual and inevitable death.

This chapter reports how these basic research findings have been transformed into a parallel project entitled Conversations about Cancer (CAC). This project conveys important messages about how cancer patients, family members, and medical experts communicate about and through cancer journeys. The foundation for CAC is *The Cancer Play*, a unique and professional theatrical production adapting *A Natural History of Family Cancer* to the stage. This production is designed for diverse audience members whose lives have somehow (directly or indirectly) been impacted by cancer, as well as an array of psychosocial and biomedical experts who are involved in diagnosing, caring for, and in other ways involved in cancer journeys. Only verbatim dialogue, from real phone conversations, is employed to provide a grounded appreciation for real-time, naturally occurring interactions produced by ordinary people in the midst of cancer. And following viewings of *The Cancer Play*, talk-back sessions are utilized to solicit feedback, stimulate meaningful discussions, and promote educational possibilities for better understanding communication and cancer.

As a unique form of 'edutainment' (Beach et al., 2012b), CAC is a sustainable health intervention and educational campaign. Anchored in basic social science research, yet harnessing the considerable power of the Arts, the CAC project is beginning to have important impacts on diverse audiences nationwide and holds considerable potential for global dissemination and influence. In what follows, we first review how communication has traditionally been conceived within public health interventions, and describes

---

[1] National Communication Association awards for *A Natural History of Family Cancer* (Beach, 2009) include the 2010–2011 Outstanding Book Award (Health Communication Division), and 2010–2011 Outstanding Scholarship Award (Language & Social Interaction Division).

how CAC's focus on actual family interactions begins to remedy these shortcomings. Second, we overview preliminary and compelling findings from Phase I viewings of *The Cancer Play*, and describe the methods we employ to design, implement, and evaluate CAC outcomes. Finally, we overview current priorities with a Phase II dissemination and effectiveness trial, including long-term goals for extending CAC into a broad array of ethnic and global populations where cancer is a predominant health threat.

CAC as a Viable Alternative to Traditional Public Health Interventions

Public health interventions have been anchored in theoretical frameworks targeting individuals' attitudes and beliefs (Brewer & Rimer, 2008). These include theories like the Health Belief Model, which is primarily concerned with perceived susceptibility, severity, barriers, benefits, cues to action, and self-efficacy (Rosenstock, Stretcher, & Becker, 1988; but see Beach, 2012). Other prominent theories include The Theory of Reasoned Action, the Transtheoretical Model, and the Socio-Ecological Model (National Cancer Institute, 2005), which also focus on perceptual dimensions of intra-personal, interpersonal, organizational, and community level influences of health behavior. Recently, public health theory has also moved toward environmental and structural interventions with theoretical frameworks like the Social Ecologic Framework and Structural Models (see, e.g., Sallis et al., 2006).

Communication in Public Health

Typically, public health interventions have framed communication not as a primary resource for tapping into social interactions (i.e., recorded conversations), or the explicit target of the desired change (i.e., altering communication skills), but as the means or channel for disseminating health interventions and findings. As Bernhardt (2004) noted, "the discipline of communication has until recently operated at the periphery of public health. Perceived as more skill than science, communication was equated only with dissemination of findings" (p. 2051). To address this issue, there has been an increased focus on large-scale health communication campaigns. One example of a health communication campaign is the VERB campaign, which used nationally paid mass media to encourage physical activity in 9–13 year-old children (Bauman, 2004). The campaign targeted the children's beliefs and norms about physical activity. The campaign also measured physical activity in the targeted communities. Mass communication was the medium, but actual communication activities per se were not the target of the campaign.

Like the VERB campaign, most health communication campaigns frame communication as essential for promoting health information but do not attempt to directly access, examine, utilize, or change communication of the participants themselves. This approach is consistent with the recurring treatments of communication in public health: "the dominant communication question of interest among healthcare researchers and practitioners focused on the individual field of influence is: Can we use messages to influence people in beneficial ways?" (Maibach, Abroms, & Marosits (2007, p. 6). However, public health communication campaigns framing communication as crafting persuasive messages have only been "modestly effective" (Maibach et al., 2007).

In Table 1 (below), a summary is provided of public health orientations toward individual perceptions and designing persuasive health messages. These approaches are contrasted with the CAC project, which directly accesses ordinary communication activities, discovers key patterns and practices organizing these events, and relies on this knowledge to structure educational interventions to enhance communication skills of ordinary participants in natural settings. Following Table 1, a brief discussion is provided of message-crafting theories and social support as prominent approaches to communication in public health.

To summarize, message-crafting approaches provide valuable information on how to design messages that are as persuasive as possible and account for the important factors of the target audience. However, these approaches do not target communication itself as a potential avenue for health behavior change or as potential resource for participants. Within these approaches, communication is limited to the 'tool' for disseminating the health message. Theories and campaigns focusing on social support examine how individuals report on ways that support from family, friends, and peers facilitates (or detracts from) healthy behavior (Heaney & Israel, 2002). Social support is divided into emotional, appraisal, informational, and instrumental support (House, 1981), but this approach does not directly examine these and related activities as interactional and thus communicative achievements. While attending to social support provides valuable insight on how relationships can foster improved health outcomes and behaviors, the role of communication as a supporting process is not fully explored.

Table 1. Public Health Approaches to Communication in Contrast to CAC

Communication in Public Health	Limitations	CAC Perspective
Message-Crafting Approaches		
Elaboration Likelihood	• Provides a description of message-processing • Emphasis on improving the persuasiveness of the message • Communication is the 'tool' used to disseminate the health message • Communication is not itself the 'target' of the change	• Anchored in and informed by Conversation Analysis (CA), a methodology that identifies and explains practices for organizing real-time, naturally occurring interaction (both ordinary/casual and institutional) • Communication understood as sets of interactional resources employed to create patterns and form relationships, not simply a 'tool' or medium for message design or intervention • Findings can be translated into communication strategies for managing social problems (e.g., cancer journeys) • Seeks to influence the communication of the participants themselves • Communication is framed as an important resource for dealing with specific dilemmas (e.g., hopes, fears, and uncertainties throughout cancer journeys)
Information Processing Paradigm	• Emphasis on creating the ideal fit with source, receiver, message and channel • Goal is persuasion / behavior change • Again, communication is used as a 'tool'	
Social Cognitive Theory	• Not a public health communication theory per se, but used to inform health messages • The theory highlights the interaction btw the individual and environment • Emphasis on creating messages that account for environmental factors (e.g:, media influences) • Does not target communication itself	
Social Marketing	• Communication to promote a particular 'product' • Use of 4 Ps • Provides tools for creating ideal promotional messages • Does not focus on communication as the target • Again communication is used as the 'tool'	

Communication in Public Health	Limitations	CAC Perspective
Stages of Change	• Not a public health communication theory per se, but used to craft health messages • Emphasizes matching the persuasion message to the stage of change • Goals is persuasion / behavior change • Communication is used as the 'tool'	
Theory of Reasoned Action / Planned Behavior	• Not a public health communication theory per se, but used to craft health messages • Explores how attitudes, beliefs, social norms, perceived behavioral control, and intention influence behavior • Communication is used as 'tool' not target	
• *Social Support*		
Social Support	• Provides an interpersonal perspective • Emphasis on support • Communication may be part of support but it is not overtly named or examined directly as interactional practices / activities • Non-communication supportive behaviors are also included	• CAC overtly examines the role of family interactions, and how social support is accomplished as various phases and challenges of the cancer journey unfold

In contrast to the message-crafting and social support approaches, the CAC project targets communication itself as naturally occurring activities within which health behaviors are displayed, adjusted, managed, and experienced. By making theatrical performances of actual communication between family members available to audience members, attention is drawn to how human interaction is an essential resource for dealing with the hopes, fears, and uncertainties of ordinary cancer journeys. Viewings of performances are educational experiences on their own merits. In addition, post-performance discussions trigger a wide array of conversations about how practices for managing cancer are similar to, and different from, their own experiences as patients, family members, and medical experts. Further, key opportunities arise not just for commiserating about shared illness experiences, but about identifying useful strategies and resources for making sense of and coping with cancer. Rather than only a 'tool' or medium for delivering isolated messages, CAC invites audiences into an unfolding and longitudinal family excursion. These behaviors realistically portray the fundamental importance and potential of conversations for navigating through the diagnosis, treatment, and prognosis of what is often a frightening and threatening disease.

Designing, Implementing, and Evaluating the Phase I CAC Project

The CAC project is grounded in a series of phone conversations, donated for purposes of a) generating basic knowledge from research findings, and b) with this information, designing possible applications for improving communication throughout cancer. As a long-term research project, *A Natural History of Family Cancer* (NH) reveals the social organization of a wide range of key communication activities inherent to managing cancer over time. The design, implementation, and evaluation of CAC are summarized below.

Creating a Forum for Audience Reactions

Since 2002, we have worked toward realizing the potential for dramatizing key moments from actual family conversations about cancer. A directed master's thesis began to raise possibilities for script production anchored in actual family phone calls (Lockwood, 2002). Interdisciplinary dialogue ensued with SDSU's theatre faculty. In 2006, through a combination of on-campus funding and community philanthropic support, an initial script was refined and 11 workshop readings and experimental stage productions occurred for nearly 1000 audience members. These events began to reveal the power of having diverse community members view and respond to an initial version of the play. Through talk-back sessions following performances, the ability to trigger and solicit powerful reactions from audience members was unequivocal: They could ask questions of the actors and production staff, share and compare their cancer experiences with those disclosed in the play, discuss the power and importance of communication for managing cancer journeys, raise communication problems and suggest practices for improvement, and offer praise and constructive comments about improving the performances. It also was emphasized that the script and performances were designed to encourage feedback, information grounded in audience experiences and allowing for both meaningful revisions and shaping future directions for the CAC project.

Overwhelmingly, just as the actors relied on actual transcriptions from real family phone calls, so too did it become clear that one key ingredient of the drama of everyday life is made evident through "real time" conversations when navigating through cancer as a family. From the moving talkback events described above, our beliefs were increasingly confirmed that the basic research findings could not only be heuristic for social and medical sciences, but employed to elicit emotional impacts about cancer, communication, and everyday life-world experiences. The strategic use of theatrical environments can heighten understandings of how peoples' lives have been directly and indirectly touched by such an insidious disease. Talkback sessions have revealed that ordinary people share common experiences, fears, and hopes about cancer despite cultural, demographic, religious, and socio-economic differences. In short, communication about cancer communication is critical: What family members actually go through, and the social realities they construct together, can be observed, heard, and responded to as a focal point of discussion and resource for subsequent reflection over time.

Designing the Phase I Feasibility Study

With the successful production of 11 CAC performances in San Diego in 2006, and based on over a decade of basic interactional research exposing communication dilemmas throughout cancer journeys, it became feasible to pursue SBIR/STTR funding through the National Cancer Institute (NCI). To accomplish this CAC project, an interdisciplinary team of health communication researchers, cancer professionals, and theatre experts has been formed. Colleagues at San Diego State University are working in partnership with Klein Buendel, Inc. (KB), a woman-owned small business firm in Golden, Colorado, that utilizes an effective mix of traditional and emerging media to educate diverse communities about health issues. A particular focus germane to CAC is the development of effective and engaging research-based health education programs, graphic design and multimedia products to motivate populations to act on information that impacts their lives.

The primary objective of our Phase I research plan was to assess the feasibility of producing and evaluating the CAC theatrical performance, and subsequent talkback session formats (including focus groups), in order to help people develop greater understandings and effective communication skills for managing their personal and family cancer journeys. We also proposed to develop protocols and procedures needed for an effectiveness trial in Phase II. Our research focus included refinement of the play script, talkback session formats, hiring professional actors and theatre experts, and developing strategies for effectively recruiting cancer patients, family members, and medical experts. Live San Diego performances were hosted by the Scripps Mercy Hospital Cancer Center, and recorded by a professional videographer. A subsequent DVD was produced, and the research protocol involved screening this DVD to cancer experts in Denver. With this design, we could compare the impacts of live performances to DVD screenings, and how cancer patients and family members responded to the play in contrast with medical experts. Accessing different populations allowed us to gain important experience in planning and hosting the CAC project in two urban populations (San Diego and Denver).

The following design features were also critical for our Phase I study:

- A protocol for creating and testing pre-post questionnaires (based on previous research) to assess audience impacts.
- Procedures for producing a guidebook to facilitate the play production including staffing, roles, tasks, budget, and strategies for managing site coordination, moderating talkback sessions, recruiting audiences, and producing the play for various community networks.
- Developing a prototype website for CAC dissemination in Phases II and III will be refined with audience and EAB input. This website will a) inform online users about the CAC project, its theatrical dissemination, and possible educational applications, b) allow users to view selected video clips of the live CAC performance in San Diego, c) invite users to sign up for continued updates about CAC progress, and d) provide opportunities for search engine optimization to monitor traffic and track Google searchers.
- Creation of an Expert Advisory Board (EAB) to integrate distinct experiences, knowledge, and cultural diversity from a cancer survivor and mother, health communication researchers, theatre professionals, a medical oncologist, a surgeon, registered nurse practitioner and breast cancer navigator, a university dean, and legal/business entrepreneurs to assist with reviewing prototype materials and guiding Phase I project development.

Implementing and Evaluating Impacts of The Cancer Play

In 2010 three live performances of *The Cancer Play* occurred at Scripps Mercy Hospital in San Diego for cancer patients and family members. Several months later, four DVD screenings of the play were shown to cancer professionals and healthcare providers (e.g., oncologists, oncology nurses, hospice care providers, social workers) in Denver cancer centers and community cancer organizations.

For this pilot study we recruited 204 audience members. Pre-post questionnaires were constructed from NH findings and related psychosocial research on family cancer journeys. Survey items included 15 opinion and 10 additional questions measuring the importance of communication between family members when managing cancer. Likert-type scales consist of 9 points, ranging from "strongly agree" (1) to "strongly disagree" (9), and were pilot tested prior to being utilized before and following live performances and DVD screenings.

Detailed methods for analyzing and assessing these findings are reported elsewhere (Beach et al., 2012a, b; Moran et al., 2012), but a summary of key impacts include the following:

- An average of 86% of all audience members agreed that the play was authentic, entertaining, appropriate, influential, uplifting and inspiring.
- Agreement increased significantly, from pre-test to post-test evaluations, for 14 of 15 measures of opinions about the importance of communication between patients and family members facing cancer. And agreement about the importance of 7 of 10 key communication activities also increased significantly.
- Results from factor analysis were equally striking. Across 15 opinion items and 10 primary communication activities, 5 primary indices/indicators revealed highly significant (<.001) changes in opinions, perceived importance, and self-efficacy.
- Comments from audience members participating in talk-back sessions and focus group meetings were overwhelmingly positive. Content analyses confirmed significant impacts across the following dimensions: perceived realism, involvement and identification with characters, being emotionally and cognitively transported into the play's drama, and ability to promote deep reflections about communication and cancer.

- For 4 of the 5 indices/indicators, audience impacts across live performances in San Diego and DVD screenings in Denver were not significant.
- Significant impacts did occur for cancer patients, family members, and cancer professionals/healthcare providers. No significant differences were discovered across these groups of individuals.

To summarize, our Phase I activities provide compelling evidence that a script grounded in naturally occurring conversations, and performed as staged readings by professional actors (even with a minimal set design), can evoke significant impacts for diverse audience members. It is possible to create and administer valid and reliable survey measures to evaluate the effectiveness of adapting basic communication research to the stage. And following performances, both talk-back and focus group discussions confirmed and further elaborated the ability of *The Cancer Play* to involve, entertain, and draw audience members into the dilemmas and resilience of a family facing cancer together over time. Whether audiences view live performances or DVD screenings, the impacts are noticeable and provide unique and sustainable opportunities to further develop innovative educational materials that will compliment the CAC theatrical production.

Phase II Effectiveness and Dissemination Trial

Phase II of this project was been funded by NCI and began in August 2012. During this 2–3 year phase, a multi-city effectiveness trial will occur to further assess CAC impacts in San Diego, Salt Lake City, Lincoln, and Boston. The four Specific Aims for this Phase II project are: 1) Refine the CAC play script and performances by professional actors, continue to utilize talents of theatre experts, and create new approaches to videography resulting in a professionally edited DVD; 2) Refine a protocol website for online access and dissemination of CAC information and products; 3) Further validate pre-post self-report measures to further assess impacts on diverse audience members; and 4) Conduct a group-randomized, pretest-posttest control, multi-city effectiveness trial to evaluate efficacy for 1800 audience members (see Beach et al., 2012a).

At each of the four sites, collaborations will occur across departments/schools of communication at major universities, comprehensive cancer centers, and community cancer organizations. So doing will provide necessary groundwork for Phase III commercialization strategies through: a) innovative educational programs for diverse cancer centers, medical groups, and health professionals; b) university and community-based play productions, and c) a documentary film.

Conclusion: Potential for Cultural and Global Adaptions of CAC

The CAC project has already revealed considerable potential for impacting and improving important facets of American society. Considerable attention needs to be given not only to the United States, but globally, regarding how cancer patients communicate throughout cancer journeys, the ebbs and flows of family relationships, abilities to work effectively with medical professionals, and overall quality of cancer journeys and care.

The potential for CAC is thus by no means limited to American culture. Critical and seemingly countless dimensions of communication and cancer are universal and applicable to a broad array of cultures continually faced with cancer challenges. For example, in March 2012, the senior author was invited to give lectures on communication and cancer at two prominent Universities in Seoul, South Korea. Working within the United States, he recognized that cancer is America's primary health fear, supported by the following statistics (American Cancer Society, 2011):

- About 1,638,910 new cancer cases were expected to be diagnosed in 2012.
- About 577,190 Americans are expected to die of cancer, more than 1,500 people a day.
- Cancer is the second most common cause of death in the US, exceeded only by heart disease, accounting for nearly 1 of every 4 deaths.
- What he did not recognize, and having not visited South Korea previously, was the impact of cancer on South Koreans (Jung et al., 2012; American Cancer Society, 2012).
- Cancer has been the leading cause of death in Korea since 1983.
- A total of 234,727 new cancer cases and 73,313 cancer deaths were projected in 2012.
- Annually, over 190,000 patients are newly diagnosed with cancer in Korea.
- One out of four deaths is due to cancer.

These statistics suggest that cancer incidence, and impacts on mortality and morbidity, are comparable to the United States. And even with countries with less threatening rates of cancer diagnosis and death, a countless number of patients, family members, and medical experts routinely communicate about the often delicate yet hopeful possibilities for treating, coping with, and utilizing available resources for healing this worldwide disease.

Currently in San Diego county, preliminary discussions are raising possibilities for adapting *The Cancer Play* to the Latino population. The protocol being envisioned, which could accommodate diverse ethnic communities affected by cancer, involves the following steps: 1) making the script and guidebooks available to community members; 2) allowing these individuals, groups, and organizations to adapt these materials (e.g., by altering the basic, verbatim script) to encompass cultural beliefs and practices; 3) recruiting local actors and organizing grass-root performances (e.g., in churches, schools, neighborhoods); and 4) utilizing these performances as opportunities to a) invite and engage conversations about shared and unique cancer experiences, b) generate strategies for creating alternative educational programs, and c) assisting both lay and professional participants to identify and implement skills and practices for improving communication skills throughout cancer journeys.

A related alternative is to adapt the CAC script, video record and edit performances, and make available to the general public DVDs for private, community, and corporate viewings. Similar to the methods employed for Phase I and II, these viewings will trigger meaningful discussions through talk-back, focus group, and related occasions whenever communication and cancer become focal points of concern and conversation. And for any culture, these CAC formats and materials can be further integrated into powerful and impactful programs for education, and training, for all cancer professionals and healthcare providers when pursuing certifications, degrees, and continuing education throughout career development.

Regardless of culture, when communication and cancer are studied directly and substantive materials can be made available to ordinary citizens, diverse implications arise for enhancing family relationships, medical education, doctoring effectively, and integrating often dichotomized relationships between primal human emotions, biomedicine, and social scientific investigations of the experience and communication of both illness and disease (e.g., see Beach, 2012).

Potential Obstacles and Possible Solutions

We have had to overcome a series of obstacles in the course of designing, implementing, and evaluating these intervention strategies during Phase I. We end this chapter by offering only a few potential problems and solutions we have devised to minimize possible negative impacts on data collection. One major set of decisions involved identifying and recruiting cancer patients, family members, and medical professionals. Assistance was requested and offered from local cancer centers that mailed/advertised flyers and forwarded emails to past and current cancer patients. And like any theatrical production, diverse social media were employed to inform lay and medical professional audience members about the live performances and DVD screenings. And questions were also raised about how many family members cancer patients might want to bring to experience *The Cancer Play*. Eventually it was determined that for the Phase I pilot study, each patient could ask a single family member to attend with them—though clearly others journey with them through cancer, and considerable potential exists for engaging entire families and friendship/work networks by viewing and discussing impacts of the play.

We emphasized that the play and script were drawn from natural phone conversations, involving actual family members, but that seemed to attract and not repel the majority of interested audience members. Yet it is important to describe to all parties that in this case study, the mother/wife/sister does progressively come to grips with and (over 13 months) succumb to terminal cancer. Though her actual death occurs hours following the last phone call, at times the family conversations lay bare end-of-life discussions that are highly emotional. Though these difficult moments are more than balanced with moments of humor, family support, and hope throughout the play, it is a potential delicacy that must be clarified at some point in the recruitment process and prior to the performances themselves. Further, we found it was important to make clear that the majority of cancer patients survive diagnosis and treatment, and thus that cancer is not tantamount to death and dying.

A related obstacle involved compensation for audience members' time and effort to attend and provide feedback about the play. In retrospect, we believe that offering $50 compensation was not adequate and have sought to remedy this potential problem by, as best possible, selecting centralized locations, arranging free parking, and even taking the DVD to actual locations where lay and professional persons routinely visit or gather for alternative occasions (e.g., hospitals, medical complexes, universities). So doing took at least some of the commuting time and mileage out of the equation. A possible strategy for future live performances and screenings would be to provide a larger compensation, especially for medical professionals such as nurses and physicians. Yet on the bright side, those that attended seemed very interested in the project and displayed considerable motivation to participate.

A final set of obstacles raised here involves two basic issues. First, what follow-up options exist for counseling and educating audience members about communication and cancer? As this Phase I pilot study did not involve a protocol for extending discussions and support—e.g., through local American Cancer Society networks and staff, or by providing resources for additional counseling or curricula—it became a notable topic and a need to highlight that is a potential and future goal of a project that will require additional funding and systematic efforts to insure quality care over time. And secondy, how were audience members to be informed that the DVD of *The Cancer Play* was not available for sale (e.g., through our prototype website, which was currently being developed) during our Phase I investigation? Product sales are not allowed during Phase I efforts, and so it became necessary to inform both individuals and organizations that the 'product/program' they were so impacted by, and interested in using for various purposes, would have to be purchased at a later date for any personal and/or institutional applications. In the end, these discussions promoted greater understandings of the roles and phases of basic research, and facilitated collaborations between academics, health professionals, and the lay public that continue to be pragmatic and useful as we conduct our Phase II investigations and seek to translate our findings in ways that improve communication throughout cancer journeys.

This project was supported by the National Cancer Institute (NCI) of the National Institutes of Health (NIH) through Grant CA144235.

Portions of this chapter were delivered by the senior author at the 25th Annual B. Aubrey Fisher Memorial Lecture, University of Utah, October 20, 2011.

References

American Cancer Society (2012). Global cancer facts & figures (2nd edition). http://www.cancer.org/Research/CancerFactsFigures/CancerFactsFigures/cancer-facts-figures-2012.

American Cancer Society (2011). Cancer facts & figures. (Available from) http://www.cancer.org/Research/CancerFactsFigures/GlobalCancerFactsFigures/global-facts-figures-2nd-ed.

Bauman, A. (2004). Commentary on the VERB Campaign—Perspectives on social marketing to encourage physical activity among youth. *Preventing Chronic Disease*, 1(3), 1–3.

Beach, W. (2009). *A Natural history of family cancer: Interactional resources for managing illness* (pp. 1–359). Cresskill: N J: Hampton Press.

Beach, W. A., Buller, M., Buller, D., Dozier, D., & Gutzmer, K. E. (2012a). The Conversations about Cancer (CAC) project: Assessing feasibility and audience impacts from viewing *The Cancer Play*. Submitted manuscript.

Beach, W.A., Buller, M., Dozier, D., Buller, D., & Gutzmer, K. (2012b). Edutainment and-family communication: An intervention strategy for triggering conversations about cancer. Submitted manuscript.

Beranowski, T., Perry, C. L., & Parcel, G. S. (1997). How individuals, environments, and health behavior interact: Social Cognitive Theory. *Health behavior and health education: Theory, research and practice* (pp. 165–184). San Francisco: Jossey-Bass.

Bernhardt, J. M. (2004). Communication at the core of effective public health. *American Journal of Public Health*, 94(12), 2051–53.

Brewer, N. T., & Rimer, B. K. (2008). Perspectives on health behavior: Theories that focus on individuals. In K. Glanz, B. K. Rimer, & K. Viswanath (Eds.), *Health behavior and health education: Theory research and practice* (4th ed., pp. 1–13). San Francisco: Jossey-Bass.

Grier, S., & Bryant, C. A. (2005). Social marketing in public health. *Annual Review of Public Health*, 26(9), 319–39.

Hall, J. G., Kosmoski, C., & Mastin, T. (2010). Tanning, skin cancer risk, and prevention: A content analysis of eight popular magazines that target female readers, 1997–2006. *Health Communication*, 25(1), 1–10.

Heaney, C. A., & Israel, B. A. (2002). Social networks and social support. In K. Glanz, B. K. Rimmer, & F. M. Lewis (Eds.), *Health behavior and health education: Theory research and practice* (3rd ed., pp. 185–209). San Francisco: Jossey-Bass.

House, J. S. (1981). *Work stress and social support*. Reading, MA: Addison-Wesley.

Jung, K.S., Park, S., Won, Y.J., Kong, H.J., Lee, J.Y., Seo, H.G., & Lee, J.S. (2012). Prediction of cancer incidence and mortality in Korea, 2012. *Cancer Research & Treatment*, 44 (1): 25–31.

Lockwood, A. S. (2002). Communication and cancer: Creating a play script from family conversations. (Unpublished master's thesis). San Diego State University, San Diego, CA.

Maibach, E. W., Abroms, L. C., & Marosits, M. (2007). Communication and marketing as tools to cultivate the public's health: A proposed "people and places" framework. *BMC Public Health*, 7(88), 1–15.

McGuire, W. J. (1985). Attitudes and attitude change. In G. Lindzey & E. Aronson (Eds.), *Handbook of social psychology* (3rd ed., pp. 233–346). New York: Random House.

Montaño, D. E., & Kasprzyk, D. (2002). The Theory of Reasoned Action and the Theory of Planned Behavior. In K. Glanz, B. Rimer, & F. M. Lewis (Eds.), *Health behavior and health education: Theory, research, and practice* (3rd ed., pp. 67–98). San Francisco: Jossey-Bass.

Moran, M., Beach, W., Dozier, D., Buller, M., Buller, D., & Gutzmer, K., et al., (2012). Focus group responses to *The Cancer Play*: Mechanisms underlying the effects of edutainment. Submitted manuscript.

National Cancer Institute. (2005). Theory at a glance: A guide to health promotion practice. National Cancer Institute. Retrieved from www.cancer.gov/cancertopics/cancerlibrary/theory.pdf

Prochaska, J. O., & DiClemente, C. C. (1983). Stages and processes of self-change of smoking: Toward an integrative model of change. *Journal of Consulting and Clinical Psychology, 51*(3), 390–95.

Rosenstock, I. M., Stretcher, V. J., & Becker, M. H. (1988). Social learning theory and the Health Belief Model. *Health Education Quarterly, 15*(2), 175–183.

Sallis, J. F., Cervero, R. B., Ascher, W., Henderson, K. A., Kraft, M. K., & Kerr, J. (2006). An ecological approach to creating active living communities. *Annual Review of Public Health, 27*, 297–322.

Chapter 7

Narrative-based Health Communication Interventions: Using Survivor Stories to Increase Breast Cancer Knowledge and Promote Mammography

Tess Thompson & Matthew W. Kreuter,
Washington University in St. Louis

Introduction: Narratives in Health Communication

In recent years, narratives have emerged as a powerful means of communicating health information. We define a narrative as "any cohesive and coherent story with an identifiable beginning, middle, and end that provides information about scene, characters, and conflict; raises unanswered questions or unresolved conflict; and provides resolution" (Hinyard & Kreuter, 2007, p. 778). Stories are, for most people, a natural and comfortable way of communicating in daily life, and they hold promise as an engaging way of communicating health information.

The term "narrative" can be used to encompass a wide variety of story-based communications. Schank and Berman (2002) identify five kinds of stories: *firsthand experiential stories, official stories, invented stories, secondhand stories,* and *culturally common stories.* Health behavior change communication most commonly employs firsthand experiential stories, invented stories, or some combination of the two. *Invented stories* are entirely fictional, although they often strive to depict realistic scenarios; *firsthand experiential stories* are the stories of real people (though they may be edited); and *composite stories* are made up of multiple authentic stories, often solicited through focus groups or other formative research, that are then fictionalized when combined into a single narrative.

The medium of a narrative may play a role in the audience's reaction (Green & Brock, 2002). Research into health narratives has examined a variety of types of stories in a variety of media, including authentic online written narratives (e.g., Betsch, Ulshöfer, Renkewitz, & Betsch, 2011), print narratives based on composite characters (e.g., Berkley-Patton et al., 2009), video narratives of composite stories delivered by actors (e.g., Ashton et al., 2010), fictional video narratives (e.g., Mazor et al., 2007), first-person video narratives edited by researchers (e.g., Houston et al., 2011a), and user-created, first-person video narratives (e.g., Chou, Hunt, Folkers, & Augustson, 2011).

In most narrative research, narratives have been compared to a control condition or non-narrative communication, not to a different version of narratives. Few studies have directly compared fictional, authentic, and composite narratives, or directly compared similar narratives conveyed in different media. Green and Brock (2002) found that labeling the same printed story "fiction" or "fact" did not affect persuasiveness, while Braverman (2008) found that audio stories containing health messages were more persuasive than the same stories in print form. In communication research more generally, visual media tend to shift an audience's attention to characteristics of the messenger (Wilson & Sherrell, 1993), accounting for more thoughts about (Sparks, Areni & Cox, 1998) and positive perceptions of the messenger (Pfau et al., 2000). In cases where a connection between the messenger and audience is especially important—for example, to build credibility and trust by showing racial or ethnic concordance between an audience and storyteller—presenting stories via visual media might have advantages over non-visual media (Wilson & Sherrell, 1993; Sparks, Areni, & Cox, 1998; Pfau et al., 2000).

Theoretical explanations for the effects of narrative vary, but three important, interconnected concepts recur in the literature: *identification* of the audience with the storytellers, *emotional response* to stories, and *engagement or transportation* into the story. The Transportation-Imagery Model (Green & Brock, 2002) suggests that narratives work by "transporting" the audience into a story through imagery and identification with the characters. Such transportation can lead to a heightened emotional response (McQueen & Kreuter, 2011), which may in turn enhance memory (Kensinger, 2008) and lead to behavior change (Hay et al., 2009). The Extended Elaboration Likelihood Model (Slater & Rouner, 2002) suggests that narrative effects may be due to a reduction in counter-arguing, and a 2007 National Cancer Institute Working Group analyzing narrative health communication proposed that narratives may help promote cancer screening by overcoming resistance to screening and by helping people process health information about screening and cancer (Kreuter et al., 2007).

Narratives are a social means of conveying information: They may provide social support through parasocial relationships between audience and storyteller, and they may be more likely than non-narrative information to be shared with others through "social proliferation" (Larkey & Hecht, 2012). Both the Precaution Adoption Process Model (Weinstein, 1998) and the Theory of Reasoned Action (Ajzen & Fishbein, 1980) emphasize the influence of other people on the adoption of new health behaviors, and stories can be one way to convey that influence. Social Cognitive Theory (Bandura, 1977) holds that behavioral modeling is an important means of learning a new behavior, and personal experience narratives can provide the audience with role models who demonstrate overcoming barriers to perform a health behavior.

Narratives may be underutilized in conveying information about cancer (Whitten, Nazione, Smith, & LaPlante, 2011). At the Health Communication Research Laboratory at Washington University in St. Louis, we have developed a program of research centered on the use of firsthand experiential video narratives about breast cancer. We have collected stories from breast cancer survivors, used them to develop a variety of health communication tools, and studied their immediate, short- and longer-term effects to better understand the mechanisms by which narrative communication works. In this chapter, we detail our experiences in order to help health professionals incorporate narratives into their work.

Case Study: Survivor Stories

Interview Process

We began by collecting stories about breast cancer from African American women in the St. Louis area. Thirty-six breast cancer survivors were recruited through breast cancer support groups and interviewed using a three-step biographic narrative interview process (Wengraf, 2001). After informed consent, women could receive optional cosmetic services on site before videotaping began (see Table 1 for an interview checklist). Women were first asked, "Tell me the story of your cancer" and given a chance to tell their story without a time limit or further prompting. After this initial telling of their story, women were then asked to elaborate on particular parts of the story, again in the form of a narrative. Finally, they were prompted to tell the story of their experience with other breast cancer-related topics that did not come up in their initial story (see Table 2). Interviews lasted 60–90 minutes, and all but two were conducted by an African-American woman who was a member of the study team. After the interviews, participants were debriefed by the interviewer (see Appendix A), and the study team conducted a group debriefing (see Appendix B).

Table 1. Step-by-Step Instructions for Storytelling Sessions

Activity	Minutes
1. Staff posts "Taping in Progress" sign on door and prepares forms for storyteller	10
2. Storyteller arrives and project team greets her	10
3. Staff administers forms: informed consent, privacy practices, tax forms	15–20
4. Staff reminds storyteller that incentive check will be mailed	15–20
5. Storyteller receives cosmetic services, if scheduled for them	10–20
6. Staff reminds everyone to turn cell phones off before taping	NA
7. Interviewer conducts interview, staff take notes using Story Notes sheet	60–90
8. Interviewer debriefs storyteller	5–10
9. Staff has storyteller sign video/audio/photo release form	5
10. If time allows between interviews, conduct staff debriefing	15–30

Table 2. Prompts to Elicit Additional Details during Biographical Interviews

Breast cancer topic	Purpose	Prompt
Pre-diagnosis context	To set the stage for survivor's pre-diagnosis awareness, attitude, feelings, and thoughts about breast cancer in general and for African American women in particular. To establish how their pre-diagnosis knowledge and awareness was formed.	I want you to think back to the time before you were diagnosed with breast cancer. Tell me what you thought about breast cancer (among African American women).
Testing process	To recount survivor's experience with the testing process and how her feelings, fears, and worries affected her decision to continue with further tests.	There is a long testing process before someone is diagnosed with cancer. Can you tell me about your experience, if you told anyone, what you were feeling, and how the uncertainty affected you?

Breast cancer topic	Purpose	Prompt
Diagnosis event	To acknowledge the feelings and emotions that many women encounter when told of a breast cancer diagnosis. To expose and correct misconceptions regarding cancer diagnosis.	Women all respond differently to hearing that they have breast cancer. Remembering the day and time you were told you had breast cancer, what was your first reaction? What did the diagnosis of breast cancer mean to you?
Self-reflection, coming to terms	To recount the survivor's decision to receive medical treatment for breast cancer. To detail the psychological, intellectual, spiritual, and emotional processes that women go through in taking action against breast cancer.	Was there a point where you said, "I'm going to fight this"? Who or what influenced your decision? Was there ever a point where you were no longer afraid of the breast cancer?
Treatment options	To recount the survivor's awareness, attitudes, feelings, and thoughts about breast cancer treatment prior to, during, and after therapy. Show how women successfully dealt with common side effects. Expose treatment myths. Demystify the health care system.	There are sometimes many treatment options given to a woman diagnosed with breast cancer. How did you decide what treatment option was the best for you? What would typically occur during a treatment session?
Coping, strategies, difficulties	To allow the survivor to relate how she was able to handle difficulties related to a breast cancer diagnosis.	Thinking about your entire experience with breast cancer, what was the most difficult part for you to handle? How did you deal with this problem?
Lives now	To allow story to come full circle and let survivors talk about awareness, attitudes, feelings, and thoughts after diagnosis and treatment.	It has been ____(mo/yrs) since you were diagnosed with breast cancer. How is your life different now than before you were diagnosed?
Final thoughts: advice for others and reflections	To end the narratives on a positive note. To provide final reflections on cancer and African American women. To summarize social, cultural, and structural obstacles to getting tested. To advance positive directions that the African American community can take in dealing with breast cancer and women.	Considering what you have learned from your experience with breast cancer, what would you want to say to African American women regarding the need for early screening and treatment of breast cancer?

We went into the process with an open mind about the kinds of stories we wanted to collect, and the broad questions of the interview protocol allowed important themes not identified a priori to emerge from the interviews. For example, we did not anticipate the stigma related to talking about cancer described by many of the participants. Our process reflects Larkey and Hecht's (2010) idea of a "culture-centric" approach to health promotion in that we drew out emic (within group) knowledge and allowed our storytellers to create, and not just illustrate, health messages.

Message Testing

The survivor interviews yielded 49 hours of recordings that were divided by the study team into 1,624 discrete story units (defined as a continuous segment of narrative that addressed a particular breast cancer topic). For each story unit, two independent coders identified the main message, rated attributes of narrative quality (emotion, dramatic tension, character development, self-disclosure, cultural appropriateness, and imagery-evoking language), and evaluated health message strength (message repetition, message centrality, explicit recommendation, behavior modeling, incentives, and overcoming obstacles).

Our initial testing (Kreuter et al., 2008) explored how viewer characteristics and story attributes affected viewers' engagement with the videos, their understanding of key cancer messages, and having positive thoughts about the stories. A community-based convenience sample of 200 African American women ages 40 and older participated in a study in which they came aboard the Neighborhood Voice mobile research facility (Alcaraz et al., 2011) and viewed three video clips. A total of 300 story clips were viewed by participants, with each clip viewed by two different women. This initial research (Kreuter et al., 2008) showed that characteristics related to the *viewers* were more important than characteristics of the stories in determining reactions to the stories. The most important predictor of being engaged in a story and having positive thoughts about it was whether the viewer liked the woman in the video and saw the woman as similar to herself. Measures of similarity and liking, combined to form the construct of "identification with a character," are useful in helping identify appropriate stories and storytellers during the audience research stage of an intervention. (For more details about the items used to measure these constructs, see Kreuter et al., 2008 and McQueen & Kreuter, 2010.)

Narrative vs. Informational Videos

The videotaped interviews were used to create a narrative DVD, *Living Proof,* that included 57 clips from 29 survivors to create a *collective narrative* that explored three of the themes that emerged from the interviews—risk of breast cancer, communication about breast cancer, and screening mammography. Based on *Living Proof,* we created a second DVD called *Facts for Life* that contained equivalent content about breast cancer but in an informational (not narrative) form, and presented by an African American female narrator (not a breast cancer survivor). Initial pilot testing among 150 African American women (Kreuter et al., 2010) found that both DVDs received similar ratings for production quality and ease of understanding.

The DVDs were evaluated in a trial (Kreuter et al., 2010) in which 489 African American women were invited onto the Neighborhood Voice van and randomized to watch either *Living Proof* or *Facts for Life*. Women were interviewed at baseline (pre-DVD), immediately post-DVD, 3 months later, and 6 months later. Participants liked the narrative video better and were more likely to remember the information from it. Among women with less than a high school education, viewing the narrative DVD was associated with higher rates of mammography at 6-month follow-up. There was also a trend towards significance among women who did not have a family member or close friend with breast cancer, which suggests that narratives may provide a substitute for first-hand experience.

Follow-up studies analyzed women's emotional responses to the two DVDs. A structural equation analysis (McQueen, Kreuter, Kalesan, & Alcaraz, 2011) found that women who saw the narrative video had stronger emotional reactions, increased engagement, and stronger identification with the source of the health messages than did women who watched the non-narrative video. In another study (Bollinger & Kreuter, 2012), fifty-nine African American women were given hand-held audience response devices to indicate their emotional reactions while watching one of the videos. Women who watched the narrative video were more likely to have strong emotional reactions to contextual details (e.g., about faith or family) than were women who saw the non-narrative video, but these emotional reactions did not detract from recall of health information. Overall, the women who saw the narrative video felt more attentive, proud, and inspired, and less upset. A separate analysis (Yoo, Kreuter, Lai, & Qu, in press) showed that sadness in particular enhanced the persuasive process. Taken together, these results show the important role emotion plays in the processing of narrative health information and suggest that emotional response should be considered in the development and selection of stories.

Tablet Applications

If narratives can help convey health information to a general screening population, they may also be effective at reaching women who have been recently diagnosed with breast cancer. A collection of our breast cancer survivor stories was used to create a tablet computer (PC) video archive to help newly diagnosed African American breast cancer patients cope with the challenges of treatment and follow-up care. A randomized controlled trial of 220 women newly diagnosed with breast cancer is currently underway to see if access to survivor stories affects quality of life, adherence to treatment, and use of surveillance mammography. Patients assigned to the intervention arm of the trial have access to a tablet computer containing a searchable archive of over 200 1–3 minute videotaped survivor stories about a dozen topics related to cancer treatment and quality of life. Patients have the tablet computer for two weeks after enrollment in the study, and again at 6 and 12 months; patients in the control arm receive usual care.

An adapted version of the tablet computer program is now also available to the general public and patients everywhere through a free application for the iPad and iPhone. The application, called *Living Proof* after the original DVD, includes over 200 video stories that are searchable either by storyteller age at diagnosis or by 18 breast cancer topics, including treatment decisions, side effects, reconstruction, and quality of life.

Lessons about Using Narratives

Our research into personal health narratives has taught us several important lessons about the use of first-person experiential stories in health communication:

- *Narratives may be especially beneficial for certain groups.* Our research found that viewing a narrative DVD increased mammography among women with less than a high school education, with a trend toward significance among women who did not have a close relationship with a cancer survivor, but mammography did not increase significantly among women in general. One advantage of stories for low education popula-

tions may be related to literacy and the increased accessibility of both stories (vs. nonnarrative information) and video (vs. print materials). For people without a direct personal connection to breast cancer, stories may serve as a substitute for first-hand experience. Additional research is needed to determine the particular audiences that may find narratives most effective.
- *Identification matters.* Our research shows that narratives worked best when viewers liked the storytellers and saw them as similar to themselves. This suggests that stories should be carefully targeted to specific groups, although further research is needed to identify specific characteristics that might be most important to match upon (e.g., demographic characteristics such race, age, sex, SES, or psychological characteristics such as attitudes or values).
- *Emotion and context matter.* Video narratives allow viewers to become emotionally engaged with health messages by presenting real stories from real people. Although it may be tempting to create streamlined stories that illustrate key health messages without "extraneous" details, doing so may reduce the audience's emotional engagement. Details unrelated to core health messages may nonetheless draw the audience in and help them connect to storytellers, thus making the audience more receptive to the health messages conveyed.
- *A culture-centric approach adds authenticity to the communication development process.* Even well-informed communication developers may not anticipate all the information that they will learn during the process of gathering real stories from real people. By using story elicitation methods that did not constrain story topics, we allowed key cancer-related themes to emerge from stories of African American cancer survivors. We also involved members of the target audience in every step of the process of developing the DVDs and the tablet databases. Such formative research and pilot testing are crucial for creating culturally relevant tools.

Important Considerations When Using Narratives

Although narrative communication can be powerful, it has drawbacks as well (Kreuter et al., 2007). When compared to non-narrative methods, authentic first-person narratives can be time-consuming and expensive to collect, which makes appropriate audience targeting crucial. Developers of narrative-based communication have less control over the content of messages than do people who create their own materials, and because storytellers may misunderstand or mis-remember health information, narratives must be carefully fact-checked for medical accuracy. Moreover, because medical knowledge and treatments evolve over time, if stories will be in use over a long period they should be re-checked periodically to ensure they reflect the current base of evidence. The selection of stories also requires careful consideration. It may be tempting to save time and money by collecting only a few stories, but limiting a project to a handful of stories may have implications for representativeness. Steiner (2007) contends that when using only one or a few stories, it can be helpful to explicitly locate a story in the "distribution" of stories (that is, explain whether the story represents a typical experience or an important outlier).

Care must also be taken to use stories in an ethical manner (Kreuter et al., 2007). When using authentic first person narratives, it is important to obtain consent from storytellers and convey clearly how stories will be edited and used, especially in the creation of composite narratives. It is important to create composite stories that are culturally sensitive and nonstigmatizing. For all narratives, one should exercise caution when removing a story from its social context. Health professionals must also consider the structural context in which people receive narrative messages and ensure that the environment supports the behavior changes encouraged by the narratives (Hinyard & Kreuter, 2007).

Although narratives may initially be more difficult to collect than non-narrative information, once obtained they may be "packaged" in different ways. Video stories can be used to create DVDs, web sites, tablet or mobile phone applications, or searchable online libraries, or they can be transformed into other media, such as brochures or articles. Further research is needed, however to determine the most appropriate media to convey narratives in various contexts and to various audiences.

We are only beginning to understand the power of narratives in health communication. Our research shows, however, that first-person experiential narratives hold great promise for engaging people emotionally, promoting positive health behaviors, and improving health in patients, families, and communities.

Appendix A
Debriefing Statement for Breast Cancer Survivors and Other Storytellers

Thank you for sharing your breast cancer experience with me. Before you leave, I would like to take the opportunity to review your storytelling session. You were first given the opportunity to tell your story uninterrupted and un-coached. This was followed by a series of questions that helped you elaborate on certain parts of your story that we felt might be especially important for women to hear. What did you like and dislike about this process? What, if anything, would you say was the best part of today's conversation? What, if anything, would you say was the worst part? Was there anything the project team including myself could have done differently to make your experience better?

Breast cancer and treatment for breast cancer is a complex subject, and we want to be sure you have the most up-to-date and accurate information. If the health professionals on our team feel there is new information you would benefit from, we will pass that information along to you.

Finally, for some women, sharing their story as a breast cancer survivor can cause them to feel emotionally or psychologically upset. This is normal, and may include feelings of sadness, anger, fear, memories, or distressful thoughts about previous treatment for cancer. If these symptoms or other symptoms occur and persist and you feel your participation in this project has caused you distress, please contact the study's Principal Investigator at [phone number] or the project manager at [phone number]. If needed, they can help refer you to the clinical services of a psychologist or psychiatrist. Before you leave, you will be given a copy of these emotional responses and the phone numbers of the study team members to call if the symptoms become troublesome.

Do you have any questions about your experience today? It has been wonderful talking with you and again I'd like to extend my appreciation and the appreciation of the entire team to you for your participation in this project.

Appendix B
The Storytelling Project's Interview Debriefing Tool

➤ This debriefing tool enables the interviewer to process the interactions with the storytellers. This is to be a cooperative effort between the interviewer and appropriate study team members involved in the interviewing process.

➤ Try to do the debriefing in the same room in which the interview took place (Wengraf, 2001, pp. 142–144). If this is not possible, at least conduct the debriefing at the end of the day in order to ensure a comprehensive recollection of events, emotions, and/or concerns.

Interview Information:

Site:
Interviewer:
Start Time:
Finish Time:
Team Members Present During Interview:

➤ Write down everything that you can remember about the conversation (Wengraf, 2001, pp. 142–144) regarding:

1. **Feelings:**

Interviewer's feelings:
Storyteller's feelings:

2. **Interview Process:**
3. **Relevant Storyteller Behavioral Characteristics (e.g., gestures):**
4. **Content (areas that contained a great deal of information):**

	Detailed Information on Topic (√)	Other Comments
Pre-Screening		
Finding a Lump		
Testing for Breast Cancer		
Diagnosis Event		
Coming to Terms		
Treatment Issues		
Relationships		
Dealing with the Health Care System		
Lives Now		
Advice for Others		
Other Topics		

5. Overall Impressions of the Conversation:

6. Interviewer Techniques:

7. Technical Problems:

8. Videography Notes:

9. Session's Procedural Issues:

Recommended Readings

Ashton, C. M., Houston, T. K., Williams, J. H., Larkin, D., Trobaugh, J., Crenshaw, K., & Wray, N. P. (2010). A stories-based interactive DVD intended to help people with hypertension achieve blood pressure control through improved communication with their doctors. *Patient Education and Counseling, 79*(2), 245–250.

Green, M.C., & Brock, T.C. (2002). Transportation-imagery model of narrative persuasion. In M. C. Green, J. J. Strange & T. C. Brock (Eds.), *Narrative impact: Social and cognitive foundations* (pp. 315–341).

Hinyard, L.J., & Kreuter, M.W. (2007). Using narrative communication as a tool for health behavior change: A conceptual, theoretical, and empirical overview. *Health Education & Behavior, 34*(5), 777–792.

Houston, T.K., Cherrington, A., Coley, H.L., Robinson, K.M., Trobaugh, J.A., Williams, J.H., & Allison, J.J. (2011b). The art and science of patient storytelling—harnessing narrative communication for behavioral interventions: The ACCE project. *Journal of Health Communication, 16*(7), 686–697.

Kreuter, M.W., Holmes, K., Hinyard, L.J., Houston, T., Woolley, S., Green, M.C., & Erwin, D.O. (2007). Narrative communication in cancer prevention and control: A framework to guide research and application. *Annals of Behavioral Medicine, 33*(3), 221–235.

Larkey, L.K., & Hecht, M. (2010). A model of effects of narrative as culture-centric health promotion. *Journal of Health Communication, 15*(2), 114–135.

Wengraf, T. (2001). *Qualitative research interviewing: Semi-structured, biographical and narrative methods.* Thousand Oaks, CA: Sage Publications.

References

Alcaraz, K.I., Weaver, N.L., Andresen, E.M., Christopher, K., & Kreuter, M.W. (2011). The neighborhood voice: Evaluating a mobile research vehicle for recruiting African Americans to participate in cancer control studies. *Evaluation & the Health Professions, 34(3),* 336–348.

Ashton, C.M., Houston, T.K., Williams, J.H., Larkin, D., Trobaugh, J., Crenshaw, K., & Wray, N.P. (2010). A stories-based interactive DVD intended to help people with hypertension achieve blood pressure control through improved communication with their doctors. *Patient Education and Counseling, 79*(2), 245–250.

Azjen, I., & Fishbein, M. (1980). *Understanding attitudes and predicting social behavior.* Englewood Cliffs, NJ: Prentice Hall.

Bandura, A. (1977). Self-efficacy: Toward a unifying theory of behavior change. *Psychology Review, 84*(2), 191–215.

Berkley-Patton, J., Goggin, K., Liston, R., Bradley-Ewing, A., & Neville, S. (2009). Adapting effective narrative-based HIV-prevention interventions to increase minorities' engagement in HIV/AIDS services. *Health Communication, 24*(3), 199–209.

Betsch, C., Ulshofer, C., Renkewitz, F., & Betsch, T. (2011). The influence of narrative v. statistical information on perceiving vaccination risks. *Medical Decision Making, 31*(5), 742–753.

Bollinger, S., & Kreuter, M.W. (2012). Real-time moment-to-moment emotional responses to narrative and informational breast cancer videos in African American women. *Health Education Research, 27*(3), 537–543.

Braverman, J. (2008). Testimonials versus informational persuasive messages: The moderating effect of delivery mode and personal involvement. *Communication Research, 35*(5):666–694.

Chou, W.Y., Hunt, Y., Folkers, A., & Augustson, E. (2011). Cancer survivorship in the age of YouTube and social media: A narrative analysis. *Journal of Medical Internet Research, 13*(1): e7.

Green, M.C., & Brock, T.C. (2002). Transportation-imagery model of narrative persuasion. In M. C. Green, J. J. Strange & T. C. Brock (Eds.), *Narrative impact: Social and cognitive foundations* (pp. 315–341).

Hay, J., Harris, J.N., Waters, E.A., Clayton, M.F., Ellington, L., Abernethy, A.D., & Prayor-Patterson, H. (2009). Personal communication in primary and secondary cancer prevention: Evolving discussions, emerging challenges. *Journal of Health Communication, 14 Suppl 1,* 18–29.

Hinyard, L.J., & Kreuter, M.W. (2007). Using narrative communication as a tool for health behavior change: A conceptual, theoretical, and empirical overview. *Health Education & Behavior, 34*(5), 777–792.

Houston, T.K., Allison, J.J., Sussman, M., Horn, W., Holt, C.L., Trobaugh, J., & Hullett, S. (2011a). Culturally appropriate storytelling to improve blood pressure: A randomized trial. *Annals of Internal Medicine, 154*(2), 77–84.

Houston, T.K., Cherrington, A., Coley, H.L., Robinson, K.M., Trobaugh, J.A., Williams, J.H., & Allison, J.J. (2011b). The art and science of patient storytelling-harnessing narrative communication for behavioral interventions: The ACCE project. *Journal of Health Communication, 16*(7), 686–697.

Kensinger, E. (2008). *Emotional memory across the adult lifespan.* London: Psychology Press.

Kreuter, M.W., Buskirk, T.D., Holmes, K., Clark, E.M., Robinson, L., Si, X., & Mathews, K. (2008). What makes cancer survivor stories work? An empirical study among African American women. *Journal of Cancer Survivorship: Research and Practice, 2*(1), 33–44.

Kreuter, M.W., Holmes, K., Alcaraz, K., Kalesan, B., Rath, S., Richert, M., & Clark, E.M. (2010). Comparing narrative and informational videos to increase mammography in low-income African American women. *Patient Education and Counseling, 81 Suppl,* S6–14.

Kreuter, M.W., Holmes, K., Hinyard, L.J., Houston, T., Woolley, S., Green, M.C., & Erwin, D.O. (2007). Narrative communication in cancer prevention and control: A framework to guide research and application. *Annals of Behavioral Medicine, 33*(3), 221–235.

Larkey, L.K., & Hecht, M. (2010). A model of effects of narrative as culture-centric health promotion. *Journal of Health Communication, 15*(2), 114–135.

Mazor, K.M., Baril, J., Dugan, E., Spencer, F., Burgwinkle, P., & Gurwitz, J.H. (2007). Patient education about anticoagulant medication: Is narrative evidence or statistical evidence more effective? *Patient Education and Counseling, 69*(1–3), 145–157.

McQueen, A., & Kreuter, M.W. (2010). Women's cognitive and affective reactions to breast cancer survivor stories: A structural equation analysis. *Patient Education and Counseling, 81 Suppl 1,* S15–S21.

McQueen, A., Kreuter, M.W., Kalesan, B., & Alcaraz, K.I. (2011). Understanding narrative effects: The impact of breast cancer survivor stories on message processing, attitudes, and beliefs among African American women. *Health Psychology, 30*(6), 674–682.

Pfau M., Holbert R., Zubric S., Pasha N., & Lin, W. (2000). Role and influence of communication modality in the process of resistance to persuasion. *Media Psychology,* 2:1–33.

Schank, R.C., & Berman, T.R. (2002). The pervasive role of stories in knowledge and action. In M.C. Green, J.J. Strange & T.C. Brock (Eds.), *Narrative impact: Social and cognitive foundations* (pp. 287–313).

Slater, M.D., & Rouner, D. (2002). Entertainment-education and elaboration likelihood: Understanding the processing of narrative persuasion. *Communication Theory, 12*(2), 173–191.

Sparks, J., Areni, C., & Cox, K. (1998). An investigation of the effects of language style and communication modality on persuasion. *Communication Monographs, 65:*108–25.

Steiner, J.F. (2007). Using stories to disseminate research: The attributes of representative stories. *Journal of General Internal Medicine, 22*(11), 1603–1607.

Weinstein, N. (1988). The precaution adoption process. *Health Psychology, 7*(4), 355–386.

Wengraf, T. (2001). *Qualitative research interviewing: Semi-structured, biographical and narrative methods.* Thousand Oaks, CA: Sage Publications.

Whitten, P., Nazione, S., Smith, S., & LaPlante, C. (2011). An examination into audience targeting and the use of storytelling or statistical evidence on breast cancer websites. *Patient Education and Counseling, 85*(2), e59–64.

Wilson, E., & Sherrell, D. (1993). Source effects in communication and persuasion research: A meta-analysis of effect size. *Journal of the Academy of Marketing Science, 21:*101–12.

Wise, M., Han, J.Y., Shaw, B., McTavish, F., & Gustafson, D.H. (2008). Effects of using online narrative and didactic information on healthcare participation for breast cancer patients. *Patient Education and Counseling, 70*(3), 348–356.

Yoo, J.H., Kreuter, M.W., Lai, C., & Qu, J. (in press) Understanding narrative effects: The role of discrete negative emotions on message processing and attitudes among low-income African American women. *Health Communication,* in press.

Chapter 8

Drama as a Rhetorical Health Communication Strategy

Anat Gesser-Edelsburg
University of Haifa

Introduction

Sociologists and social psychologists often use drama as a metaphor to demonstrate how communication-persuasion systems resemble acting. In a reverse metaphor, the art of drama can be seen as a controlled persuasion system that directs spectators' reactions. In this paradigm, theater, film and television writers function as rhetorical engineers (Shoham, 1989; Unger, 1991), whose job is to use each respective medium to convey health, cultural or political messages. Drama represents reality through the tools of the artistic medium at its disposal. The viewer, whose awareness is simultaneously inside and outside the fictional world, can be influenced by the conceptual perspective presented to him and draw conclusions about his own life. By creating a fictional boundary that protects the viewer, drama has the power to elucidate sensitive social issues in a unique and engaging way that reduces audience resistance, stimulates and destabilizes accepted social perceptions. Theater is a powerful dramatic medium because it can reach many people while maintaining intimacy and immediacy between the audience and the actor.

This chapter will present the rhetorical features that comprise the dramatic mechanism, and illustrate them through case studies of Israeli plays that raise diverse sensitive health subjects in Israel's multicultural society, such as violence against women, obesity, novice teen drivers, and illegal drug use. At the outset, this chapter will present the characteristics of drama construction from the fields of drama and rhetorical persuasion. Then, it will zoom in on a model that I label "the rhetorical change model in drama," that has the potential to become an influential tool.

Drama as the Art of Persuasion

This chapter will present the principles of drama as an instrument of influence on diverse issues and subjects. Drama as a health intervention tool is no different from other intervention dramas dealing with other social issues. Therefore the general principles explained in this chapter can be applied to the subject of public health promotion.

The Accepted Values

To understand drama as a communicative tool of intervention we must first understand the rhetorical mechanism that drives the processes of spectator influence and persuasion. Drama combines the art of rhetoric with argumentation, form with content, to achieve maximum communicative effect. In that respect drama draws its strength from the ancient Greek tradition of rhetoric, which is essentially persuasive communication. This art offered its adherents practical skills of articulate expression and theoretical insight in order to enhance communication with their audience. The sophists (the first rhetoricians) and their successors adopted as their starting point identification with their audience. Ancient rhetoricians advise orators to identify with the audience, especially when they intend to change the audience's opinions. To that end the speaker must be familiar with the audience's prevailing opinions and know how to address them.

In his book *Rhetoric*, Aristotle discusses the main component of the art of persuasion: "the maxims." He says that the speaker must address the audience's common sense not only logically but also anthropologically, by speaking to the community's accepted values, beliefs and symbols (Aristotle, 2002). Social psychologists, sociologists, media and theater practitioners have followed the principles of rhetoric and held the audience's prevailing opinions at a given time paramount in the persuasion process. The assumption is that the act of persuasion cannot occur unless the speaker addresses the listener's cultural, normative and linguistic terms of reference. Over the years, theoreticians have given the "maxims" different names, such as "commonplaces" (Billig, 1996), "social norms" (Ajzen & Fishbein, 1980; Mollen, Rimal, & Lapinski, 2010; Rimal & Real, 2005) and others; but they all refer to the same phenomenon. Like rhetoric, an effective drama speaks to the audience's prevailing opinions while addressing human subjects. Drama as rhetoric is based on communication with the audience and cannot materialize if the fictional world it represents is disengaged from the audience's emotional mentality, symbols and conventions.

Drama as rhetoric is often required to criticize and refute existing prevailing opinions. One obstacle towards creating drama that conforms to the audience's values is that the audience is often at varying stages of receptiveness for change. Addressing one subgroup in a drama scenario might miss another subgroup that is at a different stage of readiness. Another difficulty is that part of the audience might hold such deep-seated social values that it might misunderstand the play's intended message. Instead of receiving the oppositional values the playwright tries to sneak into the drama, the audience might hear only the old values it held. An example of this is Neil LaBute's play "Fat Pig," on the subject of the social image of overweight people. The play is about Tom, who falls in love with Helen, a "well-endowed" woman, and his ability to set aside all the cruelty and sarcasm of his colleagues about his relationship with an overweight woman. According to an interview with LaBute, his intention was to write a play that would be perceived by spectators as a satire on modern society and its beauty ideal. The play was performed in Israel in 2006. A study that examined whether "Fat Pig" succeeded in steering spectators to view fat people in society more positively, and whether it empowered overweight women, found it had a "boomerang effect" (Sherif & Hovland, 1961), meaning that the play had unintended consequences: the audience understood the exact opposite of the playwright's intention. Throughout the play, Tom is reluctant to be seen in public with his girlfriend Helen. At the end of the play the audience's conservative values are reaffirmed when Tom leaves Helen. The fact that the "normative" Tom leaves an overweight woman is what causes the boomerang effect; his action affirms the Western values that say overweight people are "defective" and it is they who must change and not society's values. Some of the female viewers who considered themselves overweight also felt that watching the play might encourage eating disorders (Gesser-Edelsburg & Endevelt, 2011).

The Rhetoric of Aesthetics

In his book *L'Empire rhétorique: Rhétorique et argumentation* Perelman (1977) indicates several principles of a philosophy that can be projected onto the world of drama. He argues that the test of the effectiveness of a philosophical argument is that it is persuasive, and a necessary condition for that is that it sounds real to its listeners. Likewise, drama can change positions and social conventions only when it manages to be "real" for its spectators. Any drama that strives for social change must make "fiction" (the argument or its future hypothesis) authentic in the present for its viewers. Making arguments persuasive depends on the rhetorician's ability to conjure the object up through the use of attractive visual and verbal means of repetition, symbolism, accumulation of details and synthesis. Rhetoric in drama is not limited to the literal text but also based on the narrative-aesthetic side namely: visual (lighting, pictures, colors, camera movement, graphics) and auditory (music, sound, etc.) elements that give it its artistic depth. Accordingly, the stage, cinematic or television design must be integrative to the work as a whole in order to reinforce its persuasive effect. Dramatists use aesthetics to activate the viewers' feelings of pleasure and emotional stimulation.

Aesthetic depth might pose an obstacle to the creation of persuasive drama when dramatists choose to present a critical text by way of constructing a seductive and beautiful aesthetic that draws the viewer in. In this case, instead of responding to the criticism aimed at him, the spectator may be seduced by the aesthetic stimulants and try to emulate them. One example of that is taking a violent subject and wrapping it with a beautiful and perfect aesthetic that relies on emotive music, strong and warm lighting, beautiful set design and sexy actors. All of those might cause the viewer to silence his conscience and drown in an aesthetic of beautiful violence.[1] Ultimately, instead of serving the rhetorical idea, there is a risk the drama's aesthetics will work against it.

The Spectator as Ghostwriter

The creation of the persuasion effect depends to a large extent on the way the audience decodes the text. Modern literary scholars, influenced by the field of rhetoric, view the text as a multilayered and multitiered system that guides its audience to reconstruct the dramatic work (Booth, 1961; Ingarden, 1973). The connection between the text and its reader is formed through empty spaces and negations, gaps that the reader must fill in for himself and which force him to undergo a renewed process of formulating a position (Iser, 1974). The art of theater is also composed of different layers of meaning constructed by the audience (Kaynar, 1993; Kuznicka, 1989; Shoham, 1989). In fact, the current concept of theater sees the viewer

---

1 See for example Stanley Kubrick's film *A Clockwork Orange* (Eder, 2008).

as an active partner who becomes a sort of ghost playwright/screenwriter of the dramatic work. However, since drama is complex and multilayered, the audience often responds differently from what the writers intended (Brown & Singhal, 1990). It can be stated that making the viewer an active participant in the drama can fail if the empty spaces the dramatist leaves to the viewer's imagination create a gap between the viewer and the writer's intention. The more empty spaces there are in the work the more likely the audience will fill them in ways that lead to a different interpretation than the dramatist intended.

The Mechanism of the Experience of Viewing Drama: Obstacles and Challenges

This part of the chapter presents some of the dominant rhetorical elements that direct the viewing experience: the mythical core, identification, conflict and illustration. This chapter attempts to investigate and understand the rhetorical mechanism that characterizes each element, while pointing out obstacles and challenges that should be taken into account when using drama as an intervention tool on health issues. Building the rhetorical mechanism of a drama as a tool of intervention is far more challenging than building a drama merely for "entertainment," since it also has to include a learning/educational process. The former kind of drama requires the dramatist to engineer the integration of the two components of pleasure and learning, which often pull in opposite directions. The following section will address a number of elements of the experience of viewing drama and show how to use them as tools of intervention.

The Mythical Layer

According to Gilula (1985), Freud used Sophocles' drama *Oedipus Rex* to illustrate people's deep emotional processes. Freud asked why the drama *Oedipus Rex* has attracted so many viewers since ancient times. His answer was that it is because the drama gives freedom to the unconscious, to the inner impulses hidden in the viewer's psyche (the id), impulses that conflict with social norms and values (super ego) and therefore cause anxiety. The drama allows the spectator to access emotional strata he cannot or does not want to confront, and provides an artistic cover under which he can get in touch with them and experience them, like in a fantasy or a dream (Gilula, 1985). Eli Rozik calls that primeval material the "mythical layer" of the plot

(Rozik, 1992). I will further argue that the dramatic tool enables the viewers to raise an array of questions on various subjects, questions we usually avoid.

Drama allows us to touch upon anxiety-provoking issues that are on the threshold of consciousness such as the desire to take drugs, the tendency to mix violence with sexuality, and fears and anxieties related to stigmatized diseases. Plays designed to create change might fail due to two reasons. The first is the tendency to avoid engaging deeply with the mythical layer because of the difficulty of addressing it, and resorting to superficial, unambiguous solutions, while failing to confront the viewers with their fears. The second problem is that certain dramas might arouse the mythic element too powerfully to provide tools to reduce the anxiety. In such cases the individual might choose maladaptive responses or defense mechanisms. The results would be either a failure to change or a boomerang effect.

Many dramas produced by organizations and establishments go no further than "do" and "don't" messages, without addressing the viewers' complexity and fears, thereby neutralizing the mythic core. A study of plays about drugs shown to teenagers in Israel in 2001–2002 revealed the flaws of such plays. Most of the plays chose to punish the addicted protagonist with hospitalization or death without addressing the doubts and fears that consume teenagers about drugs, such as why they are seductive, how to deal with peer pressure, what drugs do for adolescents and so on. The result was moralistic drama with a monolithic voice (Gesser-Edelsburg, Guttman, & Israelashvili, 2006; Guttman, Gesser-Edelsburg, & Israelashvili, 2008). The challenge facing dramatists is how to build a drama to serve the interventionist intentions of the organizations and establishments in the desired direction without neutralizing the mythical layer at the basis of the dramatic experience.

The Identification Element

There are various ways in which identification has been conceived in the literature. In the psychological literature some conceive identification as an imaginative event in which people experience things through someone else's point of view (Cohen, 2001). Both in the media and drama literature some authors propose that in the process of identifying with characters in a drama, viewers may feel empathy for the character or see characters as a reflection of oneself (Affron, 1991; Liebes, 1996; Livingstone, 1998). According to Kincaid (2002), identification is a "motivational force that induces members of the audience to re-conceptualize the central problem depicted in the drama and to resolve it in a similar manner in their own lives." Thomas J. Schaff discusses the different levels of awareness of the audience and characters in Shakespearian plays. He concludes that audiences feel a special affinity to characters who share their own level of awareness, not those whose level of awareness is higher than theirs, nor those whose level of awareness is lower than theirs, but those whose level of awareness is equal to their own (Schaff, 1976–77).

Drama and edutainment theorists note that the strength of drama and one of its most potent persuasive features is its ability to elicit emotional involvement with characters (Bailin, 1994; Cohen, 2001; Kincaid, 2002; Schoenmakers, 1992; Slater & Rouner, 2002; Sood, 2002). Bentley (1972) argues that there might be protected involvement where the viewer undergoes an emotional experience but remains safe in his seat. Studies (Brown, Basil, & Bocarnea, 2003; Cohen, 2001) indicate there is another kind of involvement in drama that creates a meaningful process of change in the spectator and demands him to take a clear emotional stand. In this case, the spectator moves through a range of emotions from empathy and identification to anger and rage. Rather than remaining in a voyeuristic or even alienated relation to the events on the stage, the spectator is exposed to changes of his awareness (Gesser Edelsburg, 2002; Gesser Edelsburg & Singhal, 2013). The level of the viewer's involvement in the drama is also influenced by the structure of the various genres: tragedy, comedy, tragicomedy, farce or melodrama (Bentley, 1972).

One of the main drama theoreticians who criticized the social use of the identification mechanism is Brecht. He did not assail the identification element per se but criticized the way it is used in bourgeois dramas in order to examine and explore situations to which people react as "obvious and automatic" (Brecht, 2003). The Brechtian stage wishes to shatter the viewer's narcissistic identification and ironicize the story by cutting or splitting it into gestures and making it surprising (Brecht, 2003). Feminist theories argue that the viewer's identification is likely to be a social manipulation that directs Western viewers to identify with characters who reproduce gender and ethnic stereotypes, so that the viewer falls in love with his narcissistic reflection on the stage and uses no critical mechanisms (Brewer, 1999; Case, 1988; Cixous, 1995; Diamond, 1997).

An example that illustrates this can be taken from a play about rape. *Background Games* was first produced in 1993 to critical and public acclaim. The play was warmly embraced by high schools throughout Israel, which viewed it as part of a prevention program whose goal was to raise teenagers' awareness of the gravity of the act of rape and its results. The play is rhetorically and aesthetically powerful, and manages to interest and fascinate teenagers, mainly by addressing their "common ground": their linguistic, emotional and behavioral world. However, research into the play found that its effect worked in the opposite direction of the education system's pedagogical goals. Whereas the play is supposed to fight sexual stereotypes and gender violence, it actually reproduces them. Instead of a rape scene, the rhetoric and aesthetic create an orgiastic, multi-sensual and inter-gender system of stimulants. This reinforces the prevailing masculine perception of adolescent boys as sexual creatures in need of release in whatever way possible, whereas girls who are raped are perceived as not taking care of themselves and at least partly to blame. The identification mechanism created in the play reinforced the chauvinistic, narcissistic view and did not lead to identification with the weak, victimized party. After the play, viewers were more likely to blame the victim for the occurrence of rape, attribute to rape victims a greater ability to prevent rape by behaving differently and were also more likely to believe boys could find themselves in a situation where they were lured into raping a girl (Gesser-Edelsburg, 2005).

It can therefore be stated that the way the identification mechanism exerts its influence depends to a great extent on the ways it is used: the dramatist's ideology and the rhetorical and aesthetic strategies he uses. The challenge facing the writers of interventionist drama is how to create drama that uses the emotional mechanism not to make the viewer fall in love with his own narcissistic reflection but to see the cracks and possibilities for correction both of himself and of the surrounding society.

The Conflict Element

Conflict, which can be expressed either as an internal conflict in the character's psyche or an external conflict between different characters, is caused by the meeting of clashing values, desires, and ambitions. Conflict in drama is realized by its deconstruction into the psychological, normative, and cultural barriers that prevent the person from implementing their desired behavior. Conflict appears across all the different genres and is shaped accordingly. In melodrama the conflict is external, between representations of "good" and "evil." In ancient tragedy conflict exists between man and deities. In social drama conflict is embodied by social forces that prevent the protagonist from following his conscience, and so on.

A study of plays between the years 2009–2011 about novice teen drivers in Israel[2] found that most of the plays focused on victimhood and strategies of intimidation and punishment, but failed to take a deep look at the two sides of the conflict equation: namely, the benefits of safe driving, on the one hand, and the forces that lead young drivers to take risks, on the other. For example, barriers connected to the driving culture in Israel, young people's risk perceptions, social pressure, gender perceptions regarding driving and so on. The plays lacked a theoretical basis and focused mainly on the costs of getting hurt. Additionally they failed to address the environmental, social and normative influences that motivate young people in the context of driving (Gesser Edelsburg, Baron-Epel, Hadar, & Lotam, 2013). The obstacle facing drama that seeks to create change is that the dramatists might fail to unravel the barriers that comprise the conflict and as a result the treatment of the conflict can appear to viewers as superficial and lacking credibility.

The Demonstration Element

Psychology and drama researchers have wondered how to transport the viewer from "automatic" thinking to "new" thinking. Butcher (1951) argued that the mimetic process embodied by the character of Oedipus in Sophocles' tragedy is the deep internal process of a person transforming from one existential state to another. Oedipus, and through him the spectator, undergoes a process of enlightenment. According to Aristotle, drama cannot have a "purely good" protagonist. The protagonist must have a hamartia (tragic flaw) in order for the character to undergo a meaningful transformation (Golden & Hardison, 1968). In Bandura's social cognitive theory, the "transformative character" is the character who goes from a problematic status or

---

[2] The research literature indicates a higher involvement of novice young drivers in traffic accidents than older age groups. Novice drivers are a danger to themselves, their passengers and other road users. According to figures from the Israel National Road Safety Authority, while novice drivers constitute only 15% of drivers, they cause 20% of the accidents and 21% of fatal and serious accidents. One third of the people killed in traffic accidents in recent years in Israel were killed in accidents in which young drivers were involved. There are intervention programs in Israel that address the risk behavior of young drivers.

position to a state of empowerment and change, illustrating to the viewer how he overcomes obstacles (Bandura, 2004). That act of overcoming can lead the spectator to a sense of self-efficacy and a belief in his ability to carry out a certain action just like the character (Sood, Menard, & Witte, 2004). In order for the individual's change to occur in reality as well, the drama must demonstrate how the community can undergo a transformation and empowerment and support the individual's change (Usdin, Singhal, Shongwe, Goldstein, & Shabalala, 2004).

One example of transformation can be found in plays about the Israeli-Palestinian conflict, a profound and intractable conflict that impacts the physical and mental health of both peoples. These plays raise the question whether drama can inspire change in such a politically and morally complicated situation. A study that investigated how theater represents the conflict and promotes peace and tolerance among teenagers in the years 2005–2007 mapped out and analyzed several plays on this subject from different angles. The findings indicated that in the course of viewing the plays the Israeli teenagers acquired information about the difficulties the Palestinian population has to contend with and deepened their thinking about issues and dilemmas related to the occupation. This happened mainly as a result of the humanization of the Palestinian adversary on the stage. However, the plays did not give them tools to deal with the Israeli-Palestinian conflict. Most of the plays presented the IDF soldiers' attitudes towards the Palestinian population of the occupied territories in a negative light, but did not show the audience positive models representing a different approach. Moreover, none of these plays had an Israeli character who underwent a transformation, from a character demonstrating intolerance towards the Palestinians to a character recognizing Palestinian rights and legitimacy, with whom the audience could identify and undergo a similar process. Likewise, these plays did not demonstrate a collective transformation, showing the change of a group representing the youths in the way they treat the Palestinians (Gesser-Edelsburg, 2012; Gesser-Edelsburg, 2011). Furthermore, the plays did not examine dilemmas that both sides might have in common (such as the tension between moderates and extremists in both communities), or common aspirations (such as the aspiration to live in peace). The dramatists expressed their perception of the self-construction of the "other," yet failed to incorporate that other, with its problems and aspirations, into their own self-examination. This seems to reflect the actual discourse in the complicated reality and the unreadiness of both sides

Catharsis: Satisfaction through Learning

The spectator's catharsis (emotional cleansing) occurs when the process the spectator undergoes consists not only of pleasure but also of an experience of cognitive enlightenment, or as Golden and Hardison (1968) call it, "an intellectual clarification of the events." According to Aristotle, if the plot is built solidly and coherently, then the emotional cleansing will be commensurate, even though the events in the tragedy arouse fear and compassion and are unpleasant. The fear and compassion ultimately become irrelevant when the events are "clarified" through the catharsis (Golden & Hardison, 1968).

Communication and psychology theoreticians have spoken of a meaningful transformative process in which the spectator undergoes change through the character (Bandura, 2004; Kincaid, 2002; Sood, et al., 2004). There are also interventional dramas that forge in the spectator a so-called "false catharsis" (Gesser-Edelsburg, et al., 2006). When the spectators experienced a "false catharsis," the two elements of catharsis, pleasure and learning, did not fully occur in the spectators' experience of watching. In other words, the pleasure the spectators felt from the play was a voyeuristic pleasure, devoid of emotional involvement in what was happening on the stage. That feeling of alienation precludes the existence of the second element necessary in the experiential process—the element of learning. The play did not give the spectators the tools and skills to deal with situations from their own daily lives. An example of "false catharsis" can be found in the plays cited above about drugs. A study of those plays found that all of those obstacles led the spectators to feel that what was happening to the addicts on the stage "does not belong to my world" (Gesser-Edelsburg, et al., 2006).

How to Overcome the Obstacles and Meet the Challenges: The Rhetorical Change Model in Drama

This section suggests a model for the construction of drama whose purpose is to change existing values, positions and behaviors on health issues, based on the components specified in the previous sections, along with suggestions on how to use them.

1. *The audience's accepted values and norms.* The first stage in constructing this element is identifying and characterizing the audience's positions and values. The second stage is for the writer to construct a dialogue with those positions. The dialogue should be conducted in such a way that expresses awareness and understanding of the audience's values while at the same time integrating the oppositional values it wants to convey to the spectators. The subtext (the hidden meaning of the text) is gradually revealed until it becomes the drama's manifest text. The drama is built with the additional elements of the model.

2. *The rhetoric of the aesthetic.* The drama must create a rich aesthetic world that conforms to the values the dramatist wishes to change, in order to attract and cast a positive light on a subject that might be difficult to process. The dramatist must be cautious not to attach a stimulating esthetic to the values he wishes to change. Another strategy might adopt Baudrillard's recommendation to use the refractions on the stage in order to seduce the narcissist spectator without there being anything behind the mirror that would satisfy his desire (Baudrillard, 1990). In other words, "laying a trap" for the spectator to prepare him to receive the change before the spectator activates defense mechanisms.

3. *The spectator as ghostwriter.* Being a ghostwriter gives the spectator the feeling that the dialogue is directed to him and his world. In some situations the dramatist leads the spectator to a particular reaction but the spectator reacts differently. In order to minimize the boomerang phenomenon, the dramatist should use an external mechanism of "formative evaluation" with the audience, to anticipate possible audience reactions and steer them accordingly.

4. *The mythical layer.* The mythic element arouses urges that motivate the spectator to find ways to deal with them. The alternatives proposed by the drama should be ones that can deal with those needs and urges. Dramatists should avoid jumping ahead to solutions without giving room to the audience's urges and fears. They should also avoid raising fears to such a level that the proposed solutions cannot deal with them.

5. *Identification.* Dramatists should direct the audience to identify with the character who embodies the values of the change; they should avoid illuminating the character who carries the change in an ambivalent light, to avoid the boomerang effect.

6. *Conflict.* The conflict equation pits the behavior we want to impart against the barriers that prevent it. The barriers must be presented credibly. They must be given "stage time" so that the spectator has enough time to think about them and grapple with them.

7. *Demonstration.* The drama should provide tools to help realize the change process. The process of the individual and collective change should build up throughout the drama.

8. *Catharsis.* In order for the catharsis process to occur fully, the spectator's identification should not be voyeuristic but reflective. The spectator must undergo a process of enlightenment and insight that change is in order, and be provided with tools and demonstrations or suggestions for change.

How Can Drama Be Evaluated as an Intervention Tool in Health Communication?

The evaluation tool required in order to build the drama is formative evaluation—creating the drama with audience participation at all stages, in order to try to prevent the boomerang effect. The evaluation studies currently conducted "after" the fact focus on evaluating the changes in spectators' positions and perceptions before and after viewing the drama. But only a few studies in health communication try to explore the reasons or reveal the rhetorical mechanisms that lead spectators to change or retain their positions. The question is, what is it about a specific drama that leads spectators to change or not change? I will try to propose empirical questions based on components of the Rhetorical Change Model in Drama that can serve as evaluation tools for measuring drama effectiveness (see Table 1).

Table 1. Evaluation Questions for Measuring Drama Effectiveness based on the Rhetorical Change Model in Drama

Component	Empirical Questions
Audience's prevailing values and norms	• Were the oppositional values presented coherently in the narrative? • At what moment did the spectators discover the criticism?
The rhetoric of the aesthetic	• Does the aesthetic serve the drama's concept? • Are deliberate conflicts created between the aesthetic and the drama's ideological layers? • Is that gap revealed during viewing?
The spectator as ghostwriter	• Are there proportionality and balance between the writer's intention and the open spaces he leaves to the viewer's imagination?
The mythical layer	• Is there use of an anxiety-inducing element in the drama? • Are the fears and concerns relevant to the audience? • Is there a process of revelation or does the drama go directly to offering solutions and tips?
Identification	• Did the spectators feel empathy, identification or anger, or did they remain voyeuristic and alienated? • Did the mechanism expose them to a different dialogue they had not experienced themselves during their emotional attachment with the characters? • Did the mechanism create new emotional attachments they had not experienced before viewing?
Conflict	• Are the character's barriers presented authentically? • Is the character's struggle with his barriers backed by a meaningful process that is inherent to the plot?
Demonstration	• Did the drama provide alternatives, tools or tips for overcoming obstacles? • Did the drama provide different paths for situations that appear in reality to be "dead ends" or "unmanageable"? • Did the drama manage to create an alternative that inspires the spectator with hope and strength?
Catharsis	• Did the drama encourage the viewer to undergo a cleansing personal journey that would give his life cognitive enlightenment?

Recommended Readings

Baudrillard, J. (1990). *Seduction*. New York: Saint Martin Press.
Brecht, B. (2003). Alienation effects in Chinese acting. In L. Goodman & J. de Gay (Eds.), *The Routledge reader in politics and performance* (p. 96). London and New York: Routledge.
Gesser Edelsburg, A., & Singhal, A. (2013). The Edutainment event and strategies of persuasion. *Critical Arts: South-North Cultural and Media Studies* (Special Issue on Entertainment-Education and Social Change), Vol. 27 (1): 56–74.
Perelman, C. (1977). *L'Empire rhétorique: Rhétorique et argumentation* Paris: Vrin.

References

Affron, C. (1991). Identifications. In M. Landy (Ed.), *Imitations of life* (pp. 98–117). Detroit: Wayne University Press.
Ajzen, I., & Fishbein, M. (1980). *Understanding attitudes and predicting social behavior*. Englewood Cliffs, NJ: Prentice Hall.
Aristotle. (2002). *Rhetoric*. Bnei-Brak: Sifriat Poalim.
Bailin, S. (1994). Drama as experience: A critical review. *Canadian Journal of Education*, *18*(2), 95–105.
Bandura, A. (2004). Social cognitive theory for personal and social change by entertainment-education media. In A. Singhal, M. J. Cody, E. M. Rogers & M. Sabido (Eds.), *Entertainment-Education and social change: History, research, and practice* (pp. 75–95). Mahwah, New Jersey: Lawrence Erlbaum Associates.
Baudrillard, J. (1990). *Seduction*. New York: Saint Martin Press.
Bentley, E. (1972). *The life of the drama*. New York: Atheneum.
Billig, M. (1996). *Arguing and thinking: A rhetorical approach to social psychology*. Cambridge; New York: Cambridge University Press [Editions de la Maison des sciences de l'homme].
Booth, W. C. (1961). *The rhetoric of fiction*. Chicago: The University of Chicago Press.
Brecht, B. (2003). Alienation effects in Chinese acting. In L. Goodman & J. de Gay (Eds.), *The Routledge reader in politics and performance* (p. 96). London and New York: Routledge.
Brewer, M. F. (1999). *Race sex and gender in contemporary women's theatre: The construction of 'woman.'* Brighton: Sussex Academic Press.
Brown, W. J., Basil, M. D., & Bocarnea, M. C. (2003). The influence of famous athletes on health beliefs and practices: Mark McGwire, child abuse prevention, and Androstenedione. *Journal of Health Communication, 8*(1), 41–57.
Brown, W. J., & Singhal, A. (1990). Ethical dilemmas of prosocial television. *Communication Quarterly, 38*(3), 268–280.
Butcher, S. H. (1951). Imitation as an aesthetic term. In S. H. Butcher (Ed.), *Aristotle's theory of poetry and fine art* (pp. 121–162). New York: Dover Publications, Inc.
Case, S. E. (1988). *Feminism and theatre*. London: Methuen.
Cixous, H. (1995). Aller à la mer (1977). In R. Drain (Ed.), *Twentieth-century theatre* (pp. 133–135). London: Routledge.

Cohen, J. (2001). Defining identification: A theoretical look at the identification of audiences with media characters. *Mass Communication and Society, 4*(3), 245–264.

Diamond, E. (1997). *Unmaking mimesis: Essays on feminism and theater.* London and New York: Routledge.

Gesser-Edelsburg, A. (2005). Paradoxical outcomes in an educational drama about gang rape: Ethical responsibilities of practitioners and educators. *Research in Drama Education: The Journal of Applied Theatre and Performance, 10*(2), 139–158.

Gesser-Edelsburg, A. (2012). The Israeli–Palestinian conflict through theatre: A qualitative study of Israeli high school students. *Research in Drama Education: The Journal of Applied Theatre and Performance, 17*(1), 83–101.

Gesser-Edelsburg, A., & Endevelt, R. (2011). An entertainment–education study of stereotypes and prejudice against fat women. *Health Education Journal, 70*(4), 374–382.

Gesser-Edelsburg, A., Guttman, N., & Israelashvili, M. (2006). Educational drama and the dilemma of 'false catharsis': Lessons for theory and practice from a study of anti-drug plays in Israel. *Research in Drama Education, 11*(3), 293–311.

Gesser-Edelsburg, A. (2011). Entertainment-education: Dilemmas of Israeli creators of theatre about the Israeli–Palestinian conflict in promoting peace. *Journal of Peace Education, 8*(1), 55–76.

Gesser Edelsburg, A. (2002). *Reception processes of contemporary political-social Israeli theatre.* Ph.D., Tel-Aviv University, Tel-Aviv.

Gesser Edelsburg, A., Baron-Epel, O., Hadar, L., & Lotam, T. (2013). Intervention Programs in Schools for Road Accidents Prevention Among Young Drivers—Mapping, Characterization and Evaluation of Their Effectiveness: A report to the Israel Insurance Association

Gesser Edelsburg, A., & Singhal, A. (2013). The Edutainment event and strategies of persuasion. *Critical Arts: South-North Cultural and Media Studies* (Special Issue on Entertainment-Education and Social Change), Vol. 27 (1): 56–74.

Gilula, D. (Ed.). (1985). *Oedipus the king and Sophocles: Essay collection.* Jerusalem: Keter Books.

Golden, L., & Hardison, O. B. (1968). *Aristotle's poetics: A translation and commentary for students of literature.* Englewood Cliffs, NJ: Prentice-Hall.

Guttman, N., Gesser-Edelsburg, A., & Israelashvili, M. (2008). The paradox of realism and "authenticity" in entertainment-education: A study of adolescents' views about anti-drug abuse dramas. *Health communication, 23*(2), 128–141.

Ingarden, R. (1973). *The cognition of the literary work of art* (R. A. Crowley & K. R. Olson, Trans.). Evanston, IL: Northwestern University Press.

Iser, W. (1974). *The implied reader: Patterns of communication in prose fiction from Bunyan to Beckett.* Baltimore and London: Johns Hopkins University Press.

Kaynar, G. (1993). *The implied spectator and his manifestations in four periods of the German drama.* Ph.D., Tel-Aviv University, Tel-Aviv.

Kincaid, D. L. (2002). Drama, emotion, and cultural convergence. *Communication Theory, 12*(2), 136–152.

Kuznicka, D. (1989). Ingarden on theatre. In B. Dziemidok & B. McCormick (Eds.), *On the aesthetics of Roman Ingarden: Interpretations and assessments* (pp. 283–296). Dordrecht: Kluwer Academic Publishers.

Liebes, T. (1996). Notes on the struggle to define involvement in television viewing. In L. Grossberg & E. Wartella (Eds.), *The audience and its landscaper* (pp. 177–186). Boulder, CO: Westview.

Livingstone, S. M. (1998). *Making sense of television: The psychology of audience interpretation*. New York: Routledge.

Mollen, S., Rimal, R. N., & Lapinski, M. K. (2010). What is normative in health communication research on norms? A review and recommendations for future scholarship. *Health Communication, 25*(6–7), 544–547.

Perelman, C. (1977). *L'Empire rhétorique: Rhétorique et argumentation*. Paris: Vrin.

Rimal, R. N., & Real, K. (2005). How behaviors are influenced by perceived norms. *Communication Research, 32*(3), 389–414.

Rozik, E. (1992). *The fundamentals of play analysis*. Tel-Aviv: Or-Am.

Schaff, T. J. (1976–77). Audience awareness and catharsis in drama. *Psychoanalytic Review, 63*, 529–554.

Schoenmakers, H. (1992). Aesthetic and aestheticised emotions in theatrical situations. In H. Schoenmakers (Ed.), *Performance theory reception and audience research, advances in reception and audience research 3*. Amsterdam, Netherlands: Tijdschrift voor Theaterwetenschap.

Sherif, M., & Hovland, C. I. (1961). *Social judgment: Assimilation and contrast effects in communication and attitude change*. New Haven, CT: Yale University Press.

Shoham, H. (1989). *Theatre and drama are looking for an audience*. Tel-Aviv: Or-Am.

Slater, M. D., & Rouner, D. (2002). Entertainment-education and elaboration likelihood: Understanding the processing of narrative persuasion. *Communication Theory, 12*(2), 173–191.

Sood, S. (2002). Audience involvement and entertainment-education. *Communication Theory, 12*(2), 153–172.

Sood, S., Menard, T., & Witte, K. (2004). The theory behind entertainment-education. In A. Singhal, M. J. Cody, E. M. Rogers, & M. Sabido (Eds.), *Entertainment-Education and social change: History, research, and practice* (pp. 117–149). Mahwah, New Jersey: Lawrence Erlbaum Associates, Publishers.

Unger, H. (1991). *Film and philosophy*. Tel-Aviv: Dvir Publishing House.

Usdin, S., Singhal, A., Shongwe, T., Goldstein, S., & Shabalala, A. (2004). No short cuts in entertainment-education: Designing Soul City step-by-step. In A. Singhal, M. J. Cody, E. M. Rogers & M. Sabido (Eds.), *Entertainment-Education and social change: History, research, and practice* (pp. 153–175). Mahwah, New Jersey: Lawrence Erlbaum Associates, Publishers.

Applied Communication Strategies

Chapter 9

Communication Network Analysis for the Diffusion of Health: Identifying Key Individuals

Do Kyun Kim, *University of Louisiana at Lafayette*
James W. Dearing, *Michigan State University*

Introduction

Sharing influence in human communication is a normal and everyday phenomenon. People talk to and watch each other as means of learning appropriate behavior for different social contexts, and to feel a sense of belonging. People seek feedback by communicating, nonverbal and verbal, to help them assess new ideas, new practices, new norms, and new technologies, as a sort of social sounding board. Communication is the basis for how we decide what we will try and what we won't, and how we conclude what is appropriate or beneficial and what is not. A male illegal immigrant in Botswana believes his friends when they say that "condoms have worms in them" (Kim, Chikombero, & Moroka, 2012); a young unmarried woman in the U.S. takes a risk of unwanted pregnancy because of her partner's refusal to use a condom (Williamson, 2009). As illustrated in these examples, personal influence from specific others we know, and social influence in the sense of prevalent generalized norms, are key determinants of public health. While social (or impersonal) influence is often invoked in organized health promotion efforts that rely on advertising, personal influence can sometimes be harnessed to complement social influence if we have knowledge of who influences whom for which topics. This is the topic of this chapter.

Although many people already know the ABC (Abstain, Be faithful with one sex partner, and Condomise) principles of HIV prevention, the world still experiences a high rate of new HIV infection. A major reason of declining effectiveness of HIV-prevention efforts is that individual knowledge and public advertisements are not necessarily related to behavior change at both the individual and population levels. Often, people know more than they practice about injury prevention, home safety, and occupational health. The theory of diffusion of innovations, and related theories too, explains why individuals adopt innovations, and how perceptions of societal change affect individual decisions, thus linking micro and macro levels of behavior.

According to Rogers (2003), diffusion is defined as "a process in which an innovation is communicated through certain channels over time among the members of a social system" (p. 5). Theorizing about diffusion began in the 1890s by political philosophers, sociologists, archeologists and anthropologists, especially as scholars began to notice the preponderance of imitation in society and surmise diffusion processes as the fundamental basis of the worldwide transmission and mixing of cultures. Since the 1960s, researchers have been studying the diffusion of health information and health practices. More recently, diffusion theory has been integrated with social marketing, since once lessons from diffusion scholarship are applied to intervention development, the resulting strategic steps are usefully informed by the transactional perspective that characterizes much of marketing theory, and vice versa. Due to its applicable generalized nature of theory and practice, the diffusion paradigm is an exemplar of interdisciplinary scholarship, connecting communication to agriculture, marketing and management, engineering, political science, sociology, business, economics, nursing, psychology, and social work, as well as health sciences.

Why Does an Individual Adopt an Innovation?

There are three sets of factors that, when combined, usually are sufficient to explain diffusion. First, Rogers (2003) explains part of the variance with five characteristics of innovations that help differentiate the rates of innovation adoption: 1) *relative advantage*–the degree to which an innovation is perceived as better than the idea it supersedes, 2) *compatibility*–the degree to which an innovation is perceived as being consistent with the existing values, past experiences, and needs of potential adopters, 3) *complexity*–the degree to which an innovation is perceived as difficult to understand and use, 4) *triability*–the degree to which an innovation may be experimented with on a limited basis, and 5) *observability*–the degree to which the results of an innovation are visible to others (pp. 15–16). Of these, different attributes are more or less important to different adopters; they also vary in relative importance by the type of innovation being considered for adoption. Information about these characteristics of innovations is what individuals often seek to initially understand in order to assess whether an innovation warrants their continued attention.

Second, and often overlooked by researchers who study diffusion, is the context within which an innovation is communicated to potential adopters. We define context as the timing of when an innovation is introduced, and how that introduction is framed. Rogers, in his studies of diffusion, always attended to context as a major class of factors that could make or break an innovation's chances to diffuse. This is the case both for voluntary adoption decisions and for compulsory decisions, when a government or other authority mandates or communicates incentives for adoption. Contextually, a positively perceived innovation with obvious advantages can fail to spread if it is introduced at a time when social attention is elsewhere, or "attached" through priming and framing of meanings in undesirable ways that serve to associate the innovation with negatively perceived topics.

A third factor that often helps to explain diffusion and non-diffusion is whether influential members of social networks have positive perceptions of the innovation, model its use, speak out about its advantages, and so on. An *opinion leader strategy* can accelerate positive adoption decisions within specified target populations. As a determinant component of this strategy, a communication network analysis to identify patterns of influence and connections among the members of a social system helps health professionals to design the most efficient dissemination approach for health interventions. In brief, existing trust and expertise among people is identified. The opinion leadership strategy has been used for projects with diverse purposes, such as public health promotion, poverty reduction, and public policy dissemination.

Who Are Opinion Leaders, Who Are Bridges, and What Do They Do for Diffusion?

Opinion leaders are "those individuals to whom others turn for advice and information" (Rogers, 1961, p. 9), and opinion leadership refers to "the degree to which an individual is able to influence other individuals' attitudes or overt behavior informally in a desired way with relative frequency" (Rogers, 2003, p. 388). Influence, in this sense, does not mean persuasion. Persuasion implies intent, while influence often occurs without intent. Opinion leadership can be considered a special type of social learning or modeling since so much influence occurs by observation of others' attitudes and actions.

In diffusion processes, opinion leaders tend not to be so-called innovators (the very first to adopt an innovation), but they do tend to be early relative to most social system members in deciding how to respond to an innovation. Opinion leaders perform the function of evaluating innovations

—on the basis of carefully reasoned assessments of innovation attributes—and partly, for this reason, their judgments are trusted by followers (Coleman, Katz, & Menzel, 1966; Soumerai et al., 1998). Their influence occurs through their *informal* and *interpersonal communication, both mediated and face-to-face unmediated.*

The influence of informal and interpersonal communication in the diffusion process can be compared with the two-step flow of communication hypothesis. Initially introduced by Lazarsfeld, Berelson, and Gaudet in *The People's Choice* (1948), the two-step flow hypothesis posited that "ideas often flow from radio and print to the opinion leaders and from them to the less active sections of the population" (p. 151). However, Van Den Ban's (1964) study on the diffusion of new farming methods showed that farmers' decision making during the adoption process was determined more by their personal contacts with opinion leaders, even though mass media functioned as a source of new knowledge. We first learn of innovations from mediated communication channels such as websites and Twitter. For those innovations that are perceived to be consequential—meaningful to the potential adopter in terms of how they live their lives or conduct work—potential adopters then seek out evaluative information about the innovation as well as social feedback—the truth test of trusted others' opinions. Rogers (1961, 2003) pointed out that informal and interpersonal contact is more important than media in individuals' adoption of innovations and, therefore, opinion leaders can be referred to as "adoption leaders" (1961, p. 10).

For public health intervention purposes, there is another key function played by people in social systems, that of bridging individuals whose communication relationships "bridge" or connect between groups of people in communication networks. Opinion leadership is a within-group trait; their influence tends to be local, an effect on those followers who know them well. But to diffuse, an innovation must be communicated across groups of people, too. Whereas within-group communication generally involves people with manifest similarities—they perceive commonalities among themselves—much of the challenge of diffusion is adoption of an innovation from one group to the others. This means traversing dissimilarities in perception, which is a function of relational bridges. Whereas opinion leaders can convert groups of people to adopt, bridges move innovations from group to group. Being aware of the important roles of opinion leaders and bridges, the next question concerns identification. How do we find out who they are?

How to Identify Informal Opinion Leaders and Bridging Individuals

In terms of identifying opinion leaders, Katz (1957) explained that opinion leaders could be distinguished from others in terms of three criteria: 1) "who one is"—the personification of certain values, 2) "what one knows"—expertise or competence, and 3) "whom one knows"—strategic social location in relation to others. More specifically, throughout the decades of studies, Rogers (2003) identified seven generalizable characteristics of opinion leaders: 1) greater exposure to mass media than their followers, 2) more cosmopolite than their followers; 3) greater contact with change agents than their followers; 4) greater social participation than their followers; 5) higher socioeconomic status than their followers; 6) more innovative than their followers; 7) when a social system's norms favor change, opinion leaders are more innovative, but when the system's norms do not favor change, opinion leaders are not especially innovative (pp. 316–318). Opinion leaders operate within a range of possible action; they rarely will act outside of what they perceive to be supported by current norms. They are, in other words, somewhat conservative. Weimann (1994) also synthesized attributes of opinion leaders by personal traits/personality attributes, social attributes, and sociodemographic attributes, which share similar attributes to those popularized by Katz and Rogers. One of the common lessons from these works is that opinion leaders, in being influential, not persuasive, tend not to advocate innovations. They are not champions of change. Mostly, opinion leaders "lead" by ignoring or actively rejecting innovations. They gatekeep for the system that accords them informal status and are negative as well as positive opinion leaders.

Bridges are individuals who connect groups, sometimes by communicating directly with each group's influential members. Bridges can be distinguished by not identifying with any one social group, but having relational access into multiple groups. Bridging individuals enact the pollination practices of honey bees; they go from flower to flower to flower, spreading ideas. Bridges with high degrees of access to formal authorities are referred to as policy entrepreneurs. Policy makers learn of promising practices and ideas and hear how those innovations are faring in other jurisdictions from the communicative activity of policy entrepreneurs.

These normative and overarching attributes of opinion leaders and bridges provide practitioners and change agents with a general idea of who they are. However, the question about how to actually identify them remains.

Here, communication network analysis is briefly explained concerning how it has provided researchers and practitioners of public health promotion with uniquely advantageous and specific guidelines of how to identify influentials.

Communication Network Analysis

Communication network analysis is a research method as well as a practical perspective, that provides statistical and visual estimates of network structure, groups within those networks, and how individual units are related to one another. Various software programs exist for performing network analysis. The perspective is quite established, dating to the 1920s, with considerable empirical development in the 1950s and continuing to this day especially among mathematicians, sociologists, educational researchers and increasingly public health researchers and practitioners. While personal influence can be investigated through key informant interviews, observation of how people interact with one another, and self-nomination procedures of one's own influence, network analysis based either on surveys or archival records brings sociometrics (who-to-whom relationships) to the identification of influence, groups, and network structure.

A first distinctive advantage of communication network analysis is that it depicts multidirectional communication relationships with *directions* and *strengths* of relationships (Valente, 1995). In communication network analysis, questions related to 'who talks to whom' or 'who influences whom' reveal directions, and questions asking frequency of communication with particular individuals discover strength of a communicative relationship in a group. Second, communication network analysis generates *communication network maps* visualizing communicative relationships among target populations in addition to presenting the directions and strengths of those relationships. Opinion leaders and bridges are often clearly visible by viewing network maps and confirmed through statistical assessment. Third, communication network analysis provides whole-system results, rather than probabilistic results based on random sampling. This method is based on non-probabilistic purposive data-collection by contacting most or even all members of a targeted group. Fourth, communication network analysis is progressively manipulative and able to create multiple virtual "what-if" scenarios through inclusion and exclusion of members in a communication network. Methodologically, this manipulative function of communication network analysis resembles adding and dropping variables in a hierarchical regression. In network analysis, however, the effect can be to pose the question, "What will happen to our organization when

James leaves?" or "If Kim joins the boards of these two nonprofits, will it strengthen the nonprofit network in our community?" One can then simulate the results of such action. So communication network analysis may predict structural transformation of a social system.

Although the use of opinion leader and bridge identification for diffusion strategies, facilitated by communication network analysis, has been introduced and used in many real world health communication projects, the methods of identifying opinion leaders, which significantly affect the success of a diffusion effort, have not been well synthesized. This chapter synthesizes and organizes methods of identifying opinion leaders and bridges through communication network analysis.

Communication Network Data Collection

Here this section discusses several important issues for selecting a method of communication network data collection, including:

1. Purpose of study: Is the purpose of the study to identify opinion leaders and bridges only, or the overall communication networks within which they communicate? (one or more purposes)
2. Size of target population/social system: How many individuals comprise the network of interest? (small or large network)
3. Characteristics of target population: Is this a physical community such as the inhabitants of a town, or a distributed network of similarly trained individuals such as a professional group? (lay people or homophilous professionals)
4. Access to population: Do the individuals of interest comprise a hard to reach or "hidden" population such as homeless people, sex industry workers, drug users, HIV/AIDS infected people and the like? (normal or difficult to reach group)
5. Budget: Is the research or intervention budget large enough to pay for project assistants and/or external informants? (small or large budget)
6. Time: Is the time period for data collection short or long? (time frame for intervention)
7. Existence of formative study: Is systematic formative study that provides information about the features or patterns of communication in the social system possible? (baseline or no baseline sociometric data)

8. Existence of informants: Are there well-positioned individuals who can provide local knowledge about the structure of the social system and the role of certain people or organizations? (access or no access to informants)

Methods of data collection.

Five types of communication network data collection methods have been used most frequently, including the sociometric method, informants' rating method, snowball method, observation method, and self-designating method.

Sociometric Method: Sociometric data collection has been a most frequently used method to identify opinion leaders across fields of study. This approach relies on questions administered, usually by survey, that ask about the respondent's relationships with other people, including identity, importance, and topic. Two types of questions have been usually employed. The first type is when a researcher provides exact categories that respondents consider in answering the question. An example is, "Please read each paragraph carefully and indicate the name(s) of the physician(s) that best fit each description" (Hiss, MacDonald, & Davis, 1978). The other type of question asks about more general communication, such as "Which two farmers do you talk to most frequently?" (Van Den Ban, 1964). The latter type of question is based on the idea that opinion leadership is usually constituted by informal communication.

Sociometric data collection has been used in health intervention studies with diffusion purposes, such as promotion of research-based nursing care at a community hospital (Hodnett et al., 1996); implementation of surgical practice guidelines in local hospitals (Lomas et al., 1991); physician practice promotion (Guadagnoli et al., 2000); improvement of cancer pain management in communities (Elliott et al., 1997); effect of local medical opinion leadership on quality of care for acute myocardial infarction (Soumerai et al., 1998); neurologists' adherence to specialty society-endorsed practice recommendations (Gifford et al., 1999); effectiveness of a school-based tobacco prevention program (Valente et al., 2003); and development of scales of sociometric data collection instruments (Hiss, Macdonald, & Davis, 1978; Bhandari et al., 2003).

Informants' Rating Method: Kelly (1991, 1992, 1997a, 1997b) has led a series of studies to prevent HIV/AIDS among gay men by identifying, recruiting, training, and relying on opinion leaders in gay bars. The study team asked bartenders to observe and record communicative behaviors among men in the bars over a period of time in order to identify influentials. This approach to identification has proven very effective for targeting hard-to-reach people.

For selecting valid informants, Lindlof and Taylor (2002) recommended that informants, first, were usually selected among those settings where target populations exist, as "the customary arenas of activity for those being studied (e.g., shopping malls for teens engaged in "hanging out")" (p. 15). Second, informants should be people who are knowledgeable about the culture of the intervention site. Third, they have more mobility and different roles than those who are being observed. Finally, they are more likely to be facile speakers of local language and can debrief the researcher on contextualized meanings of the local languages.

Snowball Method: Snowball sampling stems from the ethnographic research tradition. Snowball sampling can be effective in gathering data from "hidden populations," such as homeless people, prostitutes, drug addicts, and the like (Faugier & Sargeant, 1997; Spreen & Zwaagstra, 1994). Ostracized subpopulations often remain marginalized and inaccessible to many interventionists aiming at increasing awareness of health information and behavior change. A snowball sampling creates data by tracing each person one-by-one among the hidden populations. Because of the social barriers created by prejudice and discrimination toward such people having low social visibility, random sampling methods of data collection are mostly not available in research dealing with these populations. In this limited situation, the use of nonrandom methods of data collection, such as snowball sampling, has been recognized as an effective and accurate sampling technique to collect data (Morrison, 1988).

Another research situation that fits snowball sampling is when people are in a specialized field, such as prosthodontists (Leonard-Barton, 1985), or members of a certain type or strata of intact communities or organizations. According to Black and Champion (1976), the snowball method is particularly advantageous "in studying small social organizations such as small businesses or industries ... Communication methods can be uncovered and community power and decision making can be studied" (p. 159).

Even though the snowball method is feasible as a data collection method with hidden populations or special types of individuals, there are some methodological limitations related to the nonrandomness of data collection. Since researchers cannot randomly select respondents, inference about those persons not studied must be made with considerable caution (Barendregt, Poel,

& Mheen, 2005; Black & Champion, 1976; Hendricks & Blanken, 1992). In other words, the data do not represent an entire population, only specific strata of people within the population.

Observation Method: Although Rogers (2003) commented that the observation method is not frequently used to investigate opinion leadership, it has been employed for some studies appropriately. For example, in Kelly's series of studies in gay bars, bartenders were trained to systematically observe behavior among bar clients. By using participant observation coupled with ethnographic interviews, Macrí, Tagliaventi, and Bertolotti (2000) analyzed the diffusion of a new information system in a small Italian firm. For their study, participant observation was conducted during the daily working time for one and one-half months before a new information system was introduced and four and one-half months after introduction. Ethnographic interviews were conducted with various informants at the conclusion of the observations. In order to use communication network techniques and draw communication network maps, they converted their field notes to actor-by-actor interaction matrices. In the process of converting their field notes to matrices, the researchers built an initial coding (open, axial, selective) of the interactions for general interpretation of the phenomena.

Puska et al. (1986) also presented a participant observation method to select informants for their study assessing the long-term feasibility and impact of the North Karelia, India, project that employed trained lay opinion leaders. This study used the observation method as a supplementary method to augment the validity of research with other data collection methods. This study indicated that a methodological combination with an observation method could greatly enhance the validity of the research.

Self-Designating Method: The self-designating method in which survey respondents or interviewees rank themselves on influence scales has been used mostly for business studies investigating consumer influence. One of the distinctive features in consumer opinion leadership research is that considerable validity and reliability assessment has been conducted to produce effective response scales. The methodological approach of the self-designating method in business began with King and Summers' (1970) study investigating: 1) "Do opinion leaders in one topic area tend to be opinion leaders in other topic areas?" (generalizability) and 2) "Do opinion leaders tend to overlap more or less across certain combinations of topic areas instead of other combinations of topic areas?" (p. 43).

The King and Summers' study modified the Rogers and Cartano (1962) six-item scale which was not an instrument for a business study. However, they applied the six-item scale to the business context. Based on the King and Summers' (1970) instrument, many studies have developed the self-designing method of identifying respondents with opinion leader characteristics, often through data collection in large probability samples of general populations (e.g., Childers, 1986; Feick & Price, 1987; Marshall & Gitosudarmo, 1995; Flynn, Goldsmith, & Eastman, 1996; Goldsmith & De Witt, 2003).

Characteristics of Each Communication Network Data Collection Method

Sociometric and snowball data collection methods present more relational information by asking research subjects to provide names and information of others who influence them, or with whom they communicate, or those they pay attention to. For example, those methods ask questions such as "Which two farmers do you talk to most frequently?" (Van Den Ban, 1964), and "Who do you look to for new ideas or better ways of doing things concerning juvenile justice in Pennsylvania?" (Kim & Dearing, 2007). By asking such relational questions, both methods allow for the construction of data that illustrate not only directions of communication flow, but also overall advice structures of the social system. The difference between sociometric and snowball data collection, however, is that, while sociometric data collection typically relies on peoples' responses to survey questionnaires, snowball data is constructed by researchers' direct contact with each interviewee as its root on the ethnographic tradition that is a more obtrusive method. Secondly, it is through network analysis, not snowball sampling, that social networks of relationships can be graphed and interpreted. Snowball sampling more often results in personal or ego-centric networks, which can show researchers how influentials are related to each other, but not how they are positioned in an overall social network.

Informants' rating and observation data collection methods can be also used to construct relational data and to draw communication network maps. These methods may be more advantageous than other methods when a researcher has only a short period of time for data collection as opposed to methods of direct contact of target populations. Particularly, to construct relationship data by using an observational method, a researcher should train observer(s) to report opinion leaders' contact with other people or vice versa. In collecting valid data by both data collection methods, it is important to select capable informants and observer(s) who must comprehensively understand general patterns of advice or influence structure among target populations.

Data collected by a self-designating method provide only self-assessed information about their own influence to others. The question often employed for collecting the self-assessed information tends to ask about an individual's own communication with anonymous others, such as "I often persuade other people to buy new products that I like" (Goldsmith & De Witt, 2003), or their self-evaluation "My opinion on rock [fashion; environmentally friendly products] seems not to count with other people" (Flynn, Goldsmith, & Eastman, 1996). Because the self-designating method only identifies opinion leaders through self-assessment, it rarely leads to the production of relational data. For health intervention purposes, this self-assessing method is particularly useful for dealing with large target populations, such as portions of cities, and selecting individuals that are more likely to be influential with others.

Comparison of Communication Network Data Collection Methods

The selection of a communication network data collection method to identify key individuals for a health intervention should be determined by considering what is possible and what is practical as summarized above. Here Table 1 projects optimal data collection methods by given conditions/situations: 1) the sociometric method is strongly encouraged for those interventions that require investigation of both opinion leaders and communication networks simultaneously, and that deal with a moderate-sized number of individuals, small to moderate budget, and short data collection period; 2) the informants' rating method is particularly appropriate for interventions having a short period of time, willing informants, and small target populations; 3) the snowball method works well in such conditions with large target populations (e.g., communities or professional networks) when sociometric data collection is not practical or a health intervention deals with an individually and/or socially sensitive issue. The budget required for snowball sampling varies on the size of target population; the larger the population, the longer the naming process will take to turn in on itself, thus driving up costs; 4) the observation method has very similar characteristics to the snowball method, except that observation requires trained observers who should be able to see the target populations' interacting in an observable size of place. In training observers, it is critical that the observers should be able to fully understand what they have to do and how they observe research subjects in accordance with research purposes, which demands comparably high costs; 5) the self-designating method can be used only for identifying opinion leaders, since this is what the questionnaire items were developed to measure.

Table 1. Comparison of Opinion Leader Data Collection Methods by Research Conditions.

(S: Dociometric; I: Informants' rating; SB: Snowball; O:Observation; SD: Self-Designation)
(■: Strongly Encouraged, O: Very Possible, Δ: Depending on cases, X: Hard to use)

Conditions	Methods	S	I	SB	O	SD
Purpose of Study	OL* only	O	O	O	O	O
	OL*+ Ntw**	■	Δ	Δ	Δ	X
Network Size	Large	■	Δ	X	X	Δ
	Small	O	O	■	■	O
Attributes of group	Homophilous Professional	Δ	O	O	O	Δ
	Lay people	O	O	■	O	O
Budget	Large	■	O	O	■	O
	Small	■	O	X	X	■
Time	Long	O	O	■	O	O
	Short	Δ	■	X	O	■
Accessibility to target population	Hard	Δ	O	■	O	X
	Easy	O	O	O	O	O
Formative Study	Exist	O	O	O	O	O
	Non-Exist	O	X	O	O	O
Usability of Informants	Accessible	O	■	■	■	N/A***
	Not Accessible	O	X	X	X	N/A***

* OL: Identifying Opinion Leaders; ** Ntw: Identifying Networks;
***N/A: Not applicable category

Table 1 can be used to help select a data collection method (the first column in the table) by considering aspects that best characterize a given research condition. The general rule is if a research condition has an "x" mark under the method column, this match should not be considered further. A researcher can then consider the rest of the conditions and possible methods, from top to bottom in the table. The most critical condition for selecting a data collection method is listed at the top (the purpose of the study) which poses the question: Is the intent to identify opinion leaders only, or both opinion leaders and communication networks? Depending on the answer, a researcher may or may not eliminate a certain method. So Table 1 offers a way of helping to choose a data collection method through a process of elimination, beginning with five methods and ending with one for a given situation.

Identifying Opinion Leaders through Network Centrality

Using network analysis to identify key individuals relies on the asking of questions, usually in surveys, such as "Who do you communicate with about (*topic X*)?", or more directly, "List the three people whose advice about (topic X) you most value." The unique characteristic of network analysis is the set of specialized statistical measures that are used to assess each node in a network, groups in a network, and overall network structure, as well as the visual representation of the data in sociometric (who-to-whom) network maps (See Appendix 1 & 2). Network mapping is uniquely important in terms of how researchers can present their data to a wide variety of stakeholders.

Network analysis focuses on relationships among social entities (Wasserman & Faust, 1994). To identify key individuals with the purpose of then intervening to affect diffusion, measures of network centrality are particularly useful. Centrality is a measure of the structural importance of nodes (the actors in a network which can be individuals, organizations or other social aggregates such as cities or nations (Borgatti, 2006); it is a property of each unit within the network, not a measure of the network as a whole. Centrality is typically calculated with one or more of three measures: 1) *degree*, which can be assessed by in-degree and out-degree—the number of direct connections a node has and the directionality of those connections; 2) *betweenness*—how much a node controls or bridges flows of communication, advice-seeking, cooperation, collaboration, or whatever type of behavior being measured in the network via the number of other nodes; and 3) *closeness*—how fast a node can access all other nodes via a minimum number of steps. In most cases and practically speaking, by using the measure degree, individuals who have higher degrees in one or more of these three measures are more likely to be categorized by the analyst as key individuals, such as A and B in Figure 1. Figure 1 also shows structurally equivalent nodes (Borgatti, 2006). Structural equivalence is the extent to which two nodes have a common set of linkages to other nodes in a network, illustrated by nodes A and B in Figure 3. In other words, structurally equivalent nodes perform the same function in the network.

If one wants to choose two individuals with whom to intervene in a small network to help diffuse an innovation throughout the network, which two people are the optimal choices? In Figure 1, the answer is not A and B which have the highest number of contacts, but A and C, due to the presence of person D. A and B can reach other people in one step (directly) except for D; in order to reach D, both A and B require two steps, routing a message through C, while C can directly reach D. Therefore, if one can only intervene with two key players in this network to reach everyone, {A, C} or {B, C} is more efficient than {A, B} because information reaches everyone within one step (Everett & Borgatti, 1999). As demonstrated through this example, selecting key individuals for a health intervention should be strategic, depending on given conditions / situations of the intervention.

Figure 3. Communication network map IV (Source: Borgatti, 2006).

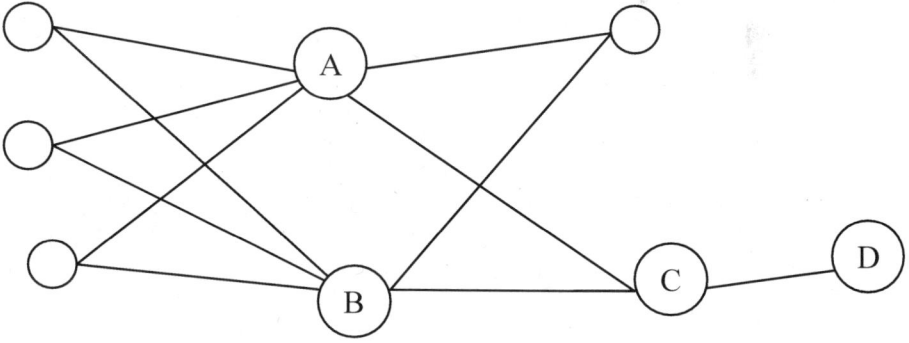

Further Suggestions

In conducting communication network data collection through surveys and analyzing the data to select key individuals for health intervention purposes, the quality of the procedure, as in all survey research, is only as good as the wording of the questions to which respondents respond. Question wording in addition to other attributes of a questionnaire also affect response rate and validity (Vehovar, Lozar, Koren, & Hlebec, 2003). This is certainly the case for network data collection. Second, since the survey method is the most frequently used method for collecting data in the social sciences, strategies to increase survey response rates should be considered when a survey method is employed to collect data. Success of communication network analysis depends on response rate (Valente et al., 2003) though multiple studies have concluded that even with response rates as low as 30 percent, essential characteristics of a network can be reliably inferred. Sensitive topics can dramatically decrease participants' response rates since the researcher is commonly asking respondents to name other people whom they communicate with. Health intervention professionals also need to consider the cultural relevance and meaning of a given topic to the target populations. For studies involving social network analysis within hidden populations or populations with unique cultures, special care needs to be taken through formative testing of the data collection instrument so that response rates will be adequate and validity of responses will be high.

Appendix 1
Communication networks among Indian farmers

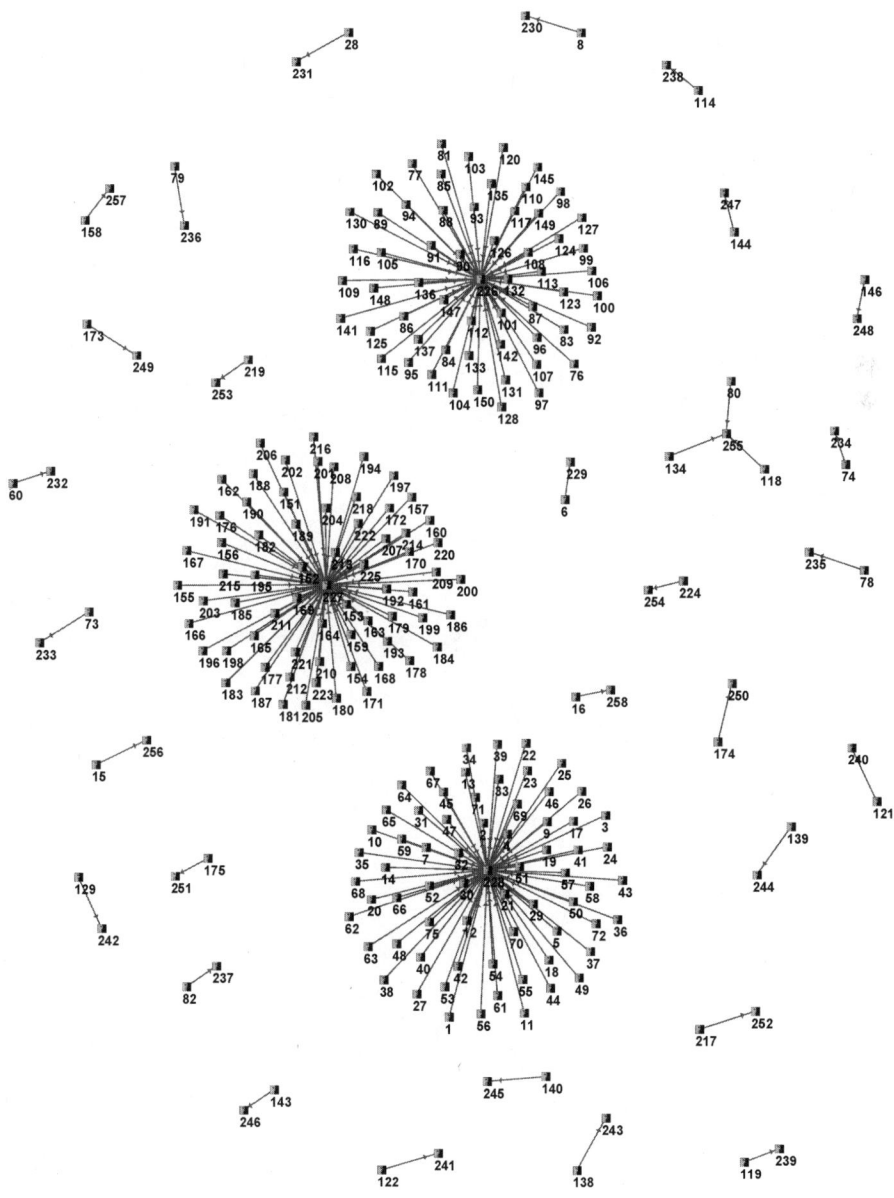

Appendix 2

Communication networks among individuals in a juvenile justice system in the U.S.

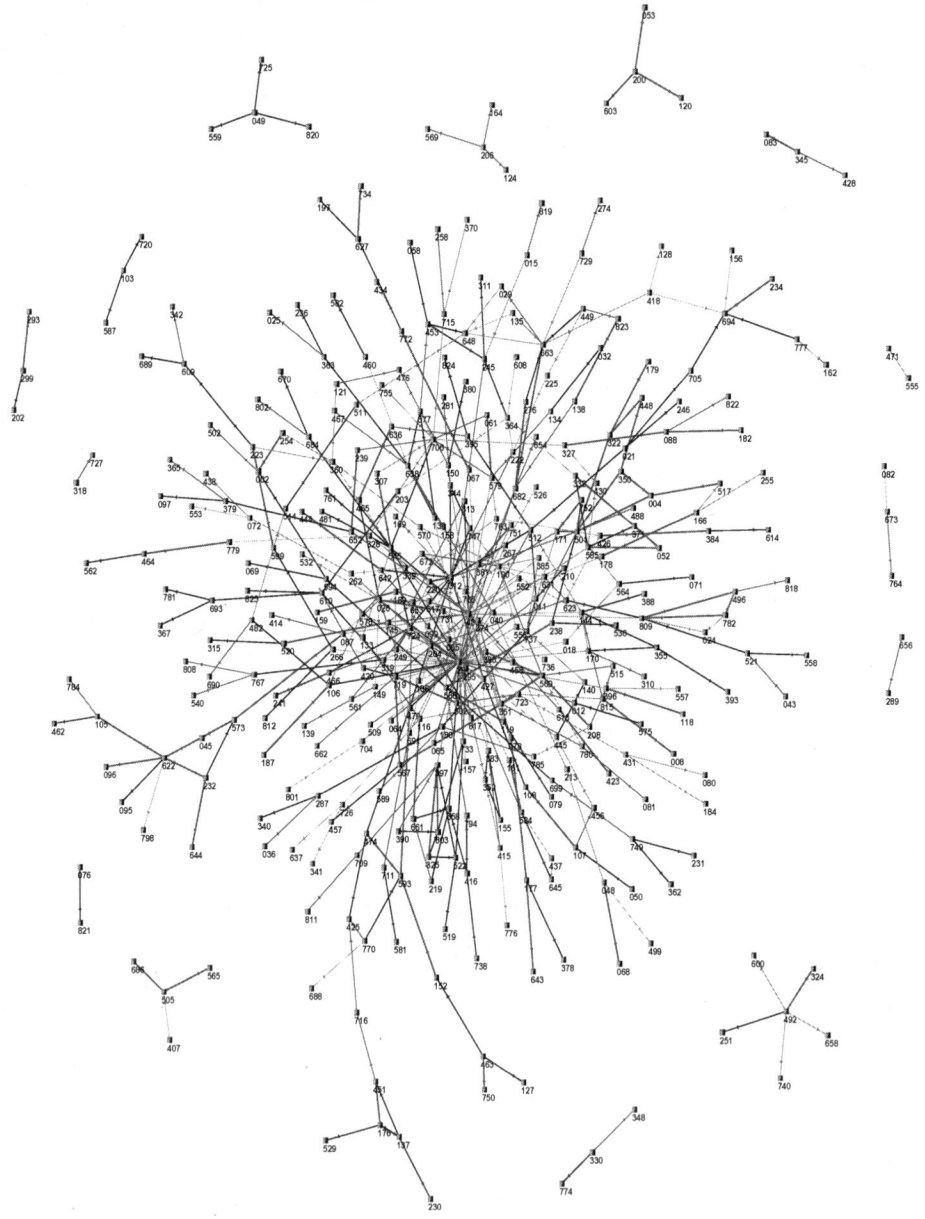

Recommended Readings

Borgatti, S. P. (2006). Identifying sets of key players in a social network. *Computational, Mathematical and Organizational Theory, 12*, 21–34.
Dearing, J. W., & Kim, D-K. (2008). Diffusion of information and innovation. *International encyclopedia of communication*. Blackwell Publishing.
Rogers, E. M. (2003). *Diffusion of innovations*. (5th ed.). New York: Free Press.
Valente, T.W. (1995). *Network models of the diffusion of innovations*. Creskill, NJ: Hampton Press.
Weimann, G. (1994). *The influentials: People who influence people*. Albany, NY: State University of New York Press.

References

Barendregt, C., Poel, A. V.D., & Mheen, D.V.D. (2005). Tracing selection effects in three non-probability samples. *European Addiction Research, 11*, 124–131.
Bhandari, M., Devereaux, P.J., Swiontkowski, M.F., Schemitsch, E.H., Shankardass, K., Sprague, S., & Guyatt, G.H. (2003). A randomized trial of opinion leader endorsement in a survey of orthopedic surgeons: Effect on primary response rates. *International Journal of Epidemiology, 32*, 634–636.
Black, J. A., & Champion, D. J. (1976). *Methods and issues in social research*. Chichester: John Wiley and Sons.
Borgatti, S. P. (2006). Identifying sets of key players in a social network. *Computational, Mathematical and Organizational Theory, 12*, 21–34.
Childers, T. (1986). Assessment of the psychometric proper tics of an opinion leadership scale. *Journal of Marketing Research, 23*, 184–188.
Coleman, J.S., Katz, E., & Menzel, H. (1966). *Medical innovation: A diffusion study*. New York: Bobbs-Merrill Company.
Elliott, T.E., David, M.M., Martin, M.O., Johnson, K.M., Braun, B.L., Elliott, B.A., & Post-White, J. (1997). Improving cancer pain management in communities: Main results from a randomized controlled trial. *Journal of Pain and Symptom Management, 13*, 191–203.
Everett, M.G., & Borgatti, S.P. (1999). The centrality of groups and classes. *Journal of Mathematical Sociology, 23*, 181–201.
Faugier, J., & Sargeant, M. (1997). Sampling hard to reach populations. *Journal of Advanced Nursing, 26*, 790–797.
Feick, L. & Price, L. (1987). The market maven: A diffuser of marketplace innovation. *Journal of Marketing, 51*, 83–97.
Flynn, L.R., Goldsmith, R.E., & Eastman, J.K. (1996). The King and Summers opinion leadership scale: Revision and refinement. *Journal of Business Research, 31*, 55–64.
Gifford, D. R., Holloway, R. G., Frankel, M. R., Albright, C. L., Meyerson, R., Griggs, R. C., & Vickrey, B. G. (1999). Improving adherence to dementia guidelines through education and opinion leaders. *Annals of internal medicine, 131*, 237–246.
Goldsmith, R. E., & De Witt, T. S. (2003), The predictive validity of an opinion leadership scale, *Journal of Marketing Theory & Practice, 11*, 28–35.

Guadagnoli, E., Soumerai, S.B., Gurwitz, J.H., Borbas, C., Shapiro, C.L., Weeks, J.C., & Morris, N. (2000). Improving discussion of surgical treatment options for patients with breast cancer: Local medical opinion leaders versus audit and performance feedback. *Breast Cancer Research and Treatment, 61,* 171–175.

Hendricks, V.M., & Blanken, P. (1992). Snowball sampling: Theoretical and practical considerations. In V. M. Hendricks, P. Blanken, & N. Adriaans (Eds.), *Snowball sampling: A pilot study on cocaine use* (pp. 17–35). Rotterdam, Den.: IVO.

Hiss, R.G., MacDonald, R., & Davis, W. K. (1978, October). *Identification of physician educational influentials in small community hospitals.* Paper presented at the seventeenth annual conference on Research in Medical Education, New Orleans, LA.

Hodnett, E.D., Kaufman, K., O'Brien-Pallas, L., Chipman, M., Watson-MacDonell, J., & Hunsburger, W. (1996). A strategy to promote research-based nursing care: Effects on childbirth outcomes. *Research in Nursing & Health, 19,* 13–20.

Katz, E. (1957). The two-step flow of communication: An up-to-date report on a hypothesis. *Public Opinion Quarterly, 21,* 61–78.

Kelly, J.A., Lawrence, J.S., Stevenson, Y.L., Hauth, A.C., Kalichman, S.C., Diaz, Y.E., Brasfield, T. L., Koob, J. J., & Morgan, M. G. (1992). Community AIDS/HIV risk reduction: The effects of endorsements by popular people in three cities. *American Journal of Public Health, 82,* 1483–1489.

Kelly, J.A., McAuliffe, T.L., Sikkema, K.J., Murphy, D.A., Somlai, A.M., Mulry, G., Miller, J.G., Stevenson, Y.L., & Fernandez, M.I. (1997a). Reduction in risk behavior among adults with severe mental illness who learned to advocate for HIV prevention. *Psychiatric Services, 48,* 1283–1288.

Kelly, J.A., Murphy, D.A., Sikkema, K.J., McAuliffe, T.L., Roffman, R.A., Soloman, L.J., Winett, R.A., Kalichman, S.C., and the Community HIV Prevention Research Collaborative (1997b). Randomized, controlled, community-level HIV-prevention intervention for sexual-risk behavior among homosexual men in US cities. *The Lancet, 350,* 1500–1505.

Kelly, J.A., St. Lawrence, J., Diaz, Y. E., Stevenson, L.Y., Hauth, A.C., Brasfield, T.L., Kalichman, S.C., Smith, J.E., & Andrew, M.E. (1991). HIV risk behavior reduction following intervention with key opinion leaders of population: An experimental analysis. *American Journal of Public Health, 81,* 168–171.

Kim, D-K., Chikombero, M., & Moroka, T. (November 2012). Innate health threat among a visibly hidden immigrant group: Field data analysis for HIV/AIDS prevention among Zimbabwean workers in Botswana. *Journal of Health Communication, 18,* 146–159.

Kim, D.K., & Dearing, J.W. (2007, November). *Communication structure in a state juvenile justice system.* Paper presented at the annual conference of the National Communication Association, Chicago, IL.

King, C.W., & Summers, J.O. (1970). Overlap of opinion leadership across consumer product categories. *Journal of Marketing Research, 7,* 43–50.

Lazarsfeld, P.F., Berelson, B., & Gaudet. H. (1948). *The people's choice: How the voter makes up his mind in a presidential campaign.* New York: Duell, Sloan and Pearce.

Leonard-Barton, D. (1985). Experts as negative opinion leaders in the diffusion of a technological innovation. *Journal of Consumer Research, 11,* 914–926.

Lindlof, T.R., & Taylor, B. C. (2002). *Qualitative communication research methods (2nd Ed.).* CA: Sage Publications.

Lomas, J., Enkin, M., Anderson, G.M., Hannah, W.J., Vayda, E., & Singer, J. (1991). Opinion leaders vs. audit and feedback to implement practice guidelines. *The Journal of the American Medical Association, 265*, 2202–2207.

Macrí, D.M., Tagliaventi, M.R., & Bertolotti, F. (2000). Sociometric location and innovation: How the social network intervenes between the structural position of early adopters and changes in the power map. *Technovation, 21*, 1–13.

Marshall, R., & Gitosudarmo, I. (1995). Variation in the characteristics of opinion leaders across cultural borders. *Journal of International Consumer Marketing, 8*, 5–22.

Morrison, V. L. (1988). Observation and snowballing: Useful tools for research into illicit drug use? *Social Pharmacology, 2*, 247–271.

Puska, R., Koskela, K., McAlister, A., Mayranen, H., Smolander, A., Moisio, S., Viri, L., Korpelainen, V., & Rogers, E.M. (1986). Use of lay opinion leaders to promote diffusion of health innovations in a community programme: Lessons learned from the North Karelia project. *Bulletin of the World Health Organization, 64*, 437–446.

Rogers, E.M. (1961). Characteristics of agricultural innovators and other adopter categories, Wooster: Ohio experiment station. *Research Bulletin, 882*.

Rogers, E. M., (2003). *Diffusion of innovations*. (5th ed.). New York: Free Press.

Rogers, E.M., & Cartano, D.G. (1962). Methods of measuring opinion leadership. *Public Opinion Quarterly, 26*, 435–441.

Soumerai, S.B, McLaughlin, T.J., Gurwitz, J.H., Guadagnoli, E.G., Hauptamn, P.J., Borbas, C., Morris, N., McLaughlin, B., Gao, X., Willison, D.J., Asinger, R., & Gobel, F. (1998). Effect of local medical opinion leadership on quality of care for acute myocardial infarction: A randomized controlled trial. *Journal of the American Medical Association, 279*, 1358–1363.

Spreen, M., & Zwaagstra, R. (1994). Personal network sampling, outdegree analysis and multilevel analysis: Introducing the network concept in studies of hidden populations. *International Sociology, 9*, 275–291.

Valente, T.W. (1995). *Network models of the diffusion of innovations*. Creskill, NJ: Hampton Press.

Valente, T.W., Hoffman, B.R., Ritt-Olsen, A., Litchman, K., & Johnson, A. (2003). Effects of a social-network method group assignment strategies on peer-led tobacco prevention programs in schools. *American Journal of Public Health, 93*, 1837–1843.

Van Den Ban, A.W. (1964). A revision of the two-step flow of communications hypothesis. *Gazette, X*, 237–249.

Vehovar, V., Manfreda, L., Koren, G., & Hlebec, V. (2003). *Methodological issues in Web data collection of ego-centered networks*. Paper presented at the annual meeting of American Association for Public Opinion Research, Nashville, TN.

Wasserman, S., & Faust, K. (1994). *Social network analysis*. Cambridge, ENG: Cambridge University Press.

Weimann, G. (1994). *The influentials: People who influence people*. Albany, NY: State University of New York Press.

Williamson, L. M., Buston, K., & Sweeting, H. (2009). Young women and limits to the normalisation of condom use: a qualitative study. *AIDS Care, 21*, 561–566.

Chapter 10

The Positive Deviance Approach to Designing and Implementing Health Communication Interventions[1]

Arvind Singhal
The University of Texas at El Paso

*"We dance round in a ring and suppose,
But the Secret sits in the middle and knows."*
—Robert Frost (1942)

During the summer of 2012, in collaboration with a dozen field researchers[2], I was privileged to be engaged in a novel type of formative research in the urban slums of New Delhi, India's capital city. Our purpose was to provide inputs to the design of a mass media health campaign to promote small family size, emphasizing delay of first child and spacing between children, focusing attention on women's and newborn child health, countering the preference for male children, and encouraging adoption of a wide range of contraceptive methods. As opposed to asking the customary deficit-based questions that guide formative research, i.e., *what are the KAP (knowledge-attitude-practice-gaps) gaps related to small family size?, what are the unmet needs of the community?*, our fieldwork instead was guided by asset-based questions: *what is working in the community with respect to small family size and with those who face the highest odds?, were there individuals,*

---

1   The present chapter draws upon the present author's work with the PD approach (Singhal, 2013; Singhal & Dura, 2009; 2012; Singhal, Buscell, & Lindberg, 2010). I am grateful to Jerry and Monique Sternin, Dr. Curt Lindberg, Prucia Buscell, Mark Munger, Muhammad Shafique, Randa Wilkinson, Dr. Lucia Dura, and other collaborators for their invaluable and collaborative inputs to my understanding of the PD approach.

2   A personal thanks to my research collaborators and colleagues at the University of Texas at El Paso (Anu Sachdev), Lady Irwin College (Dr. Sarita Anand), Institute of Home Economics (Ms. Yuki Azaad Tomar and Neeti Vaid), Mudra Institute of Communication Arts (Dr. Saumya Pant), and their dozens of alumna and current students, who participated in the India-based fieldwork utilizing PD sensibilities.

couples, and health workers who had found better solutions to problems than their peers without access to any extra resources?

Our formative research fieldwork yielded rich insights. For instance,

- We met a mother of two young girls, who effectively countered her mother-in-law's persistent desire for a male family heir by politely saying: *"We had asked Mother Goddess to bless us with girls. Now that we have two, we owe it to her to take good care of them."*

   While most young mothers in rural India would give in to their mother-in-law's wishes, our respondent had found an effective counter-argument to limit her family to only two girls.

- We met a woman who had significantly reduced her risk of getting pregnant by keeping a close track of her menstrual cycle, avoiding sex during the days she was at highest-risk for conception. During these *na na din* ("no, no days"), she employed a variety of *bahanas* (excuses) to avoid intercourse with her husband. She would, for instance, tell her husband that "I am keeping a *vrat* [fast] for a few days for your health," or "I am not feeling well these days." On her "yes, yes days," when she not at high risk for conceiving, she noted: "I go out of my way to please him."

   While most married women in rural India would not be in a position to negotiate sex with their husbands, our respondent had found creative, culturally appropriate strategies to reduce her risk for conception. After all, how could an Indian husband overrule his wife's sacred *vrat*?

- We met a health worker who employed certain uncommon practices that yielded high rates of male vasectomy. When he organized vasectomy camps in rural areas, several men who previously had agreed to have their tubes snipped, either did not show up on the appointed day, or were hesitant to be the first to undergo the procedure. Their dilly-dallying negatively impacted other participants' motivations, and many of the assembled men would dissipate, much to the chagrin of camp organizers. To overcome this problem, our health worker arranged for a few men, who were eager to undergo the vasectomy, to stride up—in open view of other men—and demand that they be the first to be snipped. And, after they had undergone their vasectomy, usually a quick and painless procedure, they would stride out with *musteid chaal* (a stallion's stride), boasting about how easy the whole thing was. Such creative orchestration of theatrical elements helped reduce the anxiety of other men, significantly boosting rates of adoption of vasectomy.

While most health workers would shrug their shoulders and embrace disappointment, our respondent found a creative way to reduce the anxiety of vasectomy prospects, i.e., presenting other men as "social proof" that there was no cause for worry.

What is most intriguing about the behavioral practices of our respondents—i.e., the invocation of Mother Goddess, the fasting strategy to forego sex, and the theatrical manifestation of "social proof"—is that they do not represent normative actions. Among their peer group, our respondents are outliers, their behaviors highly uncommon but highly effective in delivering desirable (positive) outcomes. These individuals represent what we call "positive deviants," and the (micro) behaviors they engage in are positive deviant (PD) practices.

As formative research processes for health interventions tend to be guided by needs, gaps, and deficit assessments, scholars and practitioners are rendered blind to community assets—i.e., what has been working within the community, working against all odds, and without access to any extra resources. In the present chapter, we analyze the Positive Deviance (PD) approach to social, organizational, and behavior change, arguing that often the solutions to intractable health problems lie hidden within the community. We begin by defining the positive deviance approach and then we analyze the application of PD to address *two* highly complex problems in two different settings: (1) combating malnutrition in Vietnam, and (2) reducing maternal and newborn mortality in Pakistan. We conclude by discussing the implications that the Positive Deviance (PD) approach holds for scholars and practitioners of health communication.

The Positive Deviance Approach

The *Positive Deviance* (PD) approach is based on the premise that in every community there are certain individuals or groups whose uncommon behaviors and strategies enable them to find better solutions to problems than their peers, while facing worse challenges and having access to the same resources. However, these people are ordinarily invisible to others in the community. The PD approach to social change enables communities to self-discover the positively deviant behaviors amidst them, and then find ways to act on them, and amplify them (Pascale, Sternin, & Sternin, 2010; Shafique, Sternin, & Singhal, 2010; Singhal, 2013; Singhal, Buscell, & Lindberg,

2010; Singhal & Dura, 2012; Singhal, Sternin, & Dura, 2009).

Positive Deviance to Reduce Malnutrition in Vietnam[3]

In 1990, Save the Children (USA) sent Jerry Sternin to Hanoi, Vietnam, to implement a large-scale program to combat childhood malnutrition. At that time, two-thirds of all Vietnamese children under the age of five were malnourished. The Vietnamese government had learned that results achieved by traditional supplemental feeding programs were not sustainable. Jerry Sternin, who was accompanied by his wife Monique Sternin, were challenged to come up with an approach that enabled the community, without much outside help, to take control of children's nutritional status.

As traditional methods of combating malnutrition do not yield quick and sustainable results, the Sternins wondered if the concept of positive deviance, developed a few years previously by Tufts University nutrition professor Marian Zeitlin might hold promise (Zeitlin, Ghassemi, & Mansour, 1990). While the concept of positive deviance was first broached in the nutritional literature in the 1960s, Zeitlin expanded the idea in the 1980s as she tried to understand why some children in poor households, without access to any special resources, were better nourished than others. Might combating malnutrition be helped by taking an assets-based approach? That is, focusing on what's going wrong in a community, and finding ways to amplify it?

Positive deviance sounded good in theory but the Sternins had no blueprints to launch a large-scale nutrition program. Where to begin? As childhood malnutrition rates were high in Quong Xuong District in Thanh Hoa Province, south of Hanoi, they decided to begin there. Four village communities were selected for a nutrition baseline survey. Health volunteers weighed some 2,000 children under the age of three in four villages. Their locations were mapped and a growth card for each child, with a plot of his/her age and weight, was compiled. Some 64% of the weighed children were found to be malnourished.

The Sternins then asked the question to determine whether or not there were any positive deviants, i.e., *are there any well-nourished children who come from very, very poor families*? The response: Yes, indeed, there are some children from very poor families who are healthy! Poor families in Thanh Hoa that had managed to avoid malnutrition without access to any special resources would represent the positive deviants—"positive" because

---

3   See Singhal, Sternin, and Dura (2009) and Singhal and Dura (2012).

their children were well nourished, and "deviants" because they were doing some things differently.

The next logical question was: *What were these PD families doing that others were not?* To answer this question, community members visited six of the poorest families with well-nourished children in each of the four villages. The discovery process yielded the following key PD practices:

- Family members collected tiny shrimps and crabs from paddy fields and added them to their children's meals. These foods are rich in protein and minerals.
- Family members added greens of sweet potato plants to their children's meals. These greens are rich in essential micronutrients.
- Interestingly, these foods were accessible to everyone, but most community members believed they were inappropriate for young children. Further,
- PD mothers were feeding their children smaller meals three to four times a day, rather than the two big customary twice a day; and
- PD mothers were actively feeding their children, rather than placing food in front of them, making sure there was no food wasted.
- PD mothers washed their children's hands prior to meal time.

(*Picture 1.* Community members mapping the nutritional status of children in their communities. Source: PDI, used with permission)

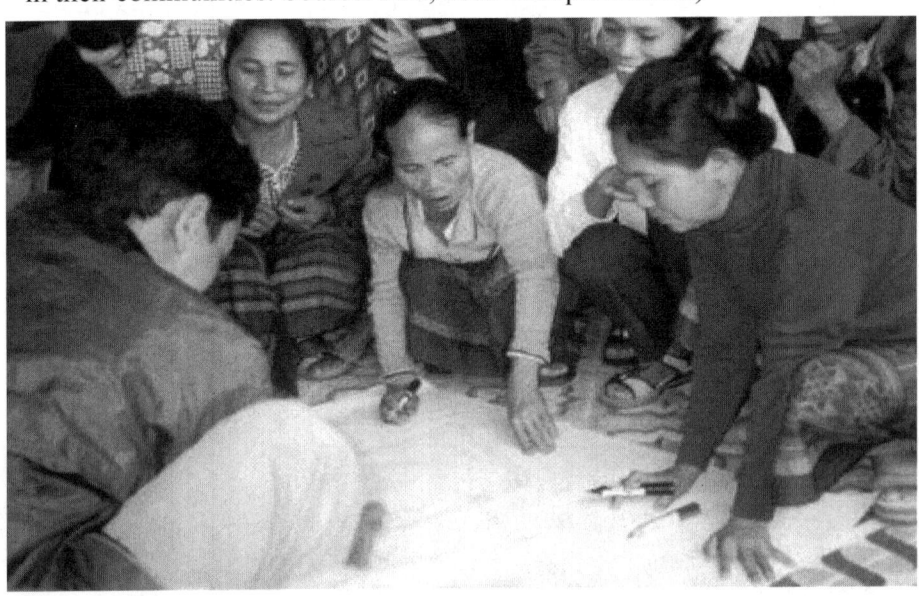

With best practices discovered, a campaign to tell the people what to do was organized, employing household visits, attractive posters, informational and educational sessions, among others. However, in spite of some modest adoption of these best practices, most of the poor households in Quong Xuong District did not adopt them. There was resistance to best practices. The Sternins, local health volunteers, and community leaders wondered how to get around it. One evening as the discussion was winding down, a skeptical village elder observed: "A thousand hearings isn't worth one seeing, and a thousand seeing isn't worth one doing." What the elder was saying was could a nutrition program be designed that emphasized *doing* more than *seeing* or *hearing*?

(*Picture 2*. Jerry Sternin (left) with mothers involved in the PD malnutrition project. Source: PDI, used with permission)

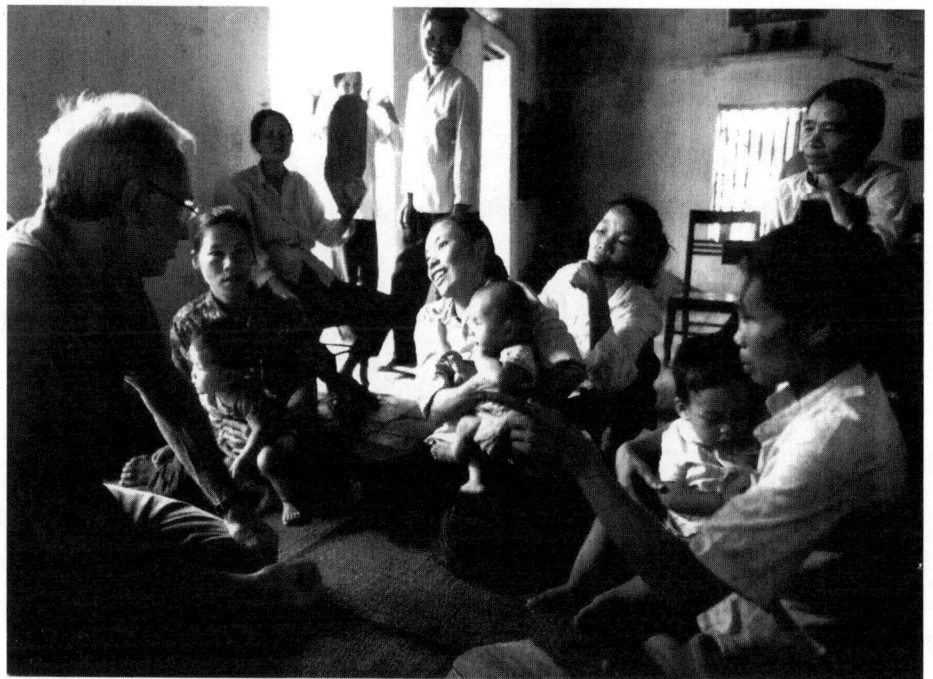

In the next few weeks, a two-week nutrition program was designed in each of the four intervention villages. Mothers whose children were malnourished were asked to forage for shrimps, crabs, and sweet potato greens. The focus was on action, picking up the shrimps and crabs, and shoots from sweet potato fields. In the company of positive deviants, mothers of malnourished children learned how to cook new recipes using the foraged ingredients. Again, the emphasis was on doing. Before these mothers fed their children, they weighed them, and plotted the data points on their growth chart. The children's hands were washed, and the mothers actively fed the children. No food was wasted. Some mothers noted their children seemed to eat more in the company of other children. When returning home, mothers were encouraged to give their children three or four small meals a day instead of the traditional two meals.

Such feeding and monitoring continued for two weeks. Mothers could visibly see their children becoming healthier. The scales were tipping! After the pilot project, which lasted two years, malnutrition had decreased by an amazing 85 percent in the PD communities. Over the next several years, the PD intervention became a nationwide program in Vietnam, helping over 2.2 million people, including over 500,000 children improve their nutritional status. A later study showed successive generations of impoverished Vietnamese children in the program villages were well-nourished (Mackintosh, Marsh, & Schroeder, 2002).

This pioneering experience in Vietnam paved the way for other PD applications to follow. Skeptics argued that PD may have worked in the field of nutrition as it was a non-contentious issue. After all, who would not want their children to be healthy? Further, with nutrition, programmatic ideas were easily trialable, and the results observable. Could the PD approach be applied to a highly intractable problem where the topic was highly sensitive, deeply ingrained in traditional structures of patriarchy and gender roles, and where prevailing beliefs and behaviors were closely connected to the harsh physical and social environment? The PD experience in Pakistan helped answer these questions.

Reducing Maternal and Newborn Mortality in Pakistan[4]

Between 2001 and 2004, the Positive Deviance approach was implemented in a phased manner in eight villages of Haripur District in Pakistan's North West Frontier Province to reduce maternal and newborn mortality. Initiated by Save the Children as part of their Saving Newborn Lives (SNL) Initiative in Pakistan, the PD process was first introduced in two experimental villages—Bagra and Banda Muneer Khan, followed by a pilot phase in Kaag and Chanjiala villages, where various PD processes, tools, and strategies

---

4   See Shafique, Sternin, and Singhal (2010) and Singhal and Dura (2012).

were refined. A larger four-village PD intervention was implemented in Garamthone, Nilorepaeen, Bhaira, and Chambapind villages. Baseline and end-line data were collected in these four interventional villages and in four comparison control villages to assess the effects of the PD intervention (Shafique, Sternin, & Singhal, 2010).

The PD approach was implemented in these eight communities of Haripur District in two phases. In Phase One, activities were initiated to foster community dialogue about the problem of newborn mortality and morbidity among community members. These were carried out separately among male and female groups to identify PD newborns and their families, discover what their demonstrably successful strategies were, and develop a plan of action. Phase Two was dedicated to community action via community-designed neighborhood activities undertaken by both male and female groups.

Given the highly taboo nature of the PD intervention—i.e., safe motherhood, pregnancy, and delivery—various participatory activities such as transect walks, focus group discussions (FGDs), social network maps, newborn mapping, and in-depth interviews were employed. During the community orientation and feedback sessions, facts and local figures about newborn and maternal care were shared, including powerful, emotive testimonies from family members who had lost a newborn or a wife, daughter-in-law, or niece during labor and delivery. A newborn mapping activity was conducted to determine how many babies had been born the year before, how many had been stillborn or died immediately after birth, after 7 days, after 28 days and within 40 days. Concurrently, explorations of common practices with women's groups around pregnancy, delivery, and immediate and subsequent post-partum care were explored using stuffed dolls as props. The dolls provided a visual representation of how the newborn was handled during the delivery process and post-delivery.

Community members were engaged to discover the uncommon yet effective behaviors and strategies to reduce maternal and newborn mortality among them, and to develop a plan of action to promote their adoption among community members. The PD team—composed of village leaders, self-identified volunteers (activists) and the NGO staff—defined a Positive Deviant (*misali kirdar*) newborn, as one who survived against heavy odds because of poverty, prematurity, and maternal history of miscarriages and anemia. Besides the newborn, family members related to the newborn were identified as PD persons, such as a father who saved money in case of obstetric emergency at delivery, a mother-in-law who prepared a delivery kit for the arriving newborn, a *dai* (midwife), who successfully resuscitated newborns that were not breathing and practiced appropriate hygiene in cutting the umbilical cord.

(*Picture 3*. Women using dolls to demonstrate common practices around pregnancy, delivery, and immediate and subsequent post-partum care.

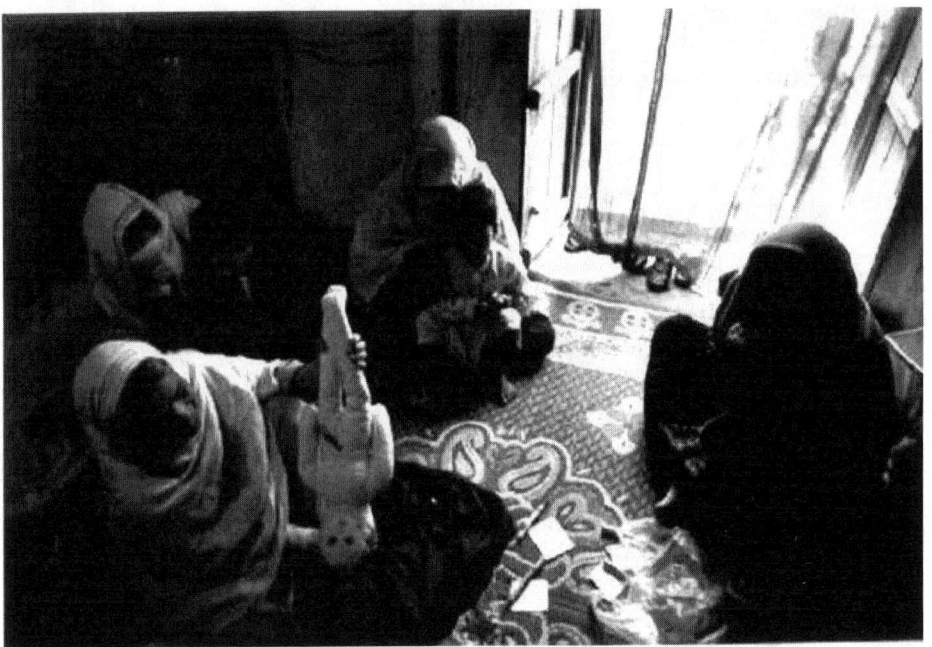

Source: PDI, used with permission)

The highly participatory PD inquiry helped discern household behaviors that increased the chances of newborn survival: the administration of tetanus toxoid vaccination and antenatal care for the mother, delivery preparedness on part of mother-in-laws and *dais*, emergency-preparedness on part of husbands, the use of clean surface for delivery, clean hands while delivering, clean cutting of umbilical cord, thermal care of newborn, exclusive breastfeeding, timely care-seeking for premature or sick babies, paternal involvement in spouse and childcare, increase in postpartum maternal diet, and others (Table 1).

The PD Inquiry also yielded rich insights on messaging strategies used by the *misali kirdars* (positive deviants). For example,

- A religious leader noted: "we don't need to bathe the baby for *azan* as when we listen to *azan* (a prayer from the Holy Quran) five times a day, we are not clean most of the time, so in the same way baby need not to be bathed before saying azan in their ears." This religious leader, and his message about delaying the bathing rituals of a newborn, was then given play in *mohallah* (neighborhood) sessions and in community Healthy Baby Fairs, thus multiplying its effects.
- A father who strongly advocates for paternal involvement in maternal health pre- and post-delivery, noted: "Giving *panjiri*, a nutritionally rich protein bar, to the pregnant woman can lead to a healthy baby and also keep mother's life out of danger. If we provide food for the mother, it will ensure the health of the baby."
- A mother-in-law explained the benefits of exclusive breastfeeding for her daughters-in-law: "The baby has no disease in the mother's womb. If breast milk were dangerous, the baby would become ill in the womb. So mother's milk is safe for the baby because it comes from the mother's body."

Once identified, PD messages were reinforced and repeated through different media, including religious and secular leaders, popular street theater, neighborhood meetings, and other means. However, the PD methodology not only focuses on the message delivery but also creates an enabling environment at the household level by involving husbands, mothers-in-law, the village health committee members, and members of Village Action Team (VAT), who collectively can facilitate and support the process of behavior change.

Table 1. Some Positive Deviance Behaviors Related to Maternal and Newborn Care

Maternal and Newborn Care Issues	Observable PD Practices
Pregnancy, Delivery, and Immediate Newborn Care	• A pregnant mother seeks antenatal consultation and tetanus toxoid injection. • A husband asked the *dai*, the traditional birth attendant, to see his wife in her 9th month of pregnancy although she was well. • A husband increased the food intake of his wife during pregnancy, especially in the last 2 months. • A husband arranged to hire a transport in case of a delivery emergency. • The family hand-stitch a small mattress (*gadeila*) for the baby to have a clean and warm surface immediately following delivery. • A husband gave the *dai* a clean blade. • A mother-in-law placed a clean plastic under the mother for delivery. • A husband ensured that nothing was applied on the umbilical cord after it was cut and tied.
Breastfeeding	• A sick and premature baby was exclusively breast-fed with no supplements and no *gutti* (a homemade pre-lacteal concoction).
Nurturing	• A father realizes that his newborn son is weak and small, and therefore a special child (*khas batcha*), requiring special care. The baby is kept warm by wrapping and his nappies are changed frequently. The child is exclusively breastfed and the quality and quantity of food for the mother is increased. The mother is made unavailable to the rest of the household so that she can exclusively care for the baby.

The discovered PD practices were openly shared with community members, separately among male and female groups. Community members had an opportunity to discuss the PD behaviors, seeing their relevance, usefulness, and practicality. Village action teams (VATs) developed a six-month plan, deciding that in cooperation with the community members a plethora of activities would be undertaken at the neighborhood level with regular bi-monthly group interaction *mohalla* (neighborhood) sessions. These meetings were facilitated by local social activists, who volunteered to carry out the community action plan, and endorsed by local religious leaders.

Each bi-monthly session was focused on a newborn and maternal care topic and highlighted certain specific PD behaviors and strategies that had been discovered during the recent PD inquiries.

In the male *mohallah* sessions, a mock bazaar was set-up where men were asked to buy what they considered a clean delivery kit for pregnant women. Discussion on each participant's purchase followed and resulted in men declaring, some anonymously, that a new razor blade was the best tool for cutting the umbilical cord. The community's respect and open support for the men's contributions and decisions helped enhance their self- and collective efficacy, leading to the emergence of a new and innovative leadership. Dozens of new male volunteers signed up to run the *mohallah* sessions initiative, multiplying the reach of the PD intervention.

In the female *mohallah* sessions, community volunteers also set up a bazaar, laying out several objects on a table and asking pregnant mothers, mothers-in-law, and *dais*, to select the five or six objects (e.g., soap bar, clean blade, clean plastic sheet, etc.) that were essential for a clean delivery kit. The selection of each object, essential or non-essential, sparked a healthy discussion about the object's relevance in delivery preparedness. New leadership emerged from these sessions to serve as volunteers and activists in improving the quality of lives of newborns and their mothers.

Several interactive games and simulated role plays were employed in the PD process to help the local Pashtun men to become more involved in the care of their wives and newborn children. Initial dialogue with community members had unequivocally revealed that male involvement in maternal and newborn care was perceived as not being "manly." One of the games used to pass on responsibility to the male Village Action team was the balloons-as-newborn game. Men were told that newborns are happy and alive as long as the balloons are afloat, but if they fall to the ground that means they are sick and may die. So, what could they do individually, as well as collectively, to minimize newborn deaths? By floating balloons, and keeping them in the air, they were "acting" on their collective communal, parental and spousal responsibilities.

A pre-post, interventional control research design involving both PD and non-PD villages pointed to significant gains in maternal and newborn care indicators. In comparison to control villages where the gains were insignificant, in the intervention villages:

(*Picture 4*. Men blowing balloons to act their way into taking care of their wives and newborns, Source: PDI, used with permission)

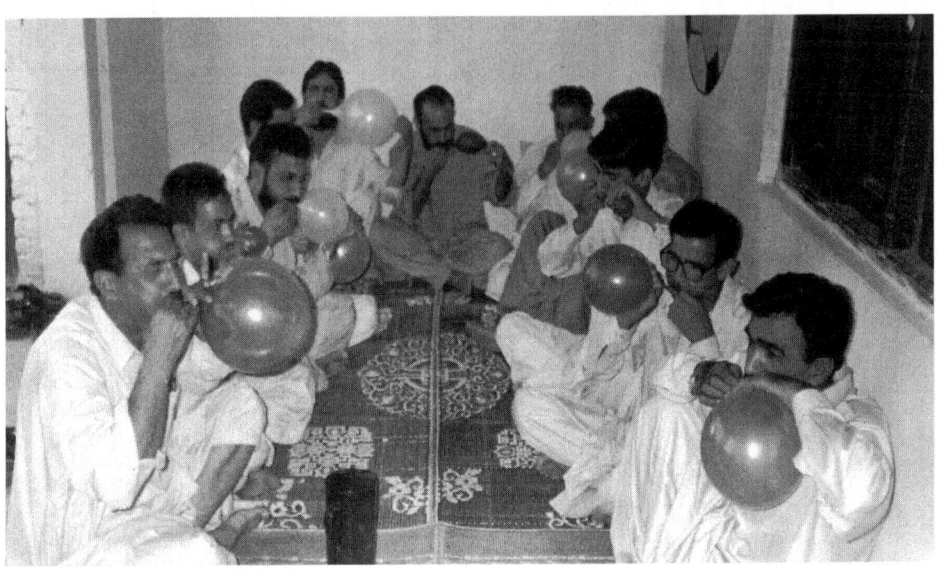

- the percentage of pregnant mothers visting antenatal clinics increased significantly from 45% to 63%
- the percentage of fathers who saved money and arranged for transport to tackle pregancy emergencies increased significantly from 45% to 62%
- the percentage of families that used a new blade to cut the baby's cord increased significantly from 19% to 33%
- the percentage of newborns whose cords did not receive unhygenic homemade remedies increased significantly from 7% to 19%
- the percentage of mothers giving homemade pre-lactal feeds in the first three days decreased significantly from 70% to 25%
- the percentage of families that bathed the baby after waiting for 24 hours post-birth increased significantly from 18% to 32%

Conclusions

In the present chapter, we drew upon a formative research study in India on family planning, and case studies on combating malnutrition in Vietnam and reducing maternal and newborn mortality in Pakistan, to make the case that often the solutions to intractable health problems reside locally and with ordinary people. This asset-based conceptualization of health interventions is known as the Positive Deviance (PD) approach—a process of change *that enables communities to discover the wisdom they already have, and finds a way to amplify it*. Over the past two decades, the PD approach has been effectively utilized to address diverse health and social problems such as combating malnutrition in Vietnam and Mali, the eradication of female genital mutilation in Egypt, curbing the trafficking of girls in Indonesia, increasing school and college retention rates in Argentina and the U.S., reducing hospital-acquired infections in the U.S., Canada, and Colombia, and promoting higher levels of condom use among commercial sex workers in Indonesia and Uganda (Pascale, Sternin, & Sternin, 2010; Singhal, Buscell, & Lindberg, 2010; Singhal & Dura, 2009).

The PD approach differs from most of the usual health communication interventions derived from the diffusion of innovations or social marketing traditions that are premised on identifying gaps and deficits and beliefs that new ideas about health come from the outside, are promoted by a change agency through expert change agents, and use top-down persuasive communication strategies to educate their client audience. The PD approach flips these long-standing tenets, positing that innovative ideas are often lurking within the system, so that the role of the change agents is to facilitate a process whereby the community can self-discover these ideas, and where dialogue and "social proof" results in a more sustainable adoption of desirable health practices. Social proof is a psychological phenomenon in which people come to believe that they can adopt a different practice because they discover people like them, in their own community, using the practice. If they can do it, others can too (Singhal & Dura, 2012). As the PD behaviors are already in practice, the solutions can be implemented without delay or access to outside resources.

Further, the PD approach challenges conventional implementation practices. Conventional learning theories assume that knowledge will change attitudes, which will in turn change practice. PD reverses that idea. PD practitioners have found action is the first step in changing attitudes. As opposed to subscribing to the notion that increased knowledge changes attitudes, and attitudinal changes change practice, PD is rooted in changing practice, as can be seen in the cooking sessions that took place in Vietnam and gender-based role-playing organized by the community in Pakistan. PD is premised on the notion that people change when that change is distilled from concrete action steps. PD believes in "acting one's way into a new way of thinking."

The PD approach holds important implications for scholars and practitioners who address global health challenges. Paradigmatically, the PD approach is situated in stark contrast to the traditional deficit-based, expert-driven, message diffusion approaches. In the PD approach, the community defines the problem, determines the presence of PDS, self-discovers the solutions, and is able to implement them right away without access to special resources. For this and other reasons, the stock of the Positive Deviance approach is bound to rise among health communication researchers and practitioners.

Recommended Readings

Pascale, R. T., Sternin, J., & Sternin, M. (2010). *The power of positive deviance: How unlikely innovators solve the world's toughest problems.* Boston, MA: Harvard University Press.

Singhal, A., Buscell, P., & Lindberg, C. (2010). *Inviting everyone: Healing healthcare through positive deviance.* Bordentown, NJ: PlexusPress.

Singhal, A., & Dura, L. (2009). *Protecting children from exploitation and trafficking: Using the Positive Deviance approach in Uganda and Indonesia.* Washington, DC: Save the Children.

References

Frost, R. (1942). The secret sits. A poem in *The Witness Tree.* http://wonderingminstrels.blogspot.com/2001/01/secret-sits-robert-frost.html. Retrieved on June 8, 2010.

Mackintosh, U., Marsh, D., & Schroeder, D. (2002). Sustained positive deviant child care practices and their effects on child growth in Viet Nam. *Food and Nutrition Bulletin* 2002; 23(4):1 6–25.

Pascale, R. T., Sternin, J., & Sternin, M. (2010). *The power of positive deviance: How unlikely innovators solve the world's toughest problems.* Boston, MA: Harvard University Press.

Shafique, M., Sternin, M., & Singhal, A. (2010). Will Rahima's firstborn survive overwhelming odds? Positive Deviance for maternal and newborn care in Pakistan. *Positive Deviance wisdom series, number 5,* pp. 1–12. Boston, MA: Tufts University, Positive Deviance Initiative.

Singhal, A. (2013). Transforming education from the inside-out: Positive Deviance to enhance learning and student retention. A chapter in Roger Hiemstra and Philippe Carré (Eds.) *International perspectives on adult learning* (pp. in press). Charlotte, NC: Information Age Publishing.

Singhal, A., Buscell, P., & Lindberg, C. (2010). *Inviting everyone: Healing healthcare through positive deviance.* Bordentown, NJ: PlexusPress.

Singhal, A., & Dura, L. (2009). *Protecting children from exploitation and trafficking: Using the Positive Deviance approach in Uganda and Indonesia.* Washington, DC: Save the Children.

Singhal, A., Sternin, J., & Dura, L. (2009). Combating malnutrition in the land of a thousand rice fields: Positive Deviance grows roots in Vietnam. *Positive Deviance wisdom series, number 1,* pp. 1–8. Boston, MA: Tufts University, Positive Deviance Initiative.

Singhal, A., & Dura, L. (2012). Positive Deviance, good for global health. A chapter in Rafael Obregon and Silvio Waisbord, (Eds.) (2012). *Handbook of Global Health Communication* (pp. 507–521). New York: Wiley.

Singhal, A., Buscell, P., & McCandless, K. (2009). Saving lives by changing relationships: Positive Deviance for MRSA prevention and control in a U.S. hospital. *Positive Deviance wisdom series, number 3,* pp. 1–8. Boston, MA: Tufts University, Positive Deviance Initiative.

Zeitlin, M., Ghassemi, H., & Mansour, M. (1990). *Positive deviance in child nutrition.* New York: UN University Press.

Chapter 11

Using Theory and Audience Research to Convey the Human Implications of Climate Change

Melinda R. Weathers, *Clemson University*
Edward Maibach, *George Mason University*
Matthew Nisbet, *American University*

Introduction

Effective public communication and engagement have played important roles in ameliorating and managing a wide range of public health problems including tobacco and substance use, cardiovascular disease, HIV/AIDS, vaccine preventable diseases, sudden infant death syndrome, and automobile injuries and fatalities (Hornik, 2002; Maibach, Abroms, & Marosits, 2007). Now, there is a rapidly growing need for the public health community to harness what has been learned about effective public communication to alert and engage the public in understanding and responding to climate change. The need is driven by three main factors:

1. The health of Americans is already being harmed by climate change, and the magnitude of this harm is likely to get much worse if effective actions are not soon taken to limit climate change, and to help communities successfully adapt to unavoidable changes in their climate. Therefore, *public health organizations and professionals have a responsibility to inform communities about these risks and how these harms can be averted.*
2. Historically, climate change public engagement efforts have focused primarily on the environmental dimensions of the threat. These efforts have mobilized an important but still relatively narrow range of Americans, but have also in some cases contributed to strong political disagreement. In contrast, *the public health community holds the potential to engage a broader range of Americans, thereby enhancing climate change understanding and decision-making capacity among members of the public, the business community, and government officials.*

3. Many of the actions that slow or prevent climate change, and that protect human health from the harms associated with climate change, also benefit health and well-being in ways unrelated to climate change. These "co-benefits" to societal action on climate change include increased physical activity, decreased obesity, reduced motor vehicle related injuries and death, reduced air and water pollution, increased social capital in and connections across communities, and reduced levels of depression. Therefore, *from a public health perspective, actions taken to address climate change are a "win-win" in that—in addition to responsibly addressing climate change—they can help us make progress on other important public health goals as well.*

In this chapter, we further elaborate on the rationale for a public health communication response to climate change, describe research we have conducted on how the public views the health risks associated with climate change, and provide practical advice to help public health organizations effectively engage Americans and their communities. This topic is timely and important because the voice of public health has been largely absent from the public dialogue on climate change, a dialogue that is often erroneously framed as an "economy vs. the environment" debate. We believe that introducing the public health voice into the public dialogue can help communities see the issues in a new light, motivating and promoting more thoughtful decision making.

Climate Change Harms Human Health

There is widespread agreement among climate scientists that the earth is warming as a result of human activity (Anderegg, Prall, Harald, & Schneider, 2010; Doran & Zimmerman, 2009), primarily due to rising levels of carbon dioxide and other heat-trapping atmospheric gases created by burning fossil fuels. It is also clear that current trends in energy use, development, and population growth will lead to continuing—and more severe—climate change over the course of this century and beyond (WHO, 2009).

Climate change harms human health, both directly and indirectly, in a variety of important ways. Direct effects can include earth system changes, including rising temperatures, increasing climate variability, increased rainfall and snowfall in some areas and drought in others, and more frequent severe weather events, all of which have considerable potential to harm human health. Heat waves, for example, can cause direct effects such as dehydration, heat exhaustion, heat stroke, and death.

Indirectly, climate change brings new challenges to the control of infectious diseases. Climate-related ecosystem changes can increase the range, seasonality, and infectivity of some vector-borne diseases (IPCC, 2007). Many of the world's most prodigious deadly infectious diseases are highly climate sensitive (via changes in temperature and rainfall) including cholera and other diarrheal diseases, and insect-borne diseases including malaria and dengue. Downpours can trigger sewage overflows, contaminating ground water that is often used for crop irrigation and drinking water. In the U.S., for example, these consequences will be particularly severe in the roughly 770 cities and towns, including New York, Chicago, Washington DC, Milwaukee, and Philadelphia, that have "combined sewer systems," an older design that carries storm water and sewage in the same pipes (IPCC, 2007).

Perhaps most seriously, the changing global climate is also affecting the basic requirements for maintaining health—including clean air and water, sufficient food, and adequate shelter—and placing other pressures on the natural, economic, and social systems that sustain health, which can contribute to poverty, population dislocation, and civil conflict (WHO, 2009). For example: mass environmental displacement and migration has the potential to disrupt the lives of hundreds of millions of people, intensifying the growing issues associated with urbanization and reverse successes in development; economic downturns and collapse erode both population health and societal development; and armed conflicts can result from resource scarcity and competition; and migration and clashes between host and migrant groups can lead to large scale loss of life and morbidity (Costello et al., 2009). The burden of all of these conditions is expected to increase as climate change advances.

In total, the direct and indirect health effects of climate change threaten to slow, halt, or in some cases reverse—possibly dramatically so—the progress made in enhancing the public's health worldwide over the past several decades. Climate change is expected to adversely affect the health of large numbers of Americans as well (TFAH, 2009; USGCRP, 2009). In fact, many communities across the U.S. are already experiencing the negative health effects associated with climate change (NIEHS, 2010).

Extreme heat can directly cause illness and death. Heat is already the leading cause of weather-related deaths in the United States, yet virtually all heat-related illness and death is preventable, if communities and individuals implement appropriate preventive measures. Between 1999 and 2003, there were more than 3,400 deaths reported deaths associated with exposure to excessive heat in the U.S. alone (Luber & Conklin, 2006). Analyses suggest that heat waves are expected to continue to increase in frequency, severity, and duration as temperatures in the U.S. continue to rise (Gutowski, 2008; Kunkel et al., 2008; USGCRP, 2009). Some American communities will be more prone to extreme heat waves than others; a study of climate change impacts in California, for example, showed that heat-related deaths in Los Angeles are projected to increase five to sevenfold over the course of this century (USGCRP, 2009). This example also illustrates the growing problem of urban heat island effect—in which cities absorb, produce, and retain more heat than the surrounding countryside—which has raised average urban air temperatures by 2 to 5°F more than surrounding areas over the past 100 years, and by up to 20°F more at night (Grimmond, 2007).

Increased temperatures can aggravate respiratory problems and disease. There has been a sharp rise in prevalence and severity of respiratory diseases in the U.S. in recent decades (WHO, 2007). Many respiratory diseases are sensitive to climate conditions. Respiratory diseases with an allergic component are climate sensitive because climate change can increase the level and duration of pollens and other air-borne allergens. Extreme heat also contributes to elevated levels of ground level ozone (a component of smog), which results in short-term decreases in lung function, and damages lung tissue; elevated ground level ozone also increases the incidence of asthma-related hospital visits and premature deaths (Confalonieri et al., 2007).

Extreme precipitation can cause injury, illness, and death. Heavy downpours (which can cause flooding) have increased in recent decades and are projected to increase further as the nation continues to warm (Gutowski, 2008; Kunkel et al., 2008). Over the last century, there was a 50% increase in the frequency of days with precipitation over four inches in the upper Midwest (Kunkel et al., 2008). Other regions, notably the South, have also seen strong increases in heavy downpours, with most of these coming in the warm season and almost all of the increase coming in the last few decades. Extreme precipitation and flooding can cause injury, illness, and deaths. For example, 2,000 Americans were killed as a result of hurricanes in 2005—more than double the average number of lives lost to hurricanes in the United States over the previous 65 years—and evacuees experienced a rise in stomach and intestinal illnesses (Ebi et al., 2008). Extreme weather events can also lead to serious indirect health effects including mental health consequences such as depression and posttraumatic stress disorder (Ebi et al., 2008).

Temperature and precipitation changes can exacerbate vector-, food-, and water-borne disease. Certain vector-, food-, and water-borne diseases are expected to occur more often and affect new populations as a result of changes in temperature and precipitation, which enable pathogens to expand into new geographic regions. People living in mountain states, for example, may become more susceptible to certain insect-borne diseases as a result of warming temperatures enabling mosquitos and other vectors to live and reproduce at higher elevations. Heavy rains and flooding can contaminate food crops with feces from nearby livestock or wild animals, increasing the likelihood of food-borne disease associated with fresh produce, and spurring outbreaks of water-borne *Cryptosporidium* and *Giardia* (Ebi et al., 2008).

Public Awareness of the Health Consequences of Climate Change Is Low

Public health officials are aware that climate change threatens health in a number of serious ways, and a majority of local public health officers across the U.S. are already seeing health impacts in their community (Maibach et al., 2008; Roser-Renouf, Elligers, Maibach, Colon, & Li, 2012). Conversely, the public is largely unaware that climate change threatens human health, much less their own health and the health of other members of their community. In surveys, without prompting, few Americans report that climate change has any connection to human health, although with prompting they are easily able to imagine such a relationship (Akerlof et al., 2010). Most members of the public, therefore, almost certainly fail to consider the health implications of climate change when they assess the issue and make decisions about how to respond.

Moreover, the majority of the public is unaware that there is a scientific consensus about human-caused climate change. While recent studies have shown that approximately 95% of active climate scientists are convinced that the planet is warming as a result of human activity (Anderegg et al., 2010; Doran & Zimmerman, 2009), only about one-third of American adults (Leiserowitz, Maibach, Roser-Renouf, & Hmielowski, 2012), and 41% of television news directors (Maibach, Wilson, & Witte, 2010) believed that "most scientists think global warming is happening."

Public health professionals have some unique opportunities to help the public and other decision makers better understand the human implications of climate change, and the scientific consensus about it. Public health professionals are uniquely positioned to explain how the rapidly emerging threats associated with climate change are connected with individual and community health. By communicating the potential of global climate change to harm human health—locally and elsewhere—and by conveying the potential to improve human health through actions that limit climate change and prevent human harm, health professionals can enhance public understanding of the full scope of the problem, and help enable appropriate responses by individuals and communities.

In addition, when climate change is framed as a public health issue, the need to invest in adaptation efforts in order to protect people and their communities becomes an important and unavoidable part of the story. The specific climate-related health risks vary by region, but the risks in most communities include reduced air quality and more extreme storms, floods and storm surges, heat events, wildfires, vector-borne diseases, and allergic reactions. Unlike limiting climate change—which is inherently a global challenge—actions to protect against health risks are inherently local. Public health officials can help citizens prioritize and choose among responses to these threats. A focus on adaptation can help move the community dialogue about climate change from the realm of global abstraction to the realm of local reality.

Framing Climate Change as a Public Health Problem May Enhance Public Engagement

Research over the past several decades has shown how experts, policymakers, and journalists "frame" an issue—i.e., how they mentally organize and discuss the issue's central ideas—greatly influences how the public understands the nature of the problem, the personal relevance or societal importance of the problem, who or what they see as being responsible for the problem, and what they feel should be done to address the problem (Nisbet, 2009; Price, Nir, & Capella, 2005; Scheufele, 1999). However, the way climate change has traditionally been framed in America—as an environmental problem—tends not to engage members of the public, at least not adequately. When climate change is framed as an environmental problem, this interpretation likely distances many people from the issue and contributes to a lack of serious and sustained public engagement necessary to develop solutions (Maibach, Nisbet, Baldwin, Akerlof, & Diao, 2010).

Framing, then, is a central process by which public health professionals can link messages and recommendations about climate change to their audience members' deeply held values and beliefs. By defining or "framing" the relevance of climate change in ways that connect to the core values of specific audience segments—and repeatedly reinforcing that information through a variety of trusted sources and networks of recruitment—purposive communication can foster enhanced public engagement with the issue.

A public health frame for climate change—i.e., making the case that climate change is a major threat to people's health and well-being—has potential to engage a much broader cross-section of the American public than has previously been engaged in the issue. Suggesting a frame that resonates with peoples' broadly shared values—such as health—helps people ground their understanding of an issue in the context of their previously existing, carefully considered, and deeply held belief systems and motivations (Price & Tewksbury, 1997; Scheufele & Tewksbury, 2007). The health frame also helps connect the complex and poorly understood topic of climate change to risks that the public already understand and accept as important, such as asthma and other respiratory problems, vulnerability to extreme heat, food-borne illness, and infectious disease. The health frame also shifts the climate debate in the U.S. from one based on environmental values to public health values which tend to cut across ideology and partisanship (Akerlof et al., 2010; Maibach, Roser-Renouf, & Leiserowitz, 2009). The public health frame also enables a new and highly respected group of voices—which includes doctors, nurses, and public health officials—to engage new segments of the public. And finally, the frame moves the location of impacts closer to home, emphasizing the risks to vulnerable people, such as children, the elderly, and the poor.

A public health frame can convey local relevance. To most Americans, the problem of climate change is global and abstract, while human health impacts are local and concrete. Large numbers of Americans believe that global warming will harm plants and animals (64%), future generations of people (65%), and people in developing countries (52%). Conversely, far fewer believe that global warming will harm themselves (29%), their family (33%), or people in their community (34%; Leiserowitz et al., 2012). In other words, people are more likely to perceive climate change impacts as a threat to plants and animals, to people in other parts of the world, and to future generations, but not as a local issue affecting themselves, their family, and their community.

Risk communication research has shown an individual's *personal* sense of risk as the most powerful motivator of behavioral change (Hale & Dillard, 1995; Witte & Allen, 2000); people are more likely to recognize and act on risks that are perceived to be close to home. Public health organizations are well positioned to demonstrate that the health risks of climate change are indeed close to home, wherever that home may be. National public health organizations can highlight the current impacts of climate change on human health in each region of the country. State and local public health organizations, in turn, can localize this information to the greatest extent possible.

By framing climate change as a local public health issue, it is possible to replace people's mental associations of climate change as being geographically and socially distant with more proximate and relevant mental associations such as the risks to children, the elderly, and the poor in their own communities and across the U.S. Americans who understand that climate change is harming people here in the U.S. (rather than only in nations far away) and now (rather than at some time in the future, if at all), are more engaged in personal actions and more supportive of climate change policies (Roser-Renouf et al., 2012). A focus on the local health consequences of climate change is likely to enhance—and sustain—public engagement on the issue, and thereby facilitate meaningful public dialogue about the problem and opportunities for solutions. Conveying local health relevance may be particularly important in encouraging public support for adaptation measures to avoid health risks associated with climate change.

In addition to enhancing public engagement, elucidating the local health risks associated with climate change is likely to engage journalists as well. Nisbet and colleagues (under review) found that when experts and their institutions pursued basic media agenda-building strategies focused on public health threats, especially when localized, the strategies lead to substantive reporting. These strategies include the release of a locally or regionally tailored study or report; the sponsorship of regional meetings; or a news conference on the part of a public health-related coalition or professional group.

A public health frame can convey additional benefits of taking action. Many actions taken to address climate change create "win-win" situations in that they create important public health benefits. For example, urban reforestation helps limit the urban heat island effect, making cities safer for vulnerable people (and more pleasant for everyone) during extreme heat events, thereby reducing heat deaths and illness. Other steps taken to address climate change also work to reduce leading causes of death and illness including obesity, physical inactivity, unhealthful diets, asthma and other chronic conditions including heart disease and cancer, and transportation-related injuries and death. Examples include programs and policies that make it easier for people to walk, cycle and take public transportation (Maibach, Steg, & Anable, 2009).

Moreover, it is a veritable truism in communication that people tend to respond better to positive information than negative information (Monahan, 1995). Therefore, highlighting the health benefits associated with taking action against climate change—including benefits that have nothing to do with climate change per se—is a useful way of accentuating the positive, giving people important additional reasons to support helpful programs, policies and individual actions. For example, the American Lung Association (2010) in California has documented the significant public health gains that Californians will enjoy if their state implements the Vision California "mixed growth" and "growing smart" initiatives. Their data show that the sustainable community and transportation development options proposed for the next two decades will help clean the air, reduce pollution-related illness and death, and avoid significant health costs, benefits that are broadly supported by all Californians.

Message Testing Demonstrates the Value of a Public Health Frame for Climate Change

Developing a clear understanding of the audience—including what they currently believe about climate change, and how those perceptions are influenced by their values—is essential to effective outreach and communication efforts by public health professionals. Research has identified six distinct groups of Americans—or audience segments—with regard to climate change (Maibach, Leiserowitz, Roser-Renouf, & Mertz, 2011; Maibach et al., 2009). These six audience segments—referred to as "Global Warming's Six Americas"—form a continuum, and each has a distinct response to the issue of climate change. On one end of the continuum is a group of people who are worried, involved and supportive of policy responses to global warming (13%), and on the other end is a similarly sized group of people (10%) who are completely unconcerned and strongly opposed to policy responses. Three of the segments (totaling 69%) are concerned about global warming and supportive of policy responses to varying degrees, one has paid little attention to the issue and is largely disengaged (6%), and two (totaling 25%) are unconcerned and unsupportive of policy responses (Leiserowitz et al., 2012). The disengaged audience includes a disproportionate number of people from low-income households many of whom likely are members of vulnerable communities.

Members of the two audience segments in the middle of the continuum—the Cautious and the Disengaged—are particularly interested in learning about the health implications of climate change. When asked what one question they would pose to an expert on global warming, if given the chance, members of these segments were most likely to ask "What harm will global warming cause?" (Maibach et al., 2009). The public health perspective on climate change is likely to be useful to all of these audiences, but especially those audiences in the middle of the continuum who are most interested in learning more about the potential impacts of climate change.

During the summer of 2009, we (EM and MN) conducted a study to systematically understand how these different segments of the public respond to information about the health risks of climate change and the benefits to health that may result from societal action on the problem (Maibach et al., 2010). Recruiting participants on the National Mall in Washington, D.C., at an outlet mall in rural Maryland, and by way of a telephone survey, we conducted open-ended interviews with 70 people—distributed more or less equally across all "Six Americas"—who resided in 29 states. During these interviews, few respondents mentioned health risks or impacts associated with climate change, suggesting that for most members of the public, this frame of reference is neither widely available in news coverage nor a salient part of interpersonal conversation.

At the end of the interview, respondents were asked to read "a brief essay about global warming" which was designed to frame climate change as a human health issue. Respondents were also given a green and a pink highlighting pen and asked to "use the green highlighter pen to mark any portions of the essay that you feel are especially clear or helpful, and use the pink highlighter pen to mark any portions of the essay that are particularly confusing or unhelpful." The one-page essay was organized into four sections: an opening paragraph that introduced the public health frame (5 total sentences); a paragraph that emphasized how human health will be harmed if action is not taken to stop, limit, and/or protect against global warming (i.e., a description of the threat; 7 sentences); a paragraph that discussed several mitigation-focused policy actions and their human health-related benefits if adopted (4 sentences); and a brief concluding paragraph intended to reinforce the public health frame (2 sentences). The health benefits mentioned included cleaner air to breathe and cleaner water to drink, healthier food to eat, fewer cars on the road, and more pedestrian- and bicycle-friendly communities. All six audience segments responded positively to the benefits section of the essay, rating this information on average as compelling and useful.

A focus group-based research study—conducted by the CDC—also found that individuals embraced information about climate change that used a health co-benefits frame (Sapru, Telfer, Luber, Price, & Ryan, 2010). Recommended behaviors were seen to benefit the individual as well as convey specific information about what the individual could do to mitigate the effects of climate change. A focus on the co-benefits of climate change prevention behaviors contained messages that convey the ways that climate change-mitigating behaviors—such as driving less, eating less processed food, and using energy-saving light bulbs—can have benefits like reduced stress, improved health, and cost savings.

In the most rigorous study conducted to date—a randomized message test experiment conducted by members of our research group (Myers, Nisbet, Maibach, & Leiserowitz, 2012)—over 1,000 nationally representative survey participants were asked to read uniquely framed news articles about climate change that emphasized either environmental, public health, or national security aspects of climate change. Across all of the "Six Americas" audience segments, the news article about the public health implications of climate change was the most likely to elicit emotional reactions consistent with support for climate change mitigation and adaptation.

Many Public Health Professionals Are Aware of the Problem, but Few Are Communicating about the Health Implications of Climate Change

A representative national survey of local public health officers conducted in 2008 found that the majority of local public health officials in the United States are aware of the growing human health risks associated with climate change (Maibach et al., 2008). Specifically, many of these health officers reported that they are already seeing the human health impacts of climate change in their jurisdiction, and that they expect these impacts will get worse over the next 20 years. The most commonly reported current climate change health impacts were heat related illnesses (56%), storm and flood related health impacts (47%), drought and fire related health impacts (47%), and vector-borne infectious diseases (42%). Over half of the health officials (56 to 73%) indicated that they anticipate these health problems will become more common over the next 20 years in their jurisdiction as a result of climate change. Overall, 60% reported that their jurisdiction would experience serious public health problems as a result of climate change over the next two decades. Relatively few of these health officials, however, had begun communicating about these risks with members of their community.

A replication of this survey in 2012 showed that little had changed over four years: rates of health impacts from climate change remained high, while little public health programming had been developed to address the issue (Roser-Renouf et al., 2012). Specifically, public health departments have significantly fewer programs now than they did four years ago in the programmatic areas that are likely to be impacted by climate change. The average number of programs within the health department addressing the health issues associated with climate change impacts decreased from 7.7 programs to 5.8 programs—a 24% decrease. Mitigation efforts have also decreased: In 2008, two-thirds of public health departments offered at least one program that promoted mitigation actions, such as conserving energy, using mass or active forms of transportation, or consuming sustainable foods; in 2012, the proportion had decreased to 45%.

An unpublished survey of public health information officers (Maibach, 2010)—conducted during a plenary presentation at the 2012 annual meeting of the National Public Health Information Coalition—showed that over three quarters of the information officers reported that they expect to see one or more serious public health problem as a result of climate change in their jurisdiction over the next 20 years (77%), and they feel that it is appropriate for their organization to communicate with external audiences about the public health implications of climate change (76%). However, less than one-third reported having communicated with external audiences about the public health implications of climate change over the past 12 months (30%), or that the issue was likely to become a higher priority in their organization over the next 12 months (29%). Among the minority who were communicating about climate change with external audiences, the most commonly reported were other government agencies (13.6%), the general public (11.2%), elected/appointed government officials (9.6%), news media (4%), and members of the business community (1.6%).

Clearly, public health professionals understand the human health implications of climate change and, to some extent, are already engaged in addressing this problem. However, much more is needed. Public health professionals are uniquely well positioned to explain how the rapidly emerging threats associated with climate change are connected with individual and community health and well-being. By communicating the potential of global climate change to harm human health, and by conveying the potential to improve human health through actions that limit climate change, they can enhance public understanding of the full scope of the problem, and help enable appropriate responses by individuals and communities.

Efforts to Activate Public Health Professionals as Climate Change Communicators

Incorporating the results of our research, we developed a climate change communication primer to serve as a training resource and guide for public health professionals. In conjunction with the California Department of Health, we trained local public health officials to use the primer during two workshops held in Los Angeles and Oakland in November 2010, and in a subsequent webinar held in April 2011. Participants at each workshop included health department directors, public information officers, communications specialists, epidemiologists, and health educators. After completing the workshops, participants were sent an electronic survey instrument to assess the effectiveness of the climate change communication primer. Overall, the primer received positive reviews. Specifically, the respondents overwhelmingly agreed that the primer would be a useful tool for their work and that of their organizations. When asked how the primer could be improved, the respondents indicated that it should be simplified as much as possible and that more information on how to communicate climate change as a human health message should be added. Based on this input from the workshop participants, the primer was finalized and was released nationally in cooperation with the American Public Health Association (APHA), National Association of County and City Health Officials (NACCHO), Association of State and Territorial Health Officials (ASTHO), Centers for Disease Control & Prevention (CDC), and the California Department of Health. Subsequently, a one day "Learning Institute" was offered at the 2011 APHA annual meeting to provide intensive support for public health professionals seeking additional training.

In the primer we make the case that public health professionals are uniquely qualified and professionally obligated to engage the public and other stakeholders in their communities on the health risks posed by climate change and the actions that can be taken to adapt to and manage these risks. We then systematically review a range of strategic and tactical recommendations. These include: those with whom public health professionals should communicating (journalists, bloggers, and community media outlets; decision makers in government, businesses, and NGOs; other professionals whose work is or will be affected by climate change; and the public, especially members of the most vulnerable communities); how to get "the message" right (framing on health; localizing; emphasizing benefits; key messages); and how to get the message out (through internal and external communication; effective partnerships; regional meetings; social media; opinion leaders; public testimony and other means). The primer can be downloaded from: http://www.climatechangecommunication.org/other-resources/health-professionals.

Public health professionals should view their work on climate change as a form of *civic education and engagement*, empowering, enabling, motivating, and educating the public around not just about the technical but also the political and social dimensions of climate change. Importantly, civic education and engagement is as much about informing the public as it is about also informing experts and decision makers. Education should be viewed as a two-way process where experts and decision makers seek input and learn from the public about preferences, needs, insights, and ideas relative to climate change solutions and policy options. There is also a need to recruit and train opinion leaders, highlight new participatory models for gathering and disseminating climate change news, and for investment in deliberative contexts such as public meetings where citizens can learn, debate, and connect (see Nisbet, 2010). With limited budgetary resources in mind, these initiatives are best focused on states, regions, or segments of the public that have the greatest need for information about climate change, either because of their political context and/or because of their vulnerability to specific climate change impacts.

Conclusion

The activities that we describe in this chapter are best considered an exploration of the premise that public health professionals should engage in climate change for a variety of reasons, not the least of which is that climate change represents a profound threat to human health and well-being. Framing theory suggests—and our research supports—the value of public communication that clarifies the public health implications of climate change. Given the magnitude of the public health threat, and the relative lack of action by our nation's leaders to address it, there is a pressing need for further research and development focused on how to motivate and enable our nation's public health leaders to embrace this issue in a manner commensurate with the threat, and the opportunity.

Acknowledgment

This chapter—and all research conducted by Ed Maibach and Matthew Nisbet described herein—was supported by a Robert Wood Johnson Foundation Health Policy Investigator Award to Drs. Maibach & Nisbet.

Recommended Readings

Leiserowitz, A., Maibach, E., Roser-Renouf, C., & Hmielowski, J. D. (2012) *Climate change in the American mind: Americans' global warming beliefs and attitudes in March 2012.* Yale University and George Mason University. New Haven, CT: Yale Project on Climate Change Communication. Available: http://environment.yale.edu/climate/files/Climate-Beliefs-March-2012.pdf

Maibach, E. W., Nisbet, M. C., Baldwin, P. K., Akerlof, K., & Diao, G. (2010). Reframing climate change as a public health issue: An exploratory study of public reactions. *BMC Public Health, 10,* 299–309.

Moser, S., & Dilling, L. (2007). *Creating a climate for change: Communicating climate change and facilitating social change.* Cambridge; New York: Cambridge University Press.

National Institute of Environmental Health Sciences. (2010). *A human health perspective on climate change: A report outlining the research needs on the human health effects of climate change.* Available: http://www.niehs.nih.gov/health/assets/docs_a_e/climatereport2010.pdf

Nisbet, M. C. (2009). Communicating climate change: Why frames matter to public engagement. *Environment, 51,* 12–23.

Additional Resources

http://communicatingscience.aaas.org/Pages/newmain.aspx
www.cdc.gov/climatechange/
www.climatechangecommunication.org/images/files/Six_Americas_June_2010(1).pdf
www.healthcanada.gc.ca
www.ipcc.ch/publications_and_data/publications_ipcc_fourth_assessment_report_wg2_report_impacts_adaptation_and_vulnerability.htm
www.thelancet.com/series/energy-and-health
www.thelancet.com/series/health-and-climate-change
www.niehs.nih.gov/health/assets/docs_a_e/climatereport2010.pdf
http://cred.columbia.edu/guide/pdfs/CREDguide_full-res.pdf

http://healthyamericans.org/reports/environment/TFAHClimateChangeWeb.pdf
http://downloads.globalchange.gov/usimpacts/pdfs/climate-impacts-report.pdf
www.who.int/globalchange/en/
www.who.int/world-health-day/toolkit/report_web.pdf

References

Akerlof, K., et al. (2010). Public perceptions of climate change as a human health risk: Surveys of the United States, Canada and Malta. *International Journal of Environmental Research and Public Health, 7,* 2559–2606.

American Lung Association. (2010). *New data shows "Smart Growth" can cut 140 premature deaths and 105,000 asthma attacks and respiratory symptoms each year.* Available: http://www.lungusa.org/associations/states/california/for-the-media/new-data-shows-smart-growth.html

Anderegg, W. L., Prall, J. W., Harald, R., & Schneider, S. (2010). Expert credibility in climate change. *Proceedings of the National Academy of Sciences, 107,* 12107–12109.

Confalonieri, U., Menne, B., Akhtar, R., Ebi, K. L., Hauengue, M., Kovats, R. S., Revich, B., & Woodward, A. (2007). Human health. In M. L. Parry, O. F. Canziani, J. P. Palutikof, P. J. van der Linden, & C. E. Hanson (Eds.), *Climate change 2007: Impacts, adaptation and vulnerability.* Cambridge: Cambridge University Press, 391–431.

Costello, A., et al. (2009). Managing the health effects of climate change. *Lancet, 373,* 1693–1733.

Doran, P., & Zimmerman, M. K. (2009). Examining scientific consensus on climate change. *EOS, Transactions American Geophysical Union, 90,* 22–23.

Ebi, K. L., et al. (2008). Effects of global change on human health. In J. L. Gamble (Ed.), *Analyses of the effects of global change on human health and welfare and human systems.* Synthesis and Assessment Product 4.6. U.S. Environmental Protection Agency, Washington, DC, 39–87.

Grimmond, S. (2007). Urbanization and global environmental change: Local effects of urban warming. *Geographical Journal, 173,* 83–88.

Gutowski, W. J. (2008). Causes of observed changes in extremes and projections of future changes. In T. R. Karl, G. A. Meehl, C. D. Miller, S. J. Hassol, A. M., Waple, & W. L. Murray (Eds.), *Weather and climate extremes in a changing climate: Regions of focus: North America, Hawaii, Caribbean, and U.S. Pacific Islands.* U.S. Climate Change Science Program, Washington, DC, 81–116.

Hale, J. L., & Dillard, J. P. (1995). Too much, too little, or just right: The role of fear in message design. In E. Maibach & R. L. Parrott (Eds.), *Designing health messages: Perspectives from communication theory and public health* (pp. 65–80). Newbury Park, CA: Sage.

Hornik, R. (2002). *Public health communication: Evidence for behavior change.* Mahwah, NJ: Lawrence Erlbaum Associates.

Intergovernmental Panel on Climate Change. (2007). *Climate change 2007. Impacts, adaptation, and vulnerability.* Cambridge, UK: University Press.

Kunkel, K. E., et al. (2008). Observed changes in weather and climate extremes. In T. R. Karl, G. A. Meehl, C. D. Miller, S. J. Hassol, A. M., Waple, & W. L. Murray (Eds.), *Weather and climate extremes in a changing climate: Regions of focus: North America, Hawaii, Caribbean, and U.S. Pacific Islands*. U.S. Climate Change Science Program, Washington, DC, 35–80.

Leiserowitz, A., Maibach, E., Roser-Renouf, C., & Hmielowski, J. D. (2012) *Climate change in the American Mind: Americans' global warming beliefs and attitudes in March 2012*. Yale University and George Mason University. New Haven, CT: Yale Project on Climate Change Communication. Available: http://environment.yale.edu/climate/files/Climate-Beliefs-March-2012.pdf

Luber, G. E., & Conklin, L. M. (2006). Heat-related deaths: United States, 1999–2003. *Morbidity and Mortality Weekly Report, 55*, 796–798.

Maibach, E. W. (October, 2010). Data collected at the annual meeting of the National Public Health Information Coalition (NPHIC), San Diego, CA.

Maibach, E. W., Abroms, L., & Marosits, M. (2007). Communication and marketing as tools to cultivate the public's health: A proposed "people and places" framework. *BMC Public Health, 7*, 88.

Maibach, E. W., Chadwick, A., McBride, D., Chuk, M., Ebi, K. L., & Balbus, J. (2008). Climate change and local public health in the United States: Preparedness, programs and perceptions of local public health department directors. *PLoS ONE, 3*, e283.

Maibach, E. W., Leiserowitz, A., Roser-Renouf, C., & Mertz, C. K. (2011). Identifying like-minded audiences for global warming public engagement campaigns: An audience segmentation analysis and tool development. *PLoS ONE, 6*, e17571.

Maibach, E. W., Nisbet, M. C., Baldwin, P. K., Akerlof, K., & Diao, G. (2010). Reframing climate change as a public health issue: An exploratory study of public reactions. *BMC Public Health, 10*, 299–309.

Maibach, E. W., Roser-Renouf, C., & Leiserowitz, A. (2009). *Global warming's six Americas 2009: An audience segmentation*. Yale Project on Climate Change: New Haven, CT. Available: http://environment.yale.edu/uploads/6Americas2009.pdf

Maibach, E. W., Steg, L., & Anable, J. (2009). Promoting physical activity and reducing climate change: Opportunities to replace short car trips with active transportation. *Preventive Medicine, 35*, 488–500.

Maibach, E. W., Wilson, K., & Witte, J. (2010). A national survey of news directors about climate change: Preliminary findings. George Mason University. Fairfax, VA: Center for Climate Change Communication. Available: http://www.climatechangecommunication.org/images/files/TV_News_Directors_&_Climate%20Change%281%29.pdf

Monahan, J. (1995). Thinking positively. Using positive affect when designing health messages. In E. Maibach & R. Parrott (Eds). *Designing health messages*. Thousand Oaks, CA: Sage Publications.

Myers, A., Nisbet, M. C., Maibach, E. W., & Leiserowitz, A. (2012). A public health frame arouses hopeful emotions about climate change. *Climatic Change* Research Letters.

National Institute of Environmental Health Sciences. (2010). *A human health perspective on climate change: A report outlining the research needs on the human health effects of cli-*

mate change. Available: http://www.niehs.nih.gov/health/assets/docs_a_e/climatereport2010.pdf

Nisbet, M. C. (2009). Communicating climate change: Why frames matter to public engagement. *Environment, 51*, 12–23.

Nisbet, M. C. (2010, December). *Civic education about climate change: Opinion-leaders, communication infrastructure, and participatory culture.* Paper presented at the National Academies' Climate Change Education Roundtable, Washington, DC.

Nisbet, M. C., Price, S., Pascual-Ferra, P., & Maibach, E. (under review). Communicating the public health relevance of climate change: A news agenda building analysis. *Science Communication.*

Price, V., Nir, L., & Capella, J. N. (2005). Framing public discussion of gay civil unions. *Public Opinion Quarterly, 69*, 179–212.

Price, V., & Tewksbury, D. (1997). News values and public opinion: A theoretical account of media priming and framing. In G. A. Barnett & F. J. Boster (Eds.), *Progress in communication science*, 13, (pp. 173–212). Greenwich, CT: Ablex.

Roser-Renouf, C., Elligers, A., Maibach, E., Colon, J., & Li, J. (2012). *Are we ready? Revisiting public health preparedness for climate change.* National Association of County and City Health Officials.

Sapru, S., Telfer, J., Luber, G., Price, S., & Ryan, C. (2010, August). *Framing climate change in terms of human health effects: Qualitative research study with emerging "green" opinion leaders.* Poster presented at the meeting of the Centers for Disease Control, Atlanta, GA.

Scheufele, D. A. (1999). Framing as a theory of media effects. *Journal of Communication 49*, 103–122.

Scheufele, D. A., & Tewksbury, D. (2007). Framing, agenda setting and priming: The evolution of three media effects models. *Journal of Communication, 57*, 9–20.

Trust for America's health. (2009). *Health problems heat up: Climate change and the public's health.* Available: http://healthyamericans.org/reports/environment/TFAHClimateChangeWeb.pdf

U.S. Global Change Research Program. (2009). *Global climate change impacts in the United States.* Cambridge, UK: University Press.

Witte, K., & Allen, M. (2000). A meta-analysis of fear appeals: Implications for effective public health campaigns. *Health Education & Behavior, 27*, 591–615.

World Health Organization. (2007). *Global surveillance, prevention and control of chronic respiratory diseases: A comprehensive approach.* Available: http://www.who.int/gard/publications/GARD_Manual/en/index.html

World Health Organization. (2009). *Protecting health from climate change: Connecting science, policy and people.* Available: http://whqlibdoc.who.int/publications/2009/9789241598880_eng.pdf

Chapter 12

Integrating the Diffusion of Innovations and Social Marketing for Designing an HIV/AIDS-Prevention Strategy among a Hard-to-Reach Population

Do Kyun Kim, *University of Louisiana at Lafayette*

Introduction

The risk of HIV/AIDS infection has been growing in Louisiana in opposition to the global trend of reduced infection rates as a result of decades of prevention efforts. The latest investigation focusing on the epidemic in Louisiana shows that 18,308 individuals are living with HIV/AIDS and 10,035 among them (55%) are diagnosed with AIDS (Louisiana Public Health Institute, 2010). In particular, the city of Baton Rouge ranked second for HIV/AIDS incidence rate among all metropolitan areas in the U.S., followed by New Orleans, which ranked third. Apparently, it is urgent to respond to the rapidly growing HIV-incidence rate in Louisiana. From the HIV/AIDS prevention aspect, one of the most vulnerable groups in terms of new infection are the members of African-American communities. In 2010, 45% of new diagnoses of HIV infection in the United States appeared among African-Americans, and they accounted for 49% of new AIDS diagnoses (Center for Disease Control and Prevention, 2012). Especially, African-American men who have sex with men (MSM) have been exposed to the greatest risk of HIV infection.

Although the risk of HIV infection among adult African-American MSM has been already well known, the risk associated with *young* African-American MSMs aged 18 to early 20s has been not much revealed mainly because of little social recognition on sexual identity among the young population and their own vulnerability to talk about their sexuality and information disparity. Many other concerns increase the level of alert related to new HIV infection among them, such as heightened sexual activity in youth, longer life expectancy that implies the infected would suffer from the infection for the rest of their lives, prevention information disparity, and little experience with their sexuality itself. Based on these concerns and the urgency of prevention efforts, this study presents an advanced health intervention strategy built upon integration of the diffusion of innovations and social marketing. This can maximize the effectiveness of HIV prevention among the hard-to-reach population, young African-American MSM populations who live in New Orleans, Louisiana. This strategy can also be applied to a diversity of health interventions targeting people with social and cultural differences.

Needs of a New Approach for HIV Prevention among Young African-American MSMs

Situation analysis gives a realistic preview related to a public health problem. First, empirically, young African-American MSMs are regarded as a hard-to-reach population whose culture and sexual activities have not been well investigated yet. Although a large amount of research has been conducted to expand understandings of African-American history and culture, there are few studies focusing on young African-Americans dealing with their homosexuality. In this information absence about young African-American MSMs, the high rates of HIV infection in Louisiana are now threatening their lives.

The lifestyle of young people in the 21st century is more open to sexual activities as the rising number of incidences of unplanned pregnancy and less stigma on premarital sex show nowadays. In addition, more experimental sexual activities are publicly discussed and personally attempted with less stigma, and risky sexual behaviors that may cause sexually transmitted diseases (STD) as well as HIV infection seem to be more prevalent among younger generations than older as the increasing number of STDs is reported. These risky sexual activities embedded in the young generation's lifestyle also make health professionals pay more attention to their sexual activities.

Information abundance can be an obstacle. The rapid development of communication technologies enables the public to be exposed to uncontrollably ample information about the topics of their interests. In terms of HIV prevention, the public can get accurate information very easily. However, they can also be exposed to inaccurate information as well. Information abundance may create obstacles mainly in two ways: information immunization and exposure to risky behaviors. Information immunization refers to the tendency of people to ignore important information due to prevalence of look-a-like information and a high frequency of information delivered. Sexual activities are already one of the most frequently discussed topics in the media as well as among the public; therefore, information about sexual activities, regardless of its accuracy, is overly abundant. Communication technologies also greatly contribute to the dissemination of information on sexual activities. Exposed to such vast amounts of information on sexual activities, the young populations' information-filtering ability becomes weakened and, therefore, they become insensitive to important messages that they should receive or simply ignore all the messages.

Information about sexual activities is not all related to disease prevention, but often contains information about risky behaviors. Information about new, but risky ways of sexual activities could stimulate young people's sexual arousal and potentially lead them to experiment with undesirable sexual activities they know of from the media. Such information is, in fact, easily accessible through any means of communication nowadays.

Coupled with these empirical obstacles, there are some theoretical obstacles in designing HIV prevention programs. Most of all, other than psychological counseling, few theories focus on an individualized intervention that concerns not a group of people as a whole, but each individual in the subject group. Whereas HIV infection is a very individual issue mostly related to personal sexual practices, the majority of HIV prevention interventions have blindly used mass communication strategies that rely on not individualized, but generalized or standardized information delivered to a mass public by mass media, such as TV, radio, and bulletin boards. Although mass communication strategies using mainly media channels may affect the target audiences' awareness, a higher awareness does not necessarily induce behavior change (Kim, Chikombero, & Moroka, 2011).

Maintaining sustainability is another task for scholars and practitioners who design HIV prevention interventions to consider. Compared with a short-term effect measured soon after conducting an intervention, sustainability of an intervention over a longer period of time has not been well studied mainly due to limited research funding on that issue. In addition, as time goes on, it is very hard to control contamination effects which make it hard to measure the effects of the intervention. Responding to these empirical and theoretical demands, the integration of diffusion of innovations and social marketing is highly suggested to overcome the weaknesses of existing interventions often designed with a single theory or perspective.

Integrating Diffusion of Innovations and Social Marketing

The design of a HIV prevention intervention among young African-American MSMs requires multifaceted considerations to be successful. Theoretically and empirically, the intervention should investigate their unique culture, behavioral attributes, patterns of communication, and socio-economic surroundings, as well as health literacy. In addition, the intervention should also consider the types and amount of resources available to facilitate the intervention. Given these considerations, this study introduces and demonstrates an intervention design based on the integration of diffusion of innovations and social marketing for HIV prevention among the hard-to-reach population.

Social marketing (SM) is based on the business marketing strategies which consider target populations as consumers of a product (Prue & Daniel, 2006). SM includes important features: First, it is a resource-oriented strategy. In other words, the design of an SM campaign is mainly based upon the availability of resources—what the campaign can utilize—at a given situation and time. Second, SM is based on the 4Ps which are Product (what the campaign offers for disease prevention), Price (monetary and non-monetary cost for the target individuals to pay), Place (where to place the product), and Promotion (strategy for dissemination of awareness and the product). Third, an SM campaign mostly uses mass communication channels to expose messages or practices to as many audience members as possible in a short period of time. Therefore, the messages disseminated are more standardized messages instead of personalized ones because they are usually designed with concerns more for the public than each individual within the target populations.

The theory of diffusion of innovation (DOI) investigates "a process in which an innovation is communicated through certain channel over time among the members of a social system" (Rogers, 2003, p. 5). An innovation in DOI is anything that is perceived as new by an individual, including a product, information, a program, a practice, or an idea. In the health communication context, an innovation is what the health intervention tries to deliver for a target population, such as information, messages, practices, and programs. The diffusion of innovations is more likely to be fast if an individual perceives an innovation as relatively advantageous, easy to use, compatible with previous experiences and values, often observed, and trialable. Another determinant for the innovation diffusion in addition to the innovation's already given characteristics is the diffusion *strategy* that is purposively designed by health intervention professionals with an analysis of potential adopters' decision patterns including their lifestyle, culture, past experience, and the level of certain individuals to others. Therefore, while the past diffusion studies usually investigated the previous diffusion patterns of innovations (see Figure 1), recent DOI studies have applied the accumulated diffusion knowledge to design, implement, and evaluate health interventions.[1] Although there are many similarities with SM, DOI has developed a more specific strategy that focuses on the use of individual influence delivered through informal opinion leaders among the target populations.

Informal opinion leaders vs. popular opinion leaders

It may be questionable if an informal opinion leader based diffusion strategy is the same as the popular opinion leader strategy that has been developed mainly by Jeffery Kelly (e.g., 1991, 1992, and 1997), who has used it for HIV/AIDS prevention campaigns since the early 1990s. There are some similarities and some differences. The popular opinion leader strategy selects opinion leaders based on their popularity. People with popularity are mostly celebrity figures in their groups, and that attribute may be important especially to catch people's attention. It is undeniable that they have certain influence on people's attitudes and behavior changes. However, it is also possible that most lay target populations may not be substantially connected to them because they are more likely to have a different lifestyle, socioeconomic status, education level, and level of communication comprehension than other target populations. When target populations perceive these discrepancies between popular opinion leaders and themselves, the effectiveness of a popular opinion leader strategy can be reduced.

In comparison with popular opinion leaders, informal opinion leaders are those who seem unaware of their influence through communication with others, but are trusted by others due to their friendliness, closeness, and expertise. They are very approachable, communicable, willing to take care of and provide advice for others, and often popular as well. Among many, the most unique characteristic of informal opinion leaders is communicability so that an individual who needs advice on a certain issue can easily and comfortably ask an informal opinion leader's opinions and experiences. Based on this characteristic, Dearing (2010) often describes people's communication networks with their informal opinion leaders as advice-seeking networks.

In terms of selecting opinion leaders for the diffusion of innovations, strategies using popular opinion leaders and informal opinion leaders also show notable differences. A popular opinion leader strategy selects seemingly influential people by asking the informants who know the target population very well and/or observing popularity. However, an informal opinion

---

1 For more detailed information, read Dearing & Kim (2007).

leader strategy employs a more sophisticated process to select opinion leaders, using network analysis as introduced in Chapter 2. For most cases, selecting informal opinion leaders takes more effort and careful analysis of network data than observing individual popularity. However, informal opinion leaders selected by the network analysis tend to have more substantial, stronger, and sustainable influence in changing target populations' attitude and, particularly, behavior change.

The influence of informal opinion leaders in changing their followers' behavior has been supported by the social cognitive theory. The social cognitive theory (Bandura, 2004) has proven that people's behavior change can be caused by mimicking what they observed, which is not necessarily based upon a psychological process or reasoning. This somewhat irrational, but simple mimicking of behavior induces behavior change, and this informality of behavior change has been referred to as the foundational mechanism of how informal opinion leaders can influence others' behavior changes (Rogers, 2003). Although some theories of rational choice can explain behavior changes induced by rational judgment and acceptance of the presented behavior, as seen in the theory of reasoned action (Ajzen & Fishbein, 1980), the major advantage of an informal opinion leader strategy is that the strategy embraces the likelihood of routine, informal, and somewhat irrational nature of human behavior change. Table 1 summarizes the major differences between informal opinion leader strategy and popular opinion leader strategy.

Table 1. Differences between informal opinion leader and popular opinion leader strategies

Informal opinion leader strategy	Popular opinion leader strategy
Close & stronger influence on behavior change	Distant influence, but effective for information diffusion
More specific influence visualized through individual communication network analysis	More overall influence (for evaluation only)
Sustainable / stable leadership	Popularity may fade out over time
Several check points of leadership (at both implementation + evaluation)	Single check point of leadership (at evaluation only)

Why combine DOI and SM

The diffusion of innovations (DOI) and social marketing (SM) have their own features and strengths. First of all, the informal opinion leader-based diffusion strategy using the influence of interpersonal communication is a better determinant for behavioral change, while the SM strategy using primarily mass media is quicker for information diffusion to the mass population. Second, DOI is a theory that presents firm principles and rules, while SM is usually known as a more practical approach which can be easily manipulated, depending on availability of resources and other external conditions. Therefore, an intervention based on DOI is regarded as a theory-based intervention, while SM is usually an evidence-based one. Third, DOI strategizes the informal opinion leadership as a means of innovation adoption, while SM mostly utilizes formal opinion leadership, such as authorities' endorsements. Fourth, DOI tends to be more tailored to an individualized strategy due to its nature of using interpersonal communication, but SM often uses standardized mass communication strategies. Related to these attributes, while a DOI strategy using interpersonal communication may be slower in the spread of health information, an SM using mass communication channels disseminates information more rapidly. Finally, while SM campaigns often cost more because they often include public events with promotional materials or collaboration with high-cost mass communication channels, the use of informal opinion leaders is very cost-effective and more sustainable due to their continuous communication with their followers. Based on these strengths and differences between SM and DOI, the health intervention that integrates these two strategies can offset the weaknesses of both strategies and maximize the effectiveness of the health intervention (Dearing et al., 1996).

Strategic Integration: A Case for HIV Prevention among the Young African-American MSM Population in New Orleans

This case is based on a health intervention grant proposal designed in collaboration between the Louisiana State Department of Health and Hospital and the author of this chapter. As addressed previously, metropolitan cities in Louisiana encounter incremental problems with HIV infection. In this situation, our task was to design an HIV-prevention intervention, targeting the young black MSM population in New Orleans. The target group was specified by age, such as post-high school ages from 18 to 30. Based on this general goal with a specific target population, our focus was on establishing not only a short-term effect, but a more sustainable health intervention for a long-term effect. With these goals in mind, we designed an intervention plan that integrated the influence of informal opinion leaders among the target population and social marketing partnering with influential external agencies preferably located in the areas where African-American communities have been established in New Orleans.

Designing a health intervention for this population in New Orleans requires careful audience and situation analyses. First of all, New Orleans has a special social atmosphere celebrating many festivals and events, such as Mardi Gras and Southern Decadence. This festival culture certainly provokes more alcohol consumption, illegal drugs, and unsafe sex among the target population. In addition, it is more likely that younger people have less concern or awareness of health risks simply because of their confidence in their own health and less experience of illness, whereas they tend to attempt high-risk behaviors for more pleasure. The economic hardship in Louisiana has been another obstacle to supply sufficient resources to promote public health. It is also nationally known that the educational level in Louisiana has been low, ranking as one of the bottom third of states (United States Education Dashboard, n.d.).

Another interesting factor in Louisiana is the religious, mainly Catholic, influence in society. In terms of the public health issue related to sexual activities, the numbers of STDs and unplanned pregnancy cases have been very high over the years in Louisiana, although risky sexual behaviors or premarital sexual relationships violate their Catholic beliefs and traditions. Some statistics show the seriousness of sexual health problems in Louisiana. For instance, Louisiana ranked 1st among 50 states in terms of P&S syphilis infection and ranked 5th in Chlamydia infection (Center for Disease Control and Prevention, 2010). Unplanned pregnancy in Louisiana has always ranked much higher than the average in both teen pregnancy (ages 15–19) and total unplanned pregnancy (The National Campaign, 2011). These very high sexual health risks, including unsafe and uncontrolled sexual activities, imply that Catholicism which has been the dominant religion in Louisiana has not been effective in reducing the number of incidences. Ironically, because of Catholicism promoting pro-life and family values, the discussion about sexual activities including not only public information, but also sex education in school has been very limited. As a side-effect of this ambivalence between religion and public health reality, the public have placed more value on new born babies, than the need for open discourses on their safe, controlled, and responsible sexual activities.

This unique religious influence in the Louisiana communities has also created unprecedented regional and social limitations in designing a health intervention as well as social movements regarding HIV/AIDS prevention among the MSM population and youth. Due to the religious reluctance toward discussing sexual activities and education, issues related to the gay community, especially about their sexual behaviors, have rarely been discussed in any social and political sectors in Louisiana. In addition, due to a high level of social stigma on homosexuality, no one wants to set the issue as a public, media, or policy agenda, which makes the young African-American MSM population a more hard-to-reach or socially hidden group in Louisiana. Accordingly, there is little data or knowledge about our target population. This reality led our intervention design to integrate diffusion of innovations utilizing the influence of interpersonal communication and social marketing partnering with external agencies and resources to combat HIV among the young African-American MSM population in New Orleans.

As two strategies are integrated, specific advantages of each strategy can be merged into one project dealing with the hard-to-reach population. Particularly, since the target population is a hard-to-reach population with a high stigma in the Catholic society, an opinion leader based interpersonal communication strategy was expected to facilitate the diffusion of information and safe sex practices to our target population individually. A social marketing strategy partnered with a recognizable external agency actively participating in public health programs, such as Walgreens—a nationwide pharmacy that also provides household goods—was considered to provide important services (e.g., HIV testing) at convenient places for our target population.

Harnessing informal opinion leaders

In order to design an intervention using informal opinion leaders among the young African-American MSM population in New Orleans, the following steps were considered:

1. Identifying informal opinion leaders by communication network analysis: Since the number of our target population is apparently large simply because New Orleans is the largest city in Louisiana and is the place

where one of the largest groups of MSM in the nation exists, how to initiate the network data collection becomes the main task in designing this part of the project. However, as other metropolitan cities in the United States, New Orleans already has multiple HIV testing centers where MSM who think they are at risk can get tested. Therefore, the clients of the testing centers can be the initial group of people who can participate in the investigation of communication networks among our target population. The communication network data collection can be extended from the testing centers' clients to their communication partners.

The network data can be collected by a simple question asked of the center's clients, such as "From whom do you get advice about your relationship with your partner in your daily lives?" and, based on their answers, the investigators can contact those who have provided advice to the clients. This data collection can be repeated until the investigator can clearly identify some key individuals in the communication networks in which the clients reside. Multiple data collection methods can be employed in this network data collection process; these include onsite surveys, mailings and online surveys, interpersonal communication with clients and their partners, and phone calls. This procedure may look much like a snowball data collection method because it starts with a relatively small group of people, the test centers' clients, and gets bigger as the data collection proceeds. (See chapter 2 of this book for learning how to specifically analyze communication network maps and identify informal opinion leaders).

2. Training informal opinion leaders (OLs): After identifying informal opinion leaders, a training session can be offered for the OLs, those who are trusted by other followers who can listen to their advice and adopt their behaviors in their daily lives. The contents of the training may not be much different from general HIV/AIDS prevention trainings. However, an important component of this training is firm recognition of their influence as informal opinion leaders. Since most of them may not fully recognize their influence in their informal communication networks, such firm recognition grows their leadership and pride as leaders of important health intervention, which consciously and unconsciously plays a role in their communication with others. Therefore, this training opportunity should remark on a clear recognition on their leadership and appreciate them as the most important people in the intervention.

3. Supporting OLs' information distribution by communicating with others and monitoring their activities: in addition to the firm recognition of their leadership role, which was emphasized from the first training session, continuous supply of information materials (e.g., brochures, fliers, and promotional items) and other prevention materials (e.g., condoms) should be given to them to help promote their active communication with their followers. If they are able to have a small group meeting, a small amount of monetary support can be also considered.

    It is expected that their communication activities may become fewer and inactive over time. Therefore, after the first training, other follow-up sessions can be offered to monitor their activities, share their experiences, and provide more means of communication. The follow-up sessions can continue their willingness to participate in this project, remind themselves as selected opinion leaders, and provide a chance to modify communication strategies between OLs and their followers, if necessary. In the follow-up sessions, the intervention designer should carefully listen to the OLs' experience about their communication with others while disseminating HIV prevention messages, analyze their motivation level and communicative initiatives, and also use the data for the future sessions as well as modifying the current project.

4. Evaluation: The evaluation of the OL strategy should investigate several outputs including 1) how many people the OLs communicate with, 2) if OLs have seen any other informal opinion leaders emerge while spreading information to the target population, 3) how the initial communication networks can be drawn and, then, modified as more people are contacted by the trained OLs, 4) if there are effective and efficient communication channels found for message delivery and behavior change promotion, 5) how much information the trained OLs retain from the training sessions after a certain period of time, 6) how their knowledge was developed by the follow-up sessions, and 7) how this communicative process of information sharing and promotion of behavior change can be implemented in the target population's daily lives after the project ends. In particular, since sustainability is a core and specific goal in this project, it is important for health intervention to keep contact with the identified informal opinion leaders.

Social marketing activities partnered with Walgreens

The social marketing part of this project considers partnering with a major external agency, Walgreens stores, that are located in the New Orleans neighborhoods with the highest HIV prevalence. This partnership can increase access to HIV testing and contribute to the identification of previously undiagnosed HIV infections among the target population. Existing HIV testing locations at local community-based organizations and Parish Health Units can also perform HIV counseling and testing. The locations, days, and times for HIV testing would be promoted and advertised by existing social marketing health campaigns and communication networks identified through this project. This project considers using the National HIV Testing Day events that are currently being planned with Kaiser and Walgreens as a kick off to this project. It was also considered to provide $5.00 Walgreens gift cards to individuals who arrive at the selected stores for HIV screening. This will incentivize the targeted communities to actually go and get tested and minimize any disruption to normal store operations and enhance the relationship with Walgreens, because people would be encouraged to shop at Walgreens in addition to getting tested for HIV. Overall, it is important that this project follows all CDC guidelines for providing HIV Prevention Counseling and Rapid Testing, including HIV Prevention Counseling, Rapid Testing and Referral Services Quality Assurance and Procedural Protocol.

Louisiana has a unique, state-administered public hospital system, comprised of ten hospitals located in the major metropolitan areas of the state which generally provide care to underserved and uninsured residents. As of 2012, each hospital has an established HIV clinic (Ryan White Part C funded HIV specialty care) and 57% of persons living with HIV (n=6,560) who had at least one medical care visit during 2010 attended one of these state administered public hospitals for their HIV care. These clinics are a critical component in the continuum of care for people living with HIV.

Once an individual is newly diagnosed with HIV at any of the Walgreens sites, he/she will be referred to the nearest HIV clinic for follow-up and treatment. There are two other Ryan White funded HIV specialty clinics in the New Orleans area which clients will also be given information about and referred to appropriately. Louisiana state law and the Louisiana standards for *HIV prevention counseling, rapid testing and referral services* (CTRS) protocol for HIV Counseling and Testing sites operating in Louisiana require that people testing HIV positive are given referrals to appropriate HIV medical care. Therefore, this project should follow Louisiana state law and CTRS protocol and ensure that all clients who test positive are referred to HIV care. In addition to making referrals to HIV care, the Walgreens Project staff should be required to follow up with positive clients to determine whether or not the referral was successful (e.g., the client attended his/her first HIV medical appointment) and to assist in overcoming any barriers that make the client unable to attend his/her first HIV care appointment.

This project also planned to use *disease intervention specialists* (DIS). DIS are to follow up with the clients and ensure that they know their HIV-positive status. They also refer the HIV positive individuals to appropriate medical care and determine whether or not their clients attend their subsequent medical appointment, in additional to providing routine HIV Partner Services that aims to inform people of their potential risk for HIV and refer them to health care facilities (Louisiana Office of Public Health, n.d) . Finally, this project is based on the surveillance system to monitor the effectiveness of linkage-to-care activities for HIV-positive clients. Table 2 explains the flow of this procedure.

Table 2. Flow Chart of Integrating Testing in this Project

- Client signs in near the pharmacy area and is assigned a number
  ↓
- HIV tester escorts client into confidential multi-purpose room for testing
  ↓
- HIV Prevention Counseling and Rapid Testing is administered
  ↓
- Client returns to waiting area near pharmacy with an ID number to wait for test
  ↓
- Client is called by given ID number when test is ready and escorted back into the multi-purpose room
  ↓
- Client is given test result. → If negative, session is over and client is given $5.00 Walgreens gift card
  ↘

  If positive, confirmatory testing is administered. Referral and follow up options are discussed. Client is given $5.00 Walgreens gift card.

The overall evaluation of this integrative intervention using both the diffusion of innovations and social marketing campaign consists of mainly two components: 1) increasing number of clients being tested as a result of recruitment of informal opinion leaders by the communication network analysis and social marketing campaigns, and 2) predicted increase of proposed tests, which is based on the analysis of the effect of this intervention. This intervention anticipated 1,500 people recruited and tested in a twelve-month period.

Conclusion

In summary, there are multiple advantages of the project integrating the diffusion of innovations and social marketing. First, this project should be able to reach a hard-to-reach target population mainly by the interpersonal communication and convenience of HIV testing, which is expected to result in greater effectiveness on HIV/AIDS prevention for a hard-to-reach population. Second, due to the sustainable nature of informal leadership and partnership with a notable external agency, the project is expected to generate a higher degree of sustainability. Third, using informal opinion leaders who communicate with their followers in the target population and their existing influence in their communication networks, the informal opinion leader based health intervention can be very cost-effective and applicable over a series of similar and different health interventions. Fourth, the integration of individualized and public strategies can generate a social synergy effect which affects not only public health promotion, but also lowering social stigma on people with HIV in a particular culture, the African-American community, having a high level of social stigma. Finally, since this project is a more relational and communicative intervention, it can be easily applicable to other projects focusing on communicative or relational health risks, such as STDs and unplanned pregnancy.

The author thanks Mr. Roger Schimberg, former staff of the Louisiana Department of Health and Hospitals for his collaboration in the process of conceptualizing this health intervention design.

Recommended Readings

Dearing, J. W., Maibach, E., & Buller, D. (2006). A convergent diffusion and social marketing approach for disseminating proven approaches to physical activity promotion. *American Journal of Preventive Medicine, 31*, S11–S23.

Dearing, J. W., Rogers, E. M., Meyer, G., Casey, M. K., Rao, N., Campo, S., Henderson, G. M. (1996). Social marketing and diffusion-based strategies for communicating with unique populations: HIV prevention in San Francisco. *Journal of Health Communication, 1*, 343–364.

Kim, D-K., Chikombero, M., & Moroka, T. (2013). Innate health threat among a visibly hidden immigrant group: Field data analysis for HIV/AIDS prevention among Zimbabwean workers in Botswana. *Journal of Health Communication, 18*, 146–59.

References

Ajzen, I., & Fishbein, M. (1980). *Understanding attitudes and predicting social behavior.* Englewood Cliffs, NJ: Prentice-Hall.

Bandura, A. (2004). Health promotion by social cognitive means. *Health Education & Behavior, 31*, 143–164.

Center for Disease Control and prevention. (2010). NCHHSTP State Profiles. Retrieve from http://www.cdc.gov/nchhstp/stateprofiles/usmap.htm on September 2, 2012

Center for Disease Control and prevention. (2012). HIV surveillance by race/ ethnicity (through 2010). Retrieved from http://www.cdc.gov/hiv/topics/surveillance/resources/slides/race-ethnicity/index.htm on September 2, 2012.

Dearing, J. W., & Kim, D-K. (2008). Diffusion of information and innovation. *International encyclopedia of communication.* Blackwell Publishing.

Dearing, J. W., Maibach, E., & Buller, D. (2006). A convergent diffusion and social marketing approach for disseminating proven approaches to physical activity promotion. American Journal of Preventive Medicine, 31, S11–S23.

Dearing, J. W., Rogers, E. M., Meyer, G., Casey, M. K., Rao, N., Campo, S., Henderson, G. M. (1996). Social marketing and diffusion-based strategies for communicating with unique populations: HIV prevention in San Francisco. *Journal of Health Communication, 1*, 343–364.

Kelly, J.A., Lawrence, J.S., Stevenson, Y.L., Hauth, A.C., Kalichman, S.C., Diaz, Y.E., Brasfield, T. L., Koob, J. J., & Morgan, M. G. (1992). Community AIDS/HIV risk reduction: The effects of endorsements by popular people in three cities. *American Journal of Public Health, 82,* 1483–1489.

Kelly, J.A., Murphy, D.A., Sikkema, K.J., McAuliffe, T.L., Roffman, R.A., Soloman, L.J., Winett, R.A., Kalichman, S.C., and the Community HIV Prevention Research Collaborative (1997). Randomized, controlled, community-level HIV-prevention intervention for sexual-risk behavior among homosexual men in US cities. *The Lancet, 350,* 1500–1505.

Kelly, J.A., St. Lawrence, J., Diaz, Y. E., Stevenson, L.Y., Hauth, A.C., Brasfield, T.L., Kalichman, S.C., Smith, J.E., & Andrew, M.E. (1991). HIV risk behavior reduction following intervention with key opinion leaders of population: An experimental analysis. *American Journal of Public Health, 81,* 168–171.

Kim, D-K., Chikombero, M., & Moroka, T. (2013). Innate health threat among a visibly hidden immigrant group: Field data analysis for HIV/AIDS prevention among Zimbabwean workers in Botswana. *Journal of Health Communication, 18,* 146–59.

Louisiana Office of Public Health (n.d.), Internet Partner Services. Retrieved from http://new.dhh.louisiana.gov/index.cfm/page/1104 on Feb. 20th, 2013.

Prue, C. E., & Daniel, K. L. (2006). Social marketing: Planning before conceiving preconception care. *Maternal & Child Health Journal*, S10, 79–84.

Rogers, E. M. (2003). *Diffusion of innovations (5th ed.)*. New York: Free Press.

The National Campaign. (2011). 50 states and national comparisons. Retrieved from http://www.thenationalcampaign.org/state-data/state-comparisions.asp on September 2, 2012.

United States Education Dashboard. (n.d.). Averaged freshmen graduation rates of public secondary schools. Retrieved from http://dashboard.ed.gov/statecomparison.aspx?i=e&id=2&wt=0 on September 2, 2012.

Community Participatory Design

Chapter 13

Community Participatory Design of Health Communication Interventions

Linda Neuhauser & S. Leonard Syme,
University of California, Berkeley
Gary L. Kreps, *George Mason University*

Introduction: Issues with Health Communication Programs

Health communication is "the central social process in the provision of health care delivery and the promotion of public health" (Kreps 1988, p. 238). A half-century of health communication research demonstrates its many important influences on promoting public health (Neuhauser & Kreps, 2003). However, research also shows that many communication efforts to promote health either fail to meet their goals, or have only modest effects (Snyder, Hamilton, Mitchell, Kiwanuka-Tondo, Fleming-Milici, & Proctor, (2004). A U.S. Institute of Medicine report (Smedley and Syme, 2003) concluded: "Behavioral and social interventions offer great promise to reduce disease morbidity and mortality, but as yet their potential to improve the public's health has been relatively poorly tapped."

The uneven results of health communication programs have been frustrating to many researchers, practitioners and policymakers and have sparked much reflection and debate about how to do better. Scholars have commented on a range of issues from weaknesses in underlying theoretical frameworks to inadequate design processes (Neuhauser & Kreps, 2003). Traditional health communication approaches are typically based on solid scientific evidence about actions that people can take to improve their health. However, such programs have tended to focus on one-way design and delivery of generic, expert messages that are not specifically relevant to people's personal characteristics or their social settings (Neuhauser & Kreps, 2010). Frequently, health communication efforts are not well adapted to people's literacy levels, languages, cultures, disabilities, social networks or other characteristics. This lack of user relevance may also explain why it has been so difficult to extend health communication efforts that have been successful in one population to have positive outcomes among others. These problems are often magnified when we attempt to replicate programs across cultures and across countries. A further issue is that health communication programs must not only show efficacy in a research project, but must also be effective, affordable and sustainable at large-scale levels to have a population impact. It is often difficult to translate approaches that researchers have designed in controlled, well-supported studies into feasible "real-world" programs when practitioners and policymakers have not been involved in the initial study.

Value of Participatory Design to Improve Health Communication

A growing body of research suggests that health communication programs are more successful if they are designed with the close participation of the intended beneficiaries and stakeholders (Hesse & Schneiderman, 2007; Neuhauser, 2001). Studies show that such programs are usually more relevant to the individual needs and social contexts of the users, and are also more feasible to implement, sustain and expand. Participatory, or user-centered design, has been defined as "an approach to the assessment, design and development of technological and organizational systems that places a premium on the active involvement of...potential or current users of the system in design and decision-making processes" (CSPR, 2000). Participatory design techniques originated in the latter half of the 20th century and are actively used in architecture, engineering, computer science, information and other technical fields.

Although participatory design is not yet the norm in health communication programs, such approaches are becoming more widely used. In particular, participatory design is now a core process in developing eHealth communication (Kreps & Neuhauser, 2010)—reflecting the strong influence of this approach in computer and informatics fields. However, even in eHealth communication, participatory design processes are not always rigorously used to understand and relate to people's specific needs and contexts (Neuhauser & Kreps; 2011).

In our view, a key problem is that researchers, practitioners and policymakers do not have enough detailed guidance about how to do participatory design that gets to the deep personal and contextual levels needed for successful communication. The purpose of this chapter is to describe the rationale, theoretical foundation, and specific methods to use participatory design for successful health communication.

Theoretical Framework for Participatory Design

Multiple theoretical models provide guidance about participatory design of health communication programs. Classic health behavior models—such as the Health Belief Model, the Learning and Conditioning model, and the Transtheoretical model—that have been widely used to guide health promotion interventions, focus primarily on individual behavioral factors rather than on important socio-cultural mediators (Neuhauser & Kreps, 2011). During the past 20 years, there has been a shift toward a "social ecological" paradigm that acknowledges the powerful social, institutional, and cultural contexts that influence people's health (Stokols, 2000). Ecological models also emphasize "systems thinking" which posit that it is important to understand and interact with all components of a system to impact health. Applying these models to research and practice requires inputs from many disciplinary perspectives across multiple sectors. For example, ecological frameworks encompass many disciplines related to health, such as public health, medicine, sociology, anthropology, policy and others. They also comprise many societal levels including individuals, families, institutions, media, and government.

By definition, a key aspect of these models is that they guide researchers and practitioners to use collaborative processes that tap into professional expertise in many professions and engage with people at many levels of society (rather than just with individuals). A related trend is the emergence of "action research" and "participatory action research" models that guide researchers, practitioners, policymakers and the lay public to collaborate on health research and programs (Stokals, 2006). Community-based participatory research (CBPR) is a popular model that emphasizes equitable and multi-step processes to engage community and academic partners in research and practice (Minkler & Wallerstein, 2008).

Design sciences models provide an important new source of guidance about participatory design in the health area. Design science is the scientific study of design initiated in the 1960s (Fuller & McHale, 1963). Design sciences, or "sciences of the artificial" are concerned "not with how things are, but with how they might be" (Simon, 1996). They are considered one of three major categories of the systematic study of knowledge (epistemology) that also include natural sciences and human sciences (Gregor, 2009). Design sciences include architecture, information systems, business and other disciplines that emphasize the process of creating something new. Such models focus on the challenges of simultaneously defining problems, studying them, and developing solutions. They include guidance for continuous evaluation and revision, rather than the traditional "before and after" approach of tradition health research. Design sciences models provide unique guidance to health research and practice that often involve complex and context-specific challenges.

Design sciences models guide researchers and practitioners to focus on engaging multiple users and stakeholders to iteratively define problems, and carefully develop, test and revise solutions over time. This process has been highly successful in developing commercial products like smart phones and tablet computers and we suggest that its participatory techniques can be equally valuable in researching health issues and designing effective programs—as they have been in the emerging eHealth field.

Six-Step Model of Participatory Design for Health Communication

We propose the following model of participatory design for health communication and other health promotion programs. This approach was developed by the Health Research for Action center at the University of California, Berkeley School of Public Health with input from many advisors and institutions, including the Center for Health and Risk Communication at George Mason University. It has guided the development and testing of many health communication programs in the U.S. and globally of the past two decades. The main steps in this process are the following:

1. Identify audiences and stakeholders and set up an advisory committee.

As we noted earlier, traditional health communication approaches have often been overly generic, rather than adapted to the specific needs of diverse groups. A key process at the outset of developing health communication programs is to define the sub-groups that are intended to benefit from the initiative. Another key step is to define not just the "end users," but also the many stakeholders that will be involved in researching, implementing, funding, and publicizing this work. Such stakeholders may include academics from multiple disciplines, health and social service providers, policymakers and staff at many government levels, foundation or private sector funders, the media, and perhaps even the general public who may influence program sustainability by voting in elections. It is often useful to establish advisory group(s) made up of members of end-users and stakeholders to advise the program research, design, evaluation and revision.

2. Conduct formative work with audiences/stakeholders using varied participatory methods.

Once the diverse end-users and stakeholders have been identified and engaged in advisory group meetings, the project team (that includes research and practice expertise) should conduct formative research to identify the major issues from the perspectives of diverse end-users and stakeholders. A literature review, of course, provides an important understanding of the state of scientific knowledge about the health issue of interest. It is also helpful for the project team to inventory existing health communication strategies and resources relevant to the planned initiative. Focus groups, in-depth interviews, case studies, surveys and other qualitative and quantitative methods can be used to gain a deeper understanding of the problems and proposed solutions from intended beneficiaries and stakeholders. One activity that we suggest is to conduct in-depth interviews with all members of the advisory committee(s) and present those data at a follow-up meeting. This helps build "ownership" as well as the formative research base.

3. Draft health communication resources and plans, adhering to principles of health literacy/cultural competency.

After users and stakeholders have defined issues and proposed health communication strategies, the project team (guided by its advisors) can begin to develop the first prototype of the health communication resource(s) and implementation plans. That initial prototype should be developed with careful attention to principles of health literacy and cultural competency so that it will be relevant to the intended beneficiary groups' literacy levels, languages, cultures, disabilities/abilities, and other needs and preferences.

We suggest several strategies to draft text materials that meet health literacy principles. One approach is to estimate the reading levels of the intended end-users. In the U.S., the average adult is estimated to read between a 6th to 8th grade level and 20% read below this level. Therefore, aiming for about a 6th grade reading level (and testing the readability level) is considered a good goal for text-based information for general American populations. However, reading levels vary greatly by country. In addition to readability, many other factors affect users' comprehension of and engagement with text-based materials. These factors are often grouped into "clear communication" or "plain language" design criteria (i.e., see: Neuhauser and Paul, 2011; US Dept of Health and Human Services: *Quick Guide to Health Literacy* and *Simply Put*). For example, the Suitability Assessment of Materials (SAM) tool provides a useful checklist to create and test easier-to-use communications (see: Neuhauser & Paul, 2011). The SAM test identifies 22 criteria related to organization of content, font size, behavioral modeling, etc. Web-based materials require navigating information with computers or other devices. The U.S. National Cancer Institute provides useful Web-usability guidance for developers on: http:www.usability.gov.

These health communication criteria also specify designing communication that is culturally appropriate for the intended users. Suggestions to create culturally relevant communication include illustrating members of the cultural groups in photos, illustrations or videos, reflecting sensitivity to cultural issues and values in the content, adapting (rather than literally translating) materials linguistically, and paying close attention to access and functional needs ("disabilities") among the intended user groups.

4. Test and iteratively revise communication prototypes and implementation with intended users and stakeholders, until these audiences approve them.

When communication developers draw on the formative research findings and use the aforementioned design principles, the initial prototype is likely to be of good quality. However, because such research and design principles are rough guidelines and cannot encompass all the factors that make health information comprehensible and motivating, it is critical to test the draft communication with the intended users and stakeholders.

Many user-centered design techniques, including focus groups, individual interviews, and usability testing can be employed to test the draft communication. *Usability testing* refers to a broad range of structured methods to engage users in designing communication materials (Nielsen, 2000). Usability tests are often one-on-one situations that involve a tester asking a user to read and navigate a draft document or web site (see *www.usability.gov*), accomplish specific tasks related to it, and to recommend changes to the text, format, and graphics. The draft is then revised with participant input.

Usability testing should continue with sub-groups of users until "saturation" is reached, meaning that additional tests no longer elicit major new issues or recommendations. The project team then examines the detailed results of the usability tests (and focus groups or other methods, if used) and determines changes to make to the prototype. After changes are made, the team conducts another round of usability tests and/or focus groups. This iterative process continues until the user groups are satisfied with the communication. In our experience, 3–5 iterations are usually sufficient if the first prototype is of good quality and the usability testing is well done.

During this step, the research team also obtains input on the prototype from the stakeholder groups either through in-depth interviews or focus groups. If an advisory group has been established, that is a ready-made source of stakeholders. We recommend seeking stakeholder input after several iterations of user testing because it is critical for stakeholders (who are often considered "experts") to see a draft that already incorporates the views of the end user—whose perspectives are often overlooked. The project team compiles key findings from the stakeholder feedback to create a revised draft.

As the prototype is iteratively tested and revised with user and stakeholder input, the research team also solicits suggestions about implementing the health communication project and about defining evaluation questions. Such questions should be included in the usability tests, focus groups, and other participatory methods. Additional relevant stakeholders, such as healthcare providers, health educators, city or county officials, media, funders and others may need to be identified and engaged at this time, if they are not already represented in the advisory group(s). Online and telephone surveys are another helpful way to engage stakeholders in implementation and evaluation planning.

5. Continuously evaluate and revise health communication programs.

Guidance from community-based participatory research, action research and design science models emphasize the need for continuous evaluation and improvement of health communication programs. For example, in design science frameworks, defining problems and solutions are concurrent and iterative activities. This approach substantially differs from the traditional methods of defining hypotheses and research questions at the outset, collecting baseline data and then outcome data after the program is implemented. In community participatory design, users and stakeholders gradually define and refine issues and solutions throughout the project. Evaluation begins with input from advisory group members, and extends to all iterations of usability and focus group testing, and other evaluation activities during and after implementation. At each of these steps, evaluation questions are likely to change, as is the project plan. Similarly, evaluation methods may need to be adjusted to answer new questions and assess a revised plan.

We recommend mixed-methods evaluation that includes qualitative and quantitative methods. The qualitative methods are necessary to gain a deep understanding of communication issues, gradually create the intervention, and explore evaluation questions. Quantitative methods provide statistical data about the program's effects. Because the initial participatory design of the program is part of the evaluation, the project team should carefully document those activities and treat them as a formal part of the evaluation. Although many researchers wait until a health communication intervention is designed before submitting a human subjects protocol to their institutional review board (IRB), we recommend that researchers submit a protocol at the first steps of participatory design activities, including usability testing. This approach recognizes participatory design activities as a key part of the research, and allows them to be reported as such in manuscripts submitted for publication—for which IRB approval is required. In addition, process evaluation should be considered an integral part of the overall participatory research, rather than simply a tool to track project activities or deliverables.

6. Extend successful programs to other populations or regions, using participatory methods.

Researchers, practitioners and policymakers are often concerned that even when a health communication program has proven successful, it is often difficult to "replicate," "expand," or "scale it up" to have a greater impact. Fortunately, just as community participatory design strategies can improve health communication programs, they are also effective to transfer them to other populations and to other locations. Translational research models increasingly focus on processes to engage diverse users and stakeholders in considering the many barriers and facilitators to scaling up health efforts (Green & Glasgow, 2006; Neuhauser et al., 2007a).

The World Health Organization (WHO) has developed the "ExpandNet" initiative to examine scaling-up issues and recommend effective strategies. In 2009, the WHO published a very useful report about scaling up health service innovations that is also applicable to extending health communication programs (WHO, 2009). Their guidance emphasizes "participatory design and management" to ensure that the program is adapted to the new socio-cultural, economic and institutional contexts. The WHO also recommends that program developers consider scaling up processes at the outset of planning a health program. Given that adapting and extending programs requires significant community participation, program developers will be more successful if they use such processes in their initial demonstration efforts.

Our experiences support the theoretical and empirical guidance from the literature and from global program reports. We have found that when we use community participatory processes from the beginning, it is much easier to use similar ones to adapt a health communication program to other population and places—including in other countries. We recommend using the same steps described above. Obviously, adapting a health communication program elsewhere will mean considering new end-users, stakeholders, contextual issues, and research questions. However, it will not change the need for strong participatory engagement at all relevant levels.

One lesson that we have learned over the years is that participatory processes are typically not well understood by decisionmakers, researchers, practitioners and end-users. For this reason, it is important to have documented participatory processes in the initial (successful) program that can be part of the plan to adapt the program to the new environment. It is also very helpful, and sometimes essential, to have a person or team (sometimes called "knowledge brokers") experienced in community participatory design to educate stakeholders via meetings/workshops about these processes and obtain their "buy-in." We have also learned that even with initial commitment to participatory design, stakeholders who make funding and/or managerial decisions may naturally revert to "top-down" approaches. In these cases, it is often necessary for the knowledge brokers to monitor the participatory processes and help make adjustments as needed. Follow-up workshops or other kinds of project staff training are helpful ways to do so.

Case Examples of the 6-Step Model: Large-Scale Health Communication Materials

The Wellness Guide: From failure to success

In 1987, the State of California (U.S.) commissioned the Center for Community Wellness at the University of California, Berkeley, School of Public Health to produce and distribute a general health and wellness resource intended for over one million diverse California residents, with special attention to low-income and vulnerable populations. At the outset, the team used the traditional approach of having researchers design and implement the project with limited input from community stakeholders and end-users. The draft resource guide contained carefully selected, evidence-based information and advice about a wide range of health and wellness issues.

Before the guide was produced and distributed large-scale, the project team pilot-tested the draft document with intended community recipients. The research team was surprised by the negative reactions to the guide. Community members criticized the choice of topics ("we have other important issues in our lives"), the tone ("it sounds condescending"), the advice ("preachy," and "it doesn't fit our lives"), the design ("we want photos of real people, like us"), and the lack of connection to local resources ("we need to know where to go for help"). The embarrassing feedback made it clear to the team that the community needed to be closely engaged in the project design.

After much soul-searching and examining guidance about participatory approaches, the project team completely reoriented its approach to be community-driven. They hired ethnically and socio-economically diverse community members as advisors (Step 1) who conducted focus groups and interviews with intended users in their area (Step 2). The team also hired writers who were experienced in communicating with multiple and hard-to-reach audiences to create an initial draft of the guide based on the input of the advisors and the formative research (Step 3). Then, the draft document was tested with the diverse groups (over 500 people) led by the community advisors until "saturation"—people were satisfied with it (Step 4). This stage involved developing and revising many drafts of the resource through a back-and-forth process with the advisors, researchers and writers. A Spanish version, *La Guía del Bienestar,* was also adapted with the participation of Spanish-language groups.

During this time, a statewide distribution plan was developed with health and social service providers who would be the implementers (Step 4). After the Wellness Guide was produced and distributed to 100,000 women who were participants in a program for low-income mothers, the project team conducted a statewide evaluation with a treatment-control design that showed positive results related to recipients' usage, satisfaction, learning, behavioral changes, and recommendations for guide revisions (Step 5) (Schwab et al.,1992; Neuhauser et al., 1998). After receiving the positive evaluation results and making recommended revisions, the state of California distributed the Wellness Guide to over one million Californians (Step 5). Several foundations funded the project team to develop versions of the Wellness Guide for Chinese-American populations and for diverse Californians with disabilities (Step 6). These versions were developed using the intensive participatory design processes of the model with the intended end-users and stakeholders. These guides were distributed to hundreds of thousands of Californians. At this time, the Center for Community Wellness transitioned into the current Health Research for Action center (HRA).

As we reflect on the development and testing of this model, we note that in the early days of this work, we had limited theoretical guidance and empirical examples of how to do community participatory design with diverse populations. Over time, we have shared our experiences and research results with other health communication colleagues around the world and learned much from them about other participatory efforts.

The Parents Kit Project: Adapting the model for other topics

After the success of the Wellness Guides, the State of California asked the Health Research for Action center in 2000 to help develop a Kit for New Parents ("Kit"). The Kit was intended to address the important problem that most new parents in California—especially those who had low-incomes or who did not speak English well—did not feel that they had the information they needed to give their children the best start in life. Our HRA center developed a *Parents Guide* using the participatory design steps with thousands of parents and hundreds of stakeholders. We also reviewed and helped develop or revise other components of the Kit, including the videos and topical pamphlets, using participatory processes.

By this time, we had carefully tested and revised the model, and guidance about health literacy and clear communication was greatly advanced over that available to us a decade earlier. From our experiences, contributions from the scientific literature, listservs about community participatory design, health literacy and other topics, we were able to refine our approach. For example, we were able to set (and test) the readability of the *Parents Guide* at a 6th to 7th grade level, in keeping with health literacy research findings in the U.S. We were also able to streamline this work to research, develop and test the *Parents Guide* in one year (Steps 1–4), whereas it had taken three years to accomplish this work on the original *Wellness Guide*.

Our HRA research team then conducted a statewide, three-year longitudinal study of the effects of the Kit. Results showed high usage (87%) and satisfaction (99%) among English- and Spanish-speaking parents. They also showed that Kit recipients gained significantly more knowledge and adopted healthier parenting and health practices than non-recipients (Neuhauser et al., 2007b) (Step 4). In California, the Kit had been distributed to over 5 million parents and is a sustainable investment, and the largest statewide parenting education program in the U.S.

The Parents Guide: Adapting the model to other states and internationally

The successful results of the Kit in California attracted attention from other U.S. states that wanted to adapt this health communication approach. With other California Kit colleagues, we worked with governors, foundations, parents, health providers and other stakeholders to adapt and extend the Kit model to four other U.S. states (Step 6). In each state, we followed our model to translate the Kit to reflect local populations and conditions. The first step was to convince state political leaders (governors) and other funders to invest in a Kit program. These decisionmakers were most interested in knowing about the scientific evidence supporting the program and about specific strategies to adapt the program to their state. They were impressed with how the approach could engage members of diverse and vulnerable populations to co-design the resources. They wanted careful attention to local health issues, laws, regulations, and referral programs. They also wanted the Kit to carry their state's "brand" and have a local "look and feel." The participatory design steps of the model were essential to fulfill these requirements.

We learned that it was necessary to follow the first five steps of the model, as it had been to develop it in California. We trained local staff in participatory design techniques, such as how to examine research evidence relevant to the state, how to identify and engage diverse sub-populations and how to select and highlight local resources. However, we found that the rigorously participatory work on the initial California Kit resulted in resources that needed relatively moderate changes to adapt them for other states. For example, because parents, experts, providers and other stakeholders had carefully chosen the major topics, few revisions were needed in each state. Major changes were needed, of course, in photos and community resource programs. Similarly, Kit distribution strategies differed greatly in each of the states. At the end of the participatory process, each state had crafted a Kit that uniquely reflected its needs and was practical to implement. Several of the states conducted evaluations showing highly positive results. Currently, the Kit is being adapted in a statewide initiative in Australia.

Extending the model to other countries: Switzerland and China

The model has also been used to develop a health communication resource for the residents of Bern, Switzerland. This health communication initiative grew out of a community-based collaborative called "Dialog Health" ("Dialog Gesunheit") established by the Medical Faculty of the University of FI-AM (fakultäre Instanz für Allgemeine Medizin) in 2003. Dialog Health hosts moderated, informal community forums to discuss issues about health and disease. The goal of Dialog Health is to create new strategies to change the health care system and promote health by means of dialogues at the level of professional and lay individuals and groups. It is "constant learning processes" intended to improve communication, self-efficacy and health literacy. It also has the objective of strengthening relationships (social capital) among population groups and the health system.

This community-based participatory approach resulted in the decision to create a health promotion resource, based on the HRA wellness guide model. HRA center staff provided advice on the model's steps and communicated with the Dialog Health team throughout the process. The project established an advisory board—called a "supra-regional think tank"—that included non-health professionals (patients and other residents) and professionals from healthcare, business and government (Step 1). During the Dialog Health forums, professionals and diverse community members selected issues for the guide, reviewed data about those topics and provided ideas about the design and community resources to include (Steps 1 & 2). The guide was created with close attention to health literacy and clear communication principles and multiple drafts were developed and revised with end-user and stakeholder input (Steps 3 & 4). The resulting *Dialog Gesundheit* guide is an attractive, easy-to-use resource covering health issues throughout the life course, with referrals to healthcare and other community organizations and information sources. The guide has been distributed to thousands of community members with positive feedback. For further information, visit: http://www.dialog-gesundheit.ch.

The model is now being adapted in Changzhou, China to benefit migrant workers who come from rural villages to work in factory zones. This effort began with several workshops led by an HRA researcher and other colleagues to describe community participatory design and the steps of the model. The Chinese project team established three advisory groups (including workers, health and social service professionals, and government officials) that identified worker health and social issues (Step 1), and conducted formative research through focus groups and a survey of factory workers (Step 2). These efforts have led to the decision to create a health and wellness guide by and for the workers, and a "wellness house" in each factory where workers, managers, and outside advisors can meet to discuss health and life issues (Step 3). These two communication strategies are now being tested and refined with workers and stakeholders (Step 4).

Conclusion

A growing body of theoretical guidance and empirical evidence strongly suggests that health communication interventions are more successful when researchers and practitioners use community participatory approaches. This has also been our experience and we have learned many lessons about systematically engaging communities. One lesson learned is that it is critically important to reach out to and engage representative and influential community members as active partners in developing, implementing, evaluating, and sustaining effective health communication intervention programs—especially when working in unfamiliar settings. Community partners include both the intended beneficiaries and a broad range of stakeholders who have essential inside information and "cultural wisdom" about the unique needs, constraints, opportunities, and available resources that will inevitably influence the success of health promotion programs. Community partners can also help guide the best ways to implement health promotion programs, given their understanding of which intervention strategies are likely to work well and which strategies are likely to be rejected. Moreover, they can personally endorse interventions and provide needed groundwork within their communities to encourage acceptance of communication programs. Community partners are much more likely to be trusted by others within their own communities than are the researchers and health promotion experts who are not native to the environments where the health promotion programs are being implemented. This familiarity and trust can help community partners gather needed evaluation data from end-users and stakeholders about the relative effectiveness of health intervention programs to guide program refinements and improvements. Ultimately, by encouraging community partners to develop a sense of ownership of communication interventions, these partners can help institutionalize and sustain health communication interventions within their communities.

Another lesson learned is that establishing community partnerships is an intricate process that involves building meaningful relationships with key organizations and individuals representing the communities where health promotion efforts are to be conducted. It is essential to identify community representatives who are interested in the goals of the project and are willing to work with the health promotion team as partners. It may take time to establish trust with partners and build commitment to the project. A critical factor in this relationship-building process is investing in community partners, letting them know how valuable their input is, and ensuring that the work they do will be respected, will be valued, and will make a difference for their communities. Maintaining effective community partnerships often demands significant efforts to nurture, encourage, and reinforce cooperation. Health intervention specialists must demonstrate through both words and actions that their community partners' ideas and efforts are important in the design and implementation of health intervention programs. Finally, we have learned that the time and effort that is put into establishing and maintaining active community partnerships—such as through our 6-step model—is well worth the work. These participatory efforts can ensure that communication intervention programs meet the needs of the individuals the interventions are designed for, that they will be accepted within the community, and they can achieve their health promotion goals over time with the intended audiences.

Recommended Readings

Minkler, M., & Wallerstein, N. (Eds). (2008). *Community based participatory research for health: process to outcomes*. (2nd edition). San Francisco: Jossey-Bass.

Neuhauser, L. (2001). Participatory design for better interactive health communication: A statewide model in the USA. *Electronic Journal of Communication* 11, nos. 3&4.

Neuhauser, L., Schwab, M., Obarski. S. K., Syme, S. L., and Bieber, M. (1998). Community participation in health promotion: Evaluation of the California Wellness Guide. *Health Promotion International,* 13(3).

Neuhauser, L., & Kreps, G.L. (2011). Participatory design and artificial intelligence: Strategies to improve health communication for diverse audiences. In N. Green, S. Rubinelli, & D. Scott. (Eds.). *Artificial Intelligence and Health Communication* (pp. 49–52). Cambridge, MA: AAAIPress. Also available at: http://www.aaai.org/ocs/index.php/SSS/SSS11/paper/viewFile/2475/2857

Neuhauser, L., Rothschild, B., Graham, C., Ivey, S., & Konishi, S. Participatory design of mass health communication in three languages for seniors and people with disabilities on Medicaid. *American Journal of Public Health.* December 2009; 99: 2188–2195.

References

Buckminster Fuller, R., & McHale, J. (1963). *World Design Science Decade, 1965–1975*, Carbondale: Southern Illinois University.

CPSR (Computer Professionals for Social Responsibility). (2000). *Participatory design*. Accessed July 1, 2012 from: http://cpsr.org/issues/pd.

Green, L. W., & Glasgow, R. E. (2006). Evaluating the relevance, generalization, and applicability of research: Issues in external validation and translation methodology. *Evaluation and the Health Professions, 29*(1), 126–153.

Gregor, S. (2009). *Building Theory in the Science of the Artificial*, Proceedings of the 4th International Conference on Design Science Research in Information Systems and Technology, (Association for Computing Machinery: New York).

Hesse, B. W., & Shneiderman, B. 2007. eHealth research from the user's perspective. *American Journal of Preventive Medicine, 32*: S97–103.

Kreps, G.L. (1988). The pervasive role of information in health and health care: Implications for health communication policy. In *Communication yearbook 11*, Ed. J.A. Anderson, 238–276. Newbury Park, CA: Sage.

Kreps, G.L. & Neuhauser, L. (2010). New directions in ehealth communication: Opportunities and challenges. *Patient Education and Counseling*. Available online 3 March 2010.

Minkler, M., & Wallerstein, N. (Eds). (2008). *Community based participatory research for health: Process to outcomes*. (2nd edition). San Francisco: Jossey-Bass.

Neuhauser, L. (2001). Participatory design for better interactive health communication: A statewide model in the USA. *Electronic Journal of Communication* 11, nos. 3&4.

Neuhauser, L, Constantine, WL, Constantine, NA, Sokal-Gutierrez, K, Obarski, SK, Clayton, L, Desai, M, Sumner, G, Syme, SL. (2007b). Promoting prenatal and early childhood health: Evaluation of a statewide materials-based intervention for parents. *American Journal of Public Health, 97*(10): 813–819.

Neuhauser, L., and G. Kreps. 2003. Rethinking communication in the e-health era. *Journal of Health Psychology, 8*: 7–22.

Neuhauser, L., & Kreps, G. (2010) Ehealth communication and behavior change: Promise and performance. *Journal of Social Semiotics*, 20:1, 9–27.

Neuhauser, L., & Kreps, G.L. (2011). Participatory design and artificial intelligence: Strategies to improve health communication for diverse audiences. In N. Green, S. Rubinelli, & D. Scott. (Eds.). *Artificial Intelligence and Health Communication* (pp. 49–52). Cambridge, MA: AAAI Press. Also available at: http://www.aaai.org/ocs/index.php/SSS/SSS11/paper/viewFile/2475/2857

Neuhauser, L., & Paul, K. (2011). Readability, comprehension and usability. In: *Communicating Risks and Benefits:An Evidence-Based User's Guide*. Silver Spring, MD: U.S. Department of Health and Human Services. Bethesda MD: Food and Drug Administration.

Neuhauser, L. Richardson, D., Mackenzie, S., & Minkler, M. (2007a). Advancing transdisciplinary and translational research practice: Issues and models of doctoral education in public health. *Journal of Research Practice, 3*(2), Article M19. Retrieved [date of access], from http://jrp.icaap.org/index.php/jrp/article/view/103/97

Neuhauser, L., Rothschild, B., Graham, C., Ivey, S., & Konishi, S. (December 2009). Participatory design of mass health communication in three languages for seniors and people with disabilities on Medicaid. *American Journal of Public Health*, 99: 2188–2195.

Neuhauser L, Schwab M, Obarski SK, Syme SL, and Bieber M. (1998). Community participation in health promotion: Evaluation of the California Wellness Guide. *Health Promotion International*, 13(3).

Nielsen, J. (2000). *Designing web usability*. Indianapolis: New Riders Publishing.

Schwab, M., and Neuhauser, L. (1994). Executive Editors, La Universidad de California *Guía del Bienestar: Su guía para mantenerse saludable en California. 3rd Edition.* University of California.

Simon, H. (1996). *The Sciences of the artificial, 3rd Ed.* Cambridge, MA: MIT Press.

Smedley, B.D., & Syme, S.L. (2000). Promoting health: Intervention strategies from social and behavioral research, Institute of Medicine. Washington, DC: National Academies Press.

Snyder, L. B., Hamilton, M. A., Mitchell, E. W., Kiwanuka-Tondo, J., Fleming-Milici, F., & Proctor, D. (2004). A meta-analysis of the effect of mediated health communication campaigns on behavior change in the United States. *Journal of Health Communication*, 9(Suppl. 1), 71–96.

Stokols, D. (2000). Social ecology and behavioral medicine: Implications for training, practice, and policy. *Behavioral Medicine, 26*, 129–138.

Stokols, D. (2006). Toward a science of transdisciplinary research. *American Journal of Community Psychology, 38*, 63–77.

US Department of Health and Human Services, Office of Disease Prevention and Health Promotion. *Quick guide to health literacy*. Retrieved from http://www.health.gov/ communication/literacy/quickguide/.

US Department of Health and Human Services, Centers for Disease Control and Prevention(CDC). *Simply Put*. Retrieved from http://www.cdc.gov/healthmarketing/pdf/Simply_Put_082010.pdf.

World Health Organization. (2009). Practical guidance for scaling up health service innovations. Geneva: WHO Press.

Chapter 14

Faith-based Community Health Interventions: Incorporating Cultural Ecology, the Social Ecological Framework, and Gender Analysis

Kari Hartwig, *Walden University*

Introduction

Public health institutions and professionals and faith-based institutions such as churches, mosques, and temples have often been engaged in a masked, jittery dance with one another in the conduct of health promotion. In this dance, no touching is allowed and the hidden faces obscure the words and meanings of the other, heightening fears and suspicions. Often at the center of the distrust is who controls the message about the health problem and how it is delivered. Although there have been many alliances between public health, medicine and faith-based institutions over the decades, the HIV and AIDS epidemic launched a resurgence of interest in public health organizations reaching out to faith communities in efforts to promote supportive HIV prevention and care messages. Globally, most people identify themselves as having some faith or religious belief (For more details, check the website at http://www.religious tolerance.org/worldrel.htm). Acknowledging both the widespread reach of religious organizations to people living at the "grassroots" and the influence of religious leaders, public health organizations, governments, and foundations have significantly increased their outreach and funding to multiple religious-based institutions. In the United States (U.S.), there are increased examples of churches partnering with public health institutions in supporting church-led "Health Ministries" covering topics such as diabetes control and prevention; healthy, nutritious cooking; heart disease; exercise programs; and stress reduction (Campbell et al., 2007; Peterson, Atwood, & Yates, 2002). Further, there is increased attention to the use of prayer as a health communication mechanism in health and healing both physically and spiritually (Hartwig, 2010; Kreps, 2012; Ucheaga & Hartwig, 2010).

In a global context of health communication, working across faith communities, public health professionals need to expand their ability to access different religious organizations and learn how best to work with them in the creation of health communication messages and interventions (Ucheaga & Hartwig, 2010). As with any communication study, identifying the sender, content of the message, the channel, audience, and measuring its impact are critical to succeed in health promotion (Lasswell, 1948; (Finnegan & Viswanath, 2002). In the global fight against AIDS, many funding organizations have supported HIV and AIDS education training with senior level Christian and Muslim leaders; in addition, they have helped national religious organizations in developing sexual health or life skills communication materials for their school curricula and worked with hospital personnel in establishing appropriate infection control protocols.

The purpose of this chapter is to provide a practical example of working with a faith community in a non-U.S. context to conduct a public health intervention. Theories and frameworks that informed its design are discussed along with samples of resources available. Although the examples in this chapter will focus on HIV/AIDS, the practical and theoretical steps provided here could be applied and adapted across multiple disease categories, faith traditions, cultures, and countries.

Theoretical Frameworks

In working across various countries, cultures, and value systems, this chapter introduces participatory methods combined with Freirian principles, cultural ecology and socio-ecological frameworks, and gender analysis. Blending these principles and frameworks allows for the evolution of a health communication intervention that is largely created and owned by the participants. Further, their participation assures that it is culturally appropriate, and incorporates their expertise of the community structures and organizations. Finally, it maximizes the potential for broader audience reach by explicitly incorporating both men and women in the design, implementation, and evaluation.

Many public health educators have built upon the principles elucidated by Brazilian educator Paulo Freire based on his work teaching illiterate farmers in the 1950s and '60s (Freire, 1970). Freire emphasized the importance of "starting where the people are" by listening to them and assisting them to identify their local problems and solutions. In the process, they become empowered for action. Wallerstein and Bernstein (1988) and others suggested that to apply these principles and practices in a public health context requires the public health specialist or educator to act as a facilitator—rather than teacher or implementer—encouraging groups to ask critical questions that explore the roots of community problems in the context of their culture and setting (Wallerstein, 1992). This perspective suggests that all communities have expertise, and the facilitator role is to move participants to utilize that expertise in solving their own problems.

The social ecological framework provides useful guidance in designing public health interventions as well. The framework takes into account local social context and suggests means of planning public health interventions and evaluations at multiple levels including individual, interpersonal, community, organizational, and policy related (McLeroy, Bibeau, Steckler, & Glanz, 1988; Stokols, Pelletier, & Fielding, 1996). Through its application, one can take a particular health outcome, analyze its determinants at various levels depending on resources and accessibility, and plan an intervention that incorporates addressing changes at multiple levels in order to reinforce opportunities for healthy behavior change. One weakness of a social ecological approach, however, is that it may not always adequately incorporate relevant aspects of culture. To address these weaknesses, this chapter includes theoretical perspectives from cultural ecology.

Cultural ecology is best known in medical geography and addresses how the relationship of population characteristics (genetics, age, and gender) interacts with habitat (natural, social, and built environments) and behavior (beliefs, social organization, and technology) to shape the health status of an individual or community (Meade & Earickson, 2000; Meade, Florin, & Gesler, 1988). It shares similarities with a social ecological perspective except that it focuses on the iterative relationship between culture, biology, physical environment, and social phenomena that affect an individual's or community's health status over time. Cultural ecology, first described by René Dubos (1965), provides a dynamic framework to describe humans' adaptations to their environments in specific geographic contexts that produce or prevent disease (Dubos, 1965).

Finally, in conducting health communication interventions in faith communities, it is critical to incorporate gender planning elements into the design, assuring that both men and women are part of the planning and implementation process. Gender planning begins with a diagnosis and understanding of men's and women's different roles and responsibilities within a community and culture (Moser, 1993). Across the major religious faith systems including Christianity, Islam, Buddhism, Hinduism, and Judaism, men tend to dominate in leadership and hierarchical positions but women make up the majority of the daily/weekly faithful who participate most often in religious ritual activities. Women also play significant leadership roles within each faith tradition although they are often overlooked. Sex segregation in religious services and activities (e.g., study groups, social outreach or evangelism) remains common in many religious organizations and/or may be practiced more regularly within a particular country or culture.

Given how religious faith is practiced in daily life, it is critical to assure that one is utilizing both formal (traditional leaders) and informal (women's group leaders, youth leaders, choir directors, etc.) communication channels. Gender planning also considers men's and women's differing productive and reproductive roles in a community; from their possible roles as parents, husbands/wives, daughters/sons, to roles as community or political leaders to various occupational roles. Each of these multiplicities of roles requires an additional channel for communication to different audiences.

Designing, Implementing, and Evaluating Your Faith-based Intervention

Step 1. Understand self and audience.

The first step in designing a faith-based intervention is to begin with role definition and clarification of the facilitators/researchers and the institution(s) you represent. Who are you? What nationalities or ethnicities do you represent? What sex, gender and/or sexual identities do you represent? What are your age mixes? What are your religious beliefs? Who or what agency or country do you represent? It is important to consider this self-reflection and how you as a team, individual, and institution are likely to be perceived initially by the faith institution you intend to work with. Based on their past experiences with universities, non-governmental organizations (NGOs), foreign consultants, local activists, etc., they will have pre-conceptions of who you are, what ideas or values you and your organization represent, and your stated and unstated objectives.

The next step is to do some research about the faith institution you plan to work with, including understanding its organizational structure, key leadership roles, and its core faith beliefs. For example, are you planning to work with a single church or mosque in one city? Or, would you want to be working with national or regional leadership from a particular faith tradition, such as all Southern Baptists or all Sunni Muslims in an area? Identifying the core components of the organizational and social structure is critical to determining where in the organizational structure to intervene and who key gatekeepers may be. What are the cultural and religious beliefs in this institution regarding men's and women's roles, the mixing of sexes, appropriate dress, the value of one's age (as an expert or facilitator)? Finally, how does this institution talk publicly about the health issue or disease you plan to address with them? Is there silence, condemnation, or already an accepting, supportive community which is trying to do a better job of reaching out to its members on this health issue?

Conducting this initial self-team-assessment and research about the institution you intend to work with will prepare you well for potential questions or concerns that may come from the faith partner institution. Note how this process incorporates aspects of gender planning, an organizational assessment of the institution and its geographic reach and a cultural assessment that respects the local context. The process of working through some of these questions may inform who participates on the public health side and how best to approach the faith institution.

Step 2. Identify individuals within the institution for training and/or partnering for the design of the intervention activity; probable communication channels and intended audience.

The type of intervention may be determined after initial talks with religious leadership about their priorities or through the process of workshop activities. Examples of interventions include editing a religious school curriculum on a particular health issue, or developing written materials to be used for lay leaders' for discussion guides, or a training on factual information about a disease/health concern and how to discuss it with peers or youth. Understanding the intended audience reach will also inform the organizational and hierarchical level within the institution that you will interact with. When inviting individuals from the religious institution to a training or to review and edit visual or written materials, it is essential to invite and include both women and men. Given their different gender roles in society and within their religious institutions, they each bring unique insights and perspectives to what will work or not work, where there is resistance and opportunity. Although each sex may think, "I know how women/men think about this issue," they are usually surprised by at least one new insight when they hear from the other sex. From here on, this chapter provides an example of designing a training for faith leaders around a particular health issue in order to simplify the steps.

Step 3. Conduct a participatory training employing Freirian principles.

Evidence from the past programs suggests that participatory methods can enhance (1) commitment and ownership of all stakeholders; (2) individual and organizational capacity; (3) relevance to local community/population needs and concerns; and (4) sustainability of program activities (Estrella & Gaventa, 1997; IDS, 1998; Zukoski & Luluquisen, 2002). Another core value that emerges from Freire's is the importance of the trainer (or public health expert) acting as a facilitator or catalyst to assist participants in critically examining their environment and deriving locally appropriate strategies for change (Wallerstein, 1992; Wallerstein & Bernstein, 1988). It will be necessary here for the trainer to develop tools and questions to assist participants in delving into the root causes of problems. After identifying root causes of the problem the next step is for the participants to begin to identify possible solutions. One example of how to do this is provided in the case study later in this chapter.

Throughout this problem identification and solution discussion, it is useful to consider developing questions that probe the different levels of the social ecological framework. For example, which individuals may be more physically/emotionally/socially at risk for this disease, based on biology, age, or social context? Who do they influence or who influences them at the interpersonal level (e.g., peers, parents, children, mentors, leaders)? Which organizations do these individuals interact with that play a direct or indirect role in shaping their behavior related to the disease risk or health promotion activity they are targeting (e.g., work places, schools, businesses, religious institutions, community organizations, etc.)? What government policies influence individual or organizational policies? What is in the physical or social environment that affects behavior? Tools and questions should be designed and pre-tested to be culturally appropriate, using language that is well understood by participants, and is gender sensitive. Working cross-culturally and across languages can be particularly challenging especially if all facilitators are not bilingual. Assuring that translations are appropriate and accurate is important.

In conducting the training, particularly with a mixed gender participant group, it is valuable to have both male and female trainers. There are likely to be times when it will be appropriate to break into single sex groups to discuss issues. This allows participants, especially women, to feel more open in their statements. In many cultures, women are socialized to not give their opinions in public, particularly in mixed sex venues. If the single sex groups are discussing common questions, it is useful to bring them back together to share their reflections. There will be inevitable overlap between the groups, but often there is a perspective that one sex brings forward that is unique and provides insight to the other. These differences may also begin new discussions as participants probe them and explore their meanings.

Step 4. Introduce concepts of evaluation and how it can be used as a tool for assessing change.

Among community organizations in both the U.S. and internationally, program evaluation is usually looked at as an external tyranny imposed by the funding agency. It often requires program implementers to complete detailed monthly or quarterly reports, summarizing process indicators (e.g., number of people trained, number of condoms distributed) and occasionally providing qualitative notes about challenges and accomplishments. The quality of these reports is often poor regardless of nationality or educational training. One of the primary reasons for poor quality monitoring and evaluation reports is that the staff who complete them do not use them or recognize their value as a tool for their own learning.

The purpose of incorporating discussion and exercises about what evaluation is and why it is done is to create a sense of value for evaluation on the part of the participants. They need to see how these numbers and stories build meaning for their own activity and outreach in their communities. Given the wide variety of faith-based organizations (e.g., a church, a Muslim hospital, a Buddhist hospice, a Hindu orphanage) and diversity of health issues, there is no generic evaluation tool for faith-based organizations. The following section however, suggests that it is possible to create tools with participants that are contextualized to that institution and the health problems it is trying to address.

Step 5. Use participatory methods to design evaluation tools and measures.

The final part of the training engages participants in defining quantitative and qualitative change indicators which reflect their local context and the change they want to see. Facilitators may need to assist participants in moving from broad conceptual change ideas to more practical types of evidence. Given the opportunity however, most participants are able to identify meaningful measures that an external consultant with little local context may never consider. As they have been instrumental in designing the measures, the participants are also more likely to use and value them.

Given the iterative nature of a participatory training event, it is ideal to conduct the training over multiple days so that the facilitators can begin to draft and develop process or intervention tools that reflect the input from participants. This also allows participants an opportunity to practice using them and recommend changes.

Next, this chapter will introduce a case study that utilized these theoretical and practical guidelines. The case study reflects a training event conducted with a faith-based NGO in Tanzania working with Lutheran church leaders in developing culturally sensitive HIV and AIDS prevention and care outreach programs and services.

Case Study

Mwangaza Teacher's Resource Centre (referred to as Mwangaza) began in 1996 as an NGO affiliated with the Evangelical Lutheran Church in Tanzania (ELCT). Its primary mission is to improve the teaching skills and methods of ELCT secondary school teachers in order to improve educational opportunities and learning for both students and teachers. In 2001, Mwangaza initiated its Integrated HIV/AIDS Program. The objective of this program is to work through its network of teachers, students, parents, and church leaders (both men and women) to lay the groundwork for community behavior change. An important feature to emphasize here is that these targeted individuals are working and living at the "grassroots" of their communities. Although some may have leadership roles in their schools or churches, they primarily live in rural villages and semi-urban areas and have not risen high in the ranks of their respective organizational hierarchies. Community behavior change is planned by identifying community leaders and peer opinion leaders to repeat consistent prevention and care messages through multiple channels, such as Bible studies, at youth drop-in centers, at the weekly markets, in clinics, through church choirs, or through other musical venues, as well as through changing the social and physical environments in which people live.

This case study featured a 3-day workshop conducted by Mwangaza with an international public health consultant with local Tanzanian Lutheran church leaders on HIV and AIDS. The purposes of the workshop were (1) to assess the effectiveness of an earlier HIV training in terms of information delivery and skill building; (2) to provide participants additional skill building opportunities to conduct their outreach activities; and (3) to develop monitoring and assessment tools with participants.

The workshop was co-designed by the Mwangaza director (Tanzanian), a Mwangaza consultant and former director (American) and the public health evaluation consultant (American), referred to hereafter as the planning team. All but one session was co-facilitated by the director and evaluation consultant. Other Mwangaza staff (male and female), all Tanzanian, and the Mwangaza consultant played multiple roles during the workshop including working as group leaders and note takers.

The workshop participants included seven men and eight women, all ELCT church leaders from the Arusha and Meru districts of Arusha region. They were selected by their diocese church leadership to participate based on their earlier participation in some HIV training and their leadership roles as pastors, evangelists, choir directors, youth leaders, and Bible study leaders. Their ages varied from early 30s to mid-50s. Ethnically, they included primarily Maasai, Warusha, and Meru, distinct tribal groups with different languages and cultural traditions. The men were either pastors or evangelists. Pastors are ordained and hold a four-year degree from a seminary whereas evangelists typically have completed only one year of seminary training. Evangelists serve as assistants to pastors and often cover those services of community outreach in remote areas underserved by ordained pastors.

The women church leaders included heads of local church women's groups and parish workers who teach Bible classes and often work with youth. In their roles as church leaders, each of these participants conducts regular outreach in their communities. Of note, none of the participants were senior level church leaders but rather they each represented the "grassroots," everyday congregations in rural or urban settings.

Preparing for the training workshop

The Mwangaza director initiated communication with the external consultant about participating in the training and evaluation workshop. A 3-day workshop date was set for May 2003. The consultant arrived one week before the workshop in order to begin intensive discussions with the rest of the planning team on the workshop objectives, agenda, format, structure, and training tools to be developed.

Defining the workshop purpose and objectives took several hours of discussion and iterative questioning of one another and what we hoped to achieve. As the facilitators discussed why we were training parents, church leaders, teachers, and students about AIDS, we returned to Mwangaza's primary objective: community behavior change to reduce risk for HIV and HIV-related stigma for those affected. Therefore, we viewed our workshop participants as both community change agents as well as monitors of community change in their neighborhoods, schools, and churches. The first workshop objective, "to learn about the impact of the HIV and AIDS training on the participants" was the easiest to articulate. To prepare for this, we reviewed together the content of the earlier AIDS training and its primary learning objectives. Additional objectives included having participants develop and practice skills in monitoring and strengthen their roles as change agents. These objectives became the guide for developing the agenda and all other tools for the training.

The draft agenda served as a working document and reference tool for the Mwangaza team to assure that (1) the objectives were appropriate; (2) the teaching or learning method fit the objectives; (3) role definition for each Mwangaza staff person involved was clear and confirmed that they would be available during those times; and (4) the outcome measures were realistic and achievable. As planning for the workshop proceeded, we were able to revise and adapt sections to make them more feasible or appropriate. Adult learning techniques also guided the format and structure of the agenda (Vella, 2002).

Developing monitoring instruments, workshop tools and exercises

As a team we discussed each learning objective and determined alternative tools and instruments that could be used. Consensus on methods was determined by our objectives, feasibility, time and financial constraints, and what we thought was reasonable for participants to learn and do. For example, to achieve the first objective, evaluating the impact of the HIV training during the workshop, we looked at the options of a questionnaire, individual interviews or focus groups. Given that our participants were church leaders/parents and our time limits, we decided that focus groups would be the best method for collecting the data. Two Tanzanian staff then worked iteratively to develop a final Swahili focus group guide. As the "end-users" were the Mwangaza staff, their buy-in or ownership of the final product was critical. Figure 1 displays the iterative development process of these instruments.

During the planning session, a number of workshop worksheets, tools, and assessment possibilities were discussed, drafted, and edited. Most of the tools were designed to stimulate the thinking of participants, provide opportunities for them to share their experiences, and empower them to be more effective in their future outreach and communication activities. A complete summary of tools and instruments developed is portrayed in Table 1. Each of these will be discussed in further detail below.

Table 1. Tools and Instruments Developed for the Workshop

Instruments	Worksheets	Tools	Other
Focus group guide (staff use)	Obstacles-Strategies	Problem-posing picture	Agenda
Interview guide (participant use)	Community resources (organizations & people)	Community mapping exercise	Workshop evaluation
Observation checklist (participant use)	Monitoring plan & target dates		Quarterly reporting form

Figure 1. Participatory process for development of training tools

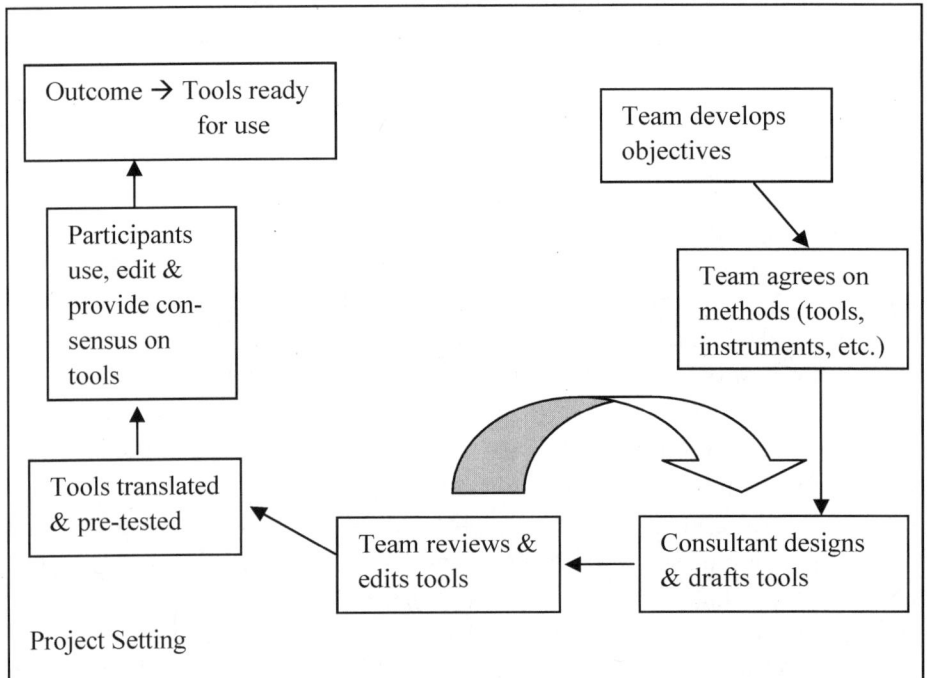

Conducting the workshop

All group sessions were co-facilitated and led by the Mwangaza director and consultant using primarily Kiswahili and some English. All of the workshop exercises were designed to either stimulate critical thinking and analysis or provide participants opportunities to practice new skills. Throughout all of the sessions, other Mwangaza staff participated as observers, small group facilitators, and note takers. At the end of each day, the staff and consultants met to debrief, review the next day's agenda, and make adjustments in the schedule where necessary.

Using the ecological framework as a guide, one of the first worksheets and group discussion sessions had participants naming obstacles to HIV prevention in their homes, churches, schools, and communities. Participants cited common themes such as lack of leadership, traditions that discouraged open discussions of sexuality, silence in the community, and fears about HIV. The issue of stigma did not get raised and so the director led a discussion on stigma and asked participants to discuss how they see it enacted.

One of the outputs of Freirian principles is the use of "problem posing pictures" to stimulate discussion and raise issues that may be observed in society but rarely discussed. The pictures may be actual photographs of a scene or a hand-made sketch. The Mwangaza staff had worked with an artist to create different "problem" scenarios in their community which were often silenced. For this workshop, they used a sketch of a man, standing in front of a crowd of people with a church in the background (see Figure 2). Typically, one begins by asking the group, "What do you see in this picture?" "What is going on?" "Have you ever seen or heard about this in your community?" "Do you think it is a problem?" After the earlier discussion on stigma, it was easy for participants to name stigma as part of the problem. The picture moved the discussion from the abstract to a more grounded reality as many participants could relate to the picture as something they had participated in or observed.

Another exercise was asking participants to draw neighborhood or community maps of where they lived and worked. This activity emerges from cultural ecology and the concepts of the natural and built environment. Each participant was from a different village or town and so they worked individually in sketching out neighborhoods, schools, churches, rivers, major roads, bus stops, and businesses. After they had developed a rudimentary map of their community, participants were asked to mark with an "X" in places of risk for HIV in their community. They could use a double or triple X to indicate places of higher risk. Typical places of risk were marketplaces and bars, but several participants also named schools and churches. These choices produced dynamic discussions and some controversy.

An environmental assessment observation checklist tool was also introduced. Participants were asked to look for both positive and negative advertising of health promotion messages in their communities and note where they saw them and how often they appeared. They first tested the tool and had a chance to discuss its use during the workshop. For example, in walking around Mwangaza's neighborhood, how many beer and cigarette advertising signs did they see? What types of health promotion posters did they see at the local clinic? The exercise proved enlightening to them as they realized how many advertisements and messages are around them all the time that they are unconsciously absorbing. It was only in noting what was there however, that they noticed the absence of positive messages, particularly about HIV.

Designing the evaluation

One of the challenges in conducting the workshop was to transfer the concepts of monitoring and evaluation and their relevance to participants. This challenge was compounded by the fact that there is no direct translation for "monitoring" and "evaluation" in Swahili. For methods where we expected participants to play an active role, such as completing an observation checklist of HIV prevention support characteristics in their communities, we built in time for them to practice these new skills and test them out with one another. A number of worksheets were also created to help each participant prepare individual work plans for monitoring.

Following the workshop

Following the workshop, the Mwangaza staff and consultant met to review the detailed notes taken during the workshop and evaluation by participants, identify what had and had not been accomplished, and discuss changes needed in the future. A workbook guide for the training and instrument components of the workshop was completed shortly after its completion as a resource for later workshops.

One of the challenges in working with a faith-based organization on the subject of HIV was the theological debates and questions that emerged about causes and the church's response. The training facilitators worked with participants to foster an environment for respectful dialogue and disagreement so that honest but difficult dialogue could ensue. The facilitators however, were careful not to take sides on theological questions even though they shared the same faith tradition, but emphasized the social and structural factors that facilitate transmission and treatment. Public health trainers working with a faith-based institution should be explicit about their own values and faith and how or if they influence the content of the training. One could deliver a "secular" training on a disease that is adapted to the faith organizations beliefs, structures, and context. Alternatively, one could create a training that incorporates explicit spiritual traditions or language of the faith with the public health messages and concepts. Ethically, it is important for public health trainers to be transparent about how they are using their own faith beliefs or that of the participants in their programming so no one from either the faith community or public health community could question their personal agenda or ethics.

Figure 2. Problem-posing picture on AIDS and stigma in the church

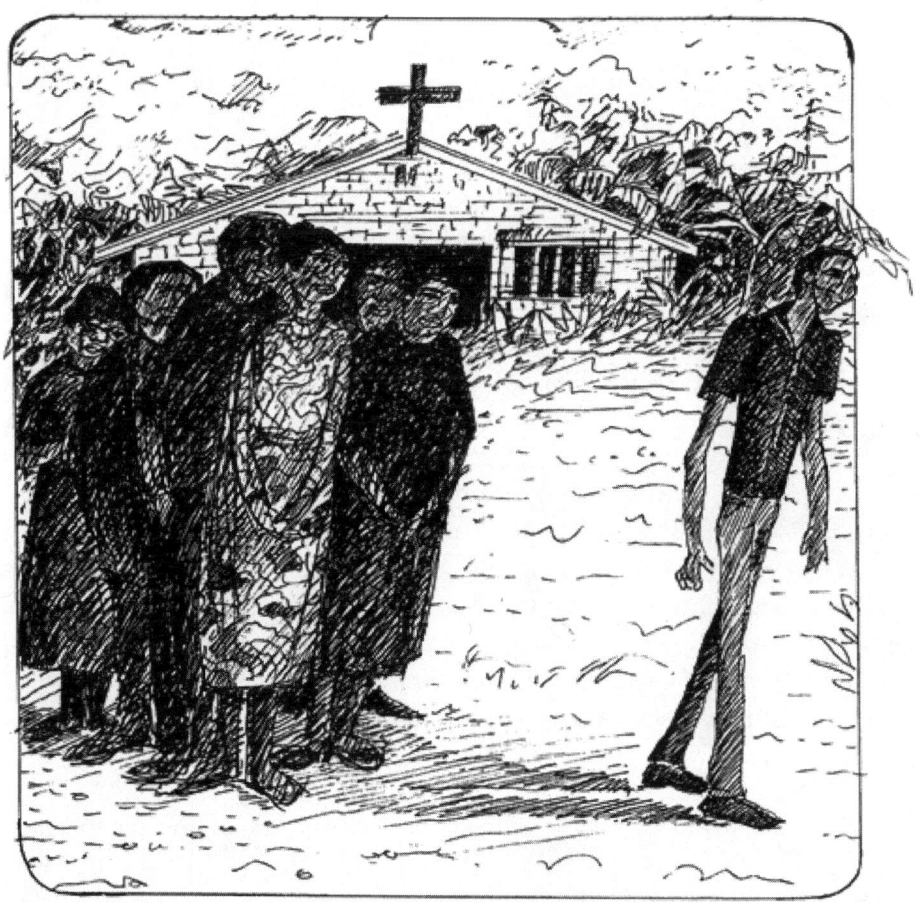

(Artist: Barbara Manger)

Other Resources

The U.S. through the United States Agency for International Development (USAID) is one of the largest global funders of international health programs, particularly HIV and AIDS prevention and care initiatives. With the expansion of funding to faith-based organizations during the George W. Bush administration, more international NGOs are expanding their work with religious organizations across the faith spectrum. It should be highlighted however, that many of these organizations were working with Muslim imams, Buddhist monks, and Catholic priests and sisters from the earliest stages of the HIV epidemic. These NGOs have developed multiple intervention and evaluation tools to work with faith-based institutions which are available through their websites. Examples of organizations and their websites include:

- Family Health International (now FHI360) http://www.fhi360.org/en/index.htm
- PATH http://www.path.org/
- PACT http://www.pactworld.org/
- Pathfinder International http://www2.pathfinder.org/site/PageServer
- World Vision http://www.worldvision.org/?open&lpos=sponsor-a-child_top_img_logo

United Nations agencies are also very active in promoting health programs and provide multiple resources at their websites including the World Health Organization, UNICEF, UNAIDS, and the United Nations Development Program (UNDP) among others.

Local NGOs, faith-based institutions, and universities within each country have rich resources for existing and past health promotion activities working through faith communities. Locally designed and created programs are often the most powerful as they arise from local realities and experiences. For example, professor Isabel Phiri, a religion professor at the University of Kwa Zulu Natal in South Africa and former chair of the Circle of Concerned African Women Theologians, designed a research intervention addressing issues of gender violence and HIV among church members (Phiri & Phiri, 2011). She used and adapted an existing assessment tool on gender violence to design a couples workshop on couples communication, sexuality, violence, and HIV risk within one church. The participatory workshop allowed couples time for skill development and open communication in order to strengthen their relationship and reduce their mutual risk for HIV in a country where more than 30% of people of reproductive age are HIV positive.

Although there is growing global attention to the problem of chronic diseases in low-income countries (Anderson & Chu, 2007), funding to support such interventions in faith communities has not been widely reported. Within the U.S., there are many examples of faith-based health promotion activities conducted in churches but few examples in other faith communities (Agadjanian & Sen, 2007; Campbell et al., 2007; Francis & Liverpool, 2009; Sutherland, Hale, & Harris, 1995; Watson et al., 2003).

There is no single formula for working with faith-based institutions. However, this chapter emphasized the importance of learning about the institution and its structure; using participatory methods; incorporating elements of cultural ecology and the social ecological framework; and explicitly incorporating male and female leaders in the design and implementation of the intervention. An important reminder for public health specialists however, as they work to partner with faith institutions is to recall that the primary mission of each faith institution is its faith. How that faith is lived out in the world spiritually, physically, socially, and in relationship with others is part of its teaching and theology. Many public health professionals, religious and non-religious, wear their secular hats when they "do" public health and worry about the judgmental attitudes of religious leaders or institutions in addressing specific health or disease issues. In the same way, public health professionals must be conscious of the possible judgmental attitudes we may bring to a faith-based group and learn to open our thinking to possibilities instead of assuming probabilities of closed doors and negative attitudes.

Recommended Readings

Phiri, I. A., Haddad, B., & Masenya, M. J. (Eds.). (2003). *African women, HIV/AIDS, and faith communities.* Cluster Publications.

The Bronx Health REACH Faith-Based Outreach. http://www.bronxhealthreach.org/our-work/faith-based-outreach-initiative/

FHI 360. Faith based initiatives. http://www.fhi360.org/en/Topics/Faith-based+Initiatives+topic+page.htm

The Center for Faith-based and Neighborhood Partnerships. U.S. Department of Health and Human Services http://www.hhs.gov/partnerships/

Engaging Faith-Based Organizations in the Response to Maternal Mortality http://www.wilsoncenter.org/event/engaging-faith-based-organizations-the-response-to-maternal-mortality

World Faiths Development Dialogue, The Berkeley Center for Religion, Peace and World Affairs, Georgetown University.
http://www.wilsoncenter.org/event/engaging-faith-based-organizations-the-response-to-maternal-mortality

Additional Resources

Resources and Tools for Building a Health Ministry, Division of Minority Health and Disparity Elimination, Department of Health, Tennessee http://health.state.tn.us/dmhde/faithresources.shtml

References

Agadjanian, V., & Sen, S. (2007). Promises and Challenges of Faith-based AIDS Care and Support in Mozambique. *American Journal of Public Health, 97*(2), 362–366.

Anderson, G. F., & Chu, E. (2007). Expanding Priorities—Confronting Chronic Disease in Countries with Low Income. *New England Journal of Medicine, 356*(3), 209–211. doi: doi:10.1056/NEJMp068182

Campbell, M. K., Hudson, M. A., Resnicow, K., Blakeney, N., Paxton, A., & Baskin, M. (2007). Church-Based Health Promotion Interventions: Evidence and Lessons Learned. *Annual Review of Public Health, 28*, 213–234.

Dubos, R. (1965). *Man adapting*. New Haven, CT: Yale University Press.

Estrella, M., & Gaventa, J. (1997). Who Counts Reality? Participatory Monitoring and Evaluation: A Literature Review. *IDS Working Paper, 70*.

Finnegan Jr., J. R., & Viswanath, K. (2002). Communication Theory and Health Behavior Change. In K. Glanz, B. K. Rimer & F. M. Lewis (Eds.), *Health Behavior and Health Education: Theory, Research, and Practice* (3rd Edition, pp. 361–388). San Francisco: Jossey-Bass.

Francis, S., & Liverpool, J. (2009). A Review of Faith-Based HIV Prevention Programs. *Journal of Religion and Health, 48*(1), 6–15. doi: 10.1007/s10943-008-9171-4

Freire, P. (1970). *Pedagogy of the Oppressed*. New York: The Seabury Press.

Hartwig, K. N., Hartwig, K.A., DiSorbo, P., Hofgren, B., Motz-Storey, L., Mmbando, P, Msurri, M., Mwangi-Powell, F., Powell, T., Smith, S. and Jacobson, M. . (2010). Scaling up a Community-based Palliative Care Program among Faith-based Hospitals in Tanzania. *Journal of Palliative Care, 26*(3), 194–201.

IDS. (1998). Participatory Monitoring and Evaluation: Learning from Change. *IDS Policy Briefing, Issue 12*(November).

Kreps, G. L. (2012). The Role of Prayer in Promoting Health and Well Being. *Journal of Communication and Relision, 35*(3).

McLeroy, K. R., Bibeau, D., Steckler, A., & Glanz, K. (1988). An ecological perspective on health promotion programs. *Health Education Quarterly, 15*(4), 351–377.

Meade, M. S., & Earickson, R. (2000). *Medical Geography* (Second Edition ed.). New York: Guilford Press.

Meade, M. S., Florin, J. W., & Gesler, W. M. (1988). *Medical Geography*. New York: The Guilford Press.

Moser, C. O. N. (1993). *Gender planning and development: Theory, practice and training.* London: Routledge Press.

Peterson, J., Atwood, J. R., & Yates, B. (2002). Key Elements for Church-Based Health Promotion Programs: Outcome-Based Literature Review. *Public Health Nursing, 19*(6), 401–411. doi: 10.1046/j.1525-1446.2002.19602.x

Phiri, I., & Phiri, M. (2011). The role of Stepping Stones Curriculum in HIV and AIDS Prevention for Church Couples in Slangspruit and Mpumalanga Townships, South Africa.

Stokols, D., Pelletier, K. R., & Fielding, J. E. (1996). The Ecology of Work and Health: Research and Policy Directions for the Promotion of Employee Health. *Health Education Quarterly, 23*(2), 137–158.

Sutherland, M., Hale, C., & Harris, G. (1995). Community Health Promotion: The Church as Partner. *The Journal of Primary Prevention, 16*(2), 201–216. doi: 10.1007/bf02407340

Ucheaga, D., & Hartwig, K. (2010). Religious Leaders' Response to AIDS in Nigeria. *Global Public Health, 5*(6), 611–625.

Vella, J. (2002). *Learning to Listen, Learning to Teach: The Power of Dialogue in Educating Adults* (Revised edition ed.). San Francisco: Jossey-Bass.

Wallerstein, N. (1992). Powerlessness, Empowerment, and Health: Implications for Health Promotion Programs. *American Journal of Health Promotion, 6*(3), 197–204.

Wallerstein, N., & Bernstein, E. (1988). Empowerment Education: Freire's Ideas Adapted to Health Education. *Health Education Quarterly, 15*(4), 379–394.

Watson, D. W., Bisesi, L., Tanamly, S., Sim, T., Branch, C. A., & Williams, E. (2003). The Role of Small and Medium-Sized African-American Churches in Promoting Healthy Life Styles. *Journal of Religion and Health, 42*(3), 191–200. doi: 10.1023/a:1024835500987

Zukoski, A., & Luluquisen, M. (2002). Participatory Evaluation: What Is It? Why Do It? What Are the Challenges? *Community-based Public Health Policy & Practice, Issue #5* (April).

Chapter 15

Designing Logos for Health Campaigns: Convergence of Semiotics and the Diffusion of Innovations

Do Kyun Kim, *University of Louisiana at Lafayette*

Introduction

Although many logos have been used in health campaigns, few studies have examined the appropriateness and effectiveness of health campaign logos. In addition, the process of creating a logo has rarely been described in practical reports of health campaigns. However, the importance of a logo as a visual representation of a health campaign much exceeds how it is considered among health professionals because it arouses the initial impression about a health campaign among the target populations and is often the most memorable image of a health campaign.

This chapter focuses on how to design health campaign logos based upon a theoretical evaluation of the red ribbon. This logo has become an important part of world-wide HIV/AIDS campaigns and has been spread to numerous target populations through as many communication channels as possible, including fliers, brochures, television, and billboards. Based on the evaluation of the red ribbon logo, this chapter contributes to designing a culturally appropriate health campaign logo.

For designing a logo especially for a global health campaign, different sense-making processes among different groups of people increase the likelihood of possible misinterpretations of the logo, which greatly affects its appropriateness and effectiveness. Theoretically, the misinterpretations of a logo among different cultures may occur due to the discrepancy of understanding between cultures as opposed to the Kantian proposition of existing universal understanding (Putnam, 1990). Similarly, Baldner (1996) argues the paradigm of "incompleteness" in the sense that it is nearly impossible for different individuals to create and perceive the same meaning out of what they experience. In addition, many cultural studies have focused on perceptional differences in public understandings that are constructed by different social systems (e.g., Markus & Kitayama, 1991; Trafimow, Triandis, & Goto, 1991), different norms (e.g., Mikulak, 2011; Ybarra & Trafimow, 1998), and different attitudes (e.g., Berry, 1969). Taking this cultural diversity in understanding an object into account, this study employs two theories—semiotics and the diffusion of innovations (DOI) to provide guidelines for designing logos for global health campaigns.

Theoretical Foundation for Logo Design

Semiotics approach to a logo

Semiotics is generally defined as the study of signs, including individual signs and grouped sign systems. According to Eco (1976), everything can be a sign if it generates and conveys meanings. Based on this definition, signs include both physically existing and non-existing objects as long as the objects have meanings (Eco, 1976; Solomon, 1988). More specifically, Mick (1986) categorizes semiotics in two ways—general semiotics and specific semiotics: General semiotics delves into the nature of meaning, and specific semiotics investigates "how does our reality—words, gestures, myths, products/services, theories—acquire meaning?" (Ransdell, 1977). The signs and meanings always work together in semiotics, as Peirce (1958–66) explains, "nothing is a sign unless it is interpreted as a sign" (p.172).

In addition, signs in semiotics are organized and combined into codes that are sign systems. Therefore, analyzing codes is an essential task for semioticians and key to understanding all types of communication having the latent rules that facilitate sign production and interpretive responses (Mick, 1986). Codes include encoding (formation) and decoding (understanding), depending on how social knowledge is dialectically communicated between authors and viewers. Related to the dialectical nature, semiotic tradition in communication has emphasized intersubjective mediation by signs and sign systems (Craig, 1999). This emphasis on intersubjectivity shifts the analytic lens from objects to relationships (Culler, 1986). In brief, semiotics deals with the nature of individual signs and meanings, and these signs and meanings are only significant when they are in relation with other signs (Babrow & Mattson, 2003).

In semiotics, a *signifier* and a *signified* coalesce into a sign. A signifier is a form or an image which a sign takes, and a signified is the concept it presents. For example, a signifier could be a red ribbon logo itself, while a signified is the concept or image of the logo as it is recognized among key populations. In other words, a sign generates its meaning with the relationship between a signifier and a particular signified, which is cultural, psychological and situational. Therefore, semiotic signs are not static, but dialectic in creating and delivering their meanings, and the communication process takes a critical role in transmitting and interpreting information among individuals and organizations with different cultures.

A logo from the diffusion perspective

While semiotics focuses more on a sign itself to create a consistent and shared meaning among the members of a social system, the theory of diffusion of innovations highlights the process in which an innovation is communicated among the target audiences. Based on the theory of diffusion of innovations, a logo newly designed for a health campaign can be identified as an innovation that is conventionally defined as "ideas, practice, or object that is perceived as new by an individual or other unit of adoption" (Rogers, 2003, p.12). An innovation is usually generated and introduced to potential adopters with four sequential steps that are need/problem, research, development, and commercialization (Rogers, 2003). In the context of health campaigns, an inventor should be motivated by a need for generating an innovation and by an existing problem to be solved. Then, the inventor needs to conduct research to determine the best strategies for creating a culturally appropriate innovation. The inventor, equipped with such specialized knowledge, should put the idea into a form that target populations are able to easily understand. If the innovation is exposed to a manufacturer who is persuaded to produce the innovation, the innovation can be introduced to mass audiences through a diversity of communication channels. Once an innovation is introduced to key audience members, it should contribute to building public knowledge about it.

In the diffusion process, the perceived attributes of an innovation greatly affect the adoption rate of the innovation. The perceived attributes consist of relative advantage, compatibility, complexity, trialability, and observability (Rogers, 2003). Relative advantage refers to the degree to which an innovation is perceived as better than the idea it supersedes. The greater the perceived relative advantage of an innovation, the more rapid its rate of adoption will be. Compatibility measures the degree to which an innovation is perceived as being consistent with the existing values, past experiences, and needs of potential adopters. An idea that is compatible with existing values and norms of a social system will be adopted more easily than those that are less compatible. Complexity refers to the degree to which an innovation is perceived as difficult to understand and use. The easier the innovation is to understand, the better it is for diffusion. Trialability explains that a new idea that can be tested out incrementally has a good chance for adoption. Observability suggests that if the results of an innovation are easily visible to others, it is likely that audiences will adopt the innovation.

Understanding culture

Peterson (1979) systematically explains culture with the following elements: 1) values: choice statements that rank behavior or goals; 2) norms: specifications of values relating to behavior in interaction; 3) beliefs: existential statements about how the world serves to justify values and norms (beliefs in turn are often justified by referencing common sense, science, religion and the like); and 4) expressive symbols: the aspects of material culture representing beliefs, and implying values and norms. As explained here, complexity and diversity may represent the core nature of culture. Then, how does culture define health?

Let's begin with a couple of simple questions. What is health? What is illness? Among health communication scholars, it is commonly accepted that health is a culturally and socially constructed concept (Airhihenbuwa, 1995; Sofolahan & Airhihenbuwa, 2013). Accordingly, the concept of health varies by the topical areas, such as physical, mental, social, spiritual and emotional health. The concept of health is also intersubjective. If a person says he/she is healthy, do other people agree? In other words, health reflects not only a self diagnosis, but also how others recognize it. From the communication perspective, health is constructed in part by the self and in part by others.

Culture has been a central issue in both theories of semiotics and diffusion of innovations (Benbaji & Fisch, 2004; Rogers, 2003). Especially, health professionals have recognized the concept of cultural relativism, which stresses the idea that each culture has its unique way of understanding things, as a key determinant to the success of their health campaigns. Based on the concept of cultural relativism, the following sections theoretically examine the appropriateness and effectiveness of the red ribbon logo, which has been used for international HIV/AIDS prevention campaigns, and provide practical guidelines for designing health campaign logos.

Analysis of the "Red Ribbon"

History of the red ribbon

What is the traditional meaning of the ribbon in the public sphere? The use of the ribbon originated from a 19th-century Civil War song in the U.S. It was first not a red, but a yellow ribbon. The content of the song is about people's sentiment about a prisoner's homecoming from Andersonville Prison. In 1973, American singers, Tony Orlando and Dawn, revived the aspiration of the old song in their number one hit, "Tie a Yellow Ribbon Round the Ole Oak Tree" (American Family Traditions, 2006). This history indicates that the public display of a (yellow) ribbon was a sign of loyalty to family, friends or loved ones who are welcome at home.

The first time the red ribbon appeared in the public consciousness was after American police officer Enrique "Kiki" Camarena died in the line of duty while he was investigating a major drug cartel in Mexico in 1985. After his death, parents who were concerned with alcohol and drug abuse formed coalitions, and those coalitions took the red ribbon as their logo in memory of Camarena's death. Along with this movement, the National Family Partnership organized the first nationwide Red Ribbon Campaign in 1988 (Texas Department of State Health Services, 2006).

The first time the red ribbon was used for an AIDS campaign was in 1991. Inspired by the tradition of the yellow ribbon, the use of a red ribbon for an AIDS campaign was started by the Visual AIDS Artists Caucus. According to Visual AIDS (2006), the artists in the group created this red ribbon to demonstrate compassion for people who were living with HIV/AIDS and their caregivers, and many international health campaign organizations including UNAIDS used the red ribbon as a representative symbol for solidarity with HIV-positive people and those living with AIDS in fighting against the disease (HIV-WEB, 2004). According to HIV-Web (2004), the red color in the ribbon is explained to be:

- Red like love, as a symbol of passion and tolerance towards those affected.
- Red like blood, representing the pain caused by the many people that died of AIDS.
- Red like the anger about the helplessness by which we are facing a disease for which there is still no chance for a cure.
- Red as a sign of warning against carelessly ignoring the biggest problems of our time.

While HIV-Web and other agents of international AIDS campaigns provide the explanation about the meanings of "red," there is no information about the choice of "ribbon." Therefore, why they have chosen the "ribbon" as a logo of an international health campaign still remains a question.

Theoretical Analysis

What is a "red ribbon"? Semantically, "red ribbon" consists of two words. Hence, before analyzing the "red ribbon," it is reasonable to speculate "red" and "ribbon" separately first. In general, a ribbon as an object is a traditional symbol of prettiness or beauty across different cultures, usually attached to something for decoration. The ribbon is also commonly perceived as a feminine symbol. Then, what is "red"? Red is a primary color and usually regarded as a color of passion, love, anger, blood, heat, and fire.

Based on these general meanings of "red" and "ribbon", how is the linguistic significance of "red ribbon" constructed? When "red" and "ribbon" are combined, grammatically, the "red" becomes an adjective of the noun, "ribbon," signifying the "ribbon" as the stronger in meaning. In other words, "red" loses its own strength in creating a meaning or image and become supportive to "ribbon" to strengthen the meaning of "ribbon." According to this socio-linguistic and grammatical analysis, it can be supported that AIDS and "red ribbon" have little intrinsic/extrinsic relationship. Due to this semantic weakness, the appropriateness of the "(red) ribbon" as a logo for international AIDS campaigns is highly questionable, and the use of the red ribbon as a symbol of the international AIDS campaigns is still at risk of creating misinterpretation of the logo.

Visually, the ribbon has no knot and, therefore, seems to lose its shape very easily (See Figure 1). This weak shape does not create a strong image worthy of the collaboration of the international society, whereas being tied together tightly may create the image of a strong international collaboration against HIV/AIDS. Second, a symbol that presents the concept of "international" should embrace the idea of diversity as the word *international* means diversity, rather than singularity. Because of internationally diverse cultures, social environments, and abilities, the strategies to combat HIV/AIDS internationally should be also diversified to create collaborative power to combat the disease. In this respect, the singular color for an international health campaign does not present or embrace diversity in any means. Even though

HIV/AIDS is a serious universal epidemic, this disease should not be treated in a singular way, but in culturally appropriate ways.

Figure 1. Red ribbon logo for international HIV/AIDS campaign

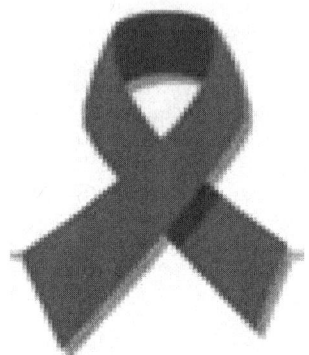

In addition to the problems of a weak tie and the red color, the idea of the red ribbon itself presents the logo's cultural inappropriateness because the ribbon has been used very narrowly only in Western countries, while a large portion of the campaign's target populations live in Africa and Southeast Asia. Due to the Western origin of the logo, people in non-Western cultures may not understand what the ribbon represents.[1] Although it might be a reasonable argument that many people in this century of globalization know what a ribbon is, this assumption could be a hasty conclusion also rooted in the Western perspective. For people who see the red ribbon for the first time, they are likely to perceive it as a symbol of beauty or an unknown object that does not imply messages intended by HIV/AIDS campaigns.

The red ribbon logo also presents specific risks in the process of diffusion. The first risky factor is related to accuracy in delivering intended health messages because of the ambiguous ways it may be perceived as a representation of female beauty, and the limited use of red ribbons in target audiences' daily lives, especially in non-Western countries. Empirically, for a person who is very sexually active and has multiple sex partners, therefore, a high risk to be infected by HIV, the interpretation of the red color, circled

---

1 This information was gathered by interviews with Ohio University's faculty members, who have studied and actively participated in international health campaigns and graduate students who came from Ghana, Kenya, Sudan, Botswana, Thailand, India, the Philippines, Malaysia, South Korea, China, and Japan.

shape, and pretty image could encourage her/him to have more sexual relationships with more partners. If it happens, the AIDS campaign will surely fail. This concern is not too much of an exaggerated example, but highly possible for a society where such ribbons have not been recognized. The interpretation about a certain image, such as the red ribbon, definitely varies by cultures and individuals (DeBar et al., 2009). Therefore, the use of the red ribbon contains a high risk of distorting the desirable messages delivered by health campaigns and possibly promoting undesirable sexual behaviors.

The second risk factor is a more communicative problem related to narrativity that refers to delivering intended health messages through people's life stories or storytelling. Traditionally, one of the most effective ways of spreading ideas and messages is by word of mouth. The narrative strategy has been an important part of social marketing as well as diffusion of innovations as they have emphasized the interpersonal contact as one of the most effective means of spreading ideas and information. To create a desirable buzz, a logo should be able to invoke people telling their own stories related to the (image of) logo and spreading the stories to others. The stories that are communicated among people should be related to desirable health messages that the health campaign planners intended. However, it is questionable how much the red ribbon is likely to create or remind target populations of stories related to HIV/AIDS prevention and safe sex.

Third, the red ribbon is a culturally incompatible symbol in many parts of the world. This incompatibility with a strange object most likely creates unexpected consequences, which critically endangers the goals of health campaigns. Again, people in different cultures think differently and understand things in different ways. Since the red ribbon stemmed from a Western idea, this post-colonial logo would not be understood by people of different cultures, but create serious communication noise talking about this logo in unintended ways (Shannon & Weaver, 1949).

Overall, the red ribbon logo has been used internationally for HIV/AIDS prevention campaigns and seems to be a very convenient logo so that many people pin it to their clothing and find it easily noticeable because of its simple shape. However, a logo as a representative figure of a health campaign has a special and important role that is to deliver *health messages* accurately and effectively with a culturally relevant understanding of the meaning. That is why we need a theoretical consideration based on semiotics and the diffusion of innovations in designing a health campaign logo. In fact, the simple shape has been used for many different campaigns with different colors internationally, although such undistinguishable use of the same shape with different colors confuses viewers about what those different ribbon logos symbolize. If this red ribbon is a symbol for fashion design, it is definitely a successful symbol. However, the red ribbon as a health campaign logo raises many questions as pointed out above.

Guidelines for Designing Health Campaign Logos

In practice, most health logos are usually designed at the clients' requests or by experienced medical illustrators (Finan, 2002). However, there are few guidelines about how the logos are created with purposes of using them for health campaigns. In spite of the importance of logos for promoting intended health messages by health campaigns, health campaign professionals have paid little attention to designing their health campaign logos. Based on what the theories of semiotics and diffusion of innovations advise and the lessons from the analysis of the red ribbon logo, this chapter provides important suggestions for designing health campaign logos.

Specifically, this study mainly considered the following three aspects for designing health campaign logos: 1) a logo should be able to generate communication that is to deliver intended messages by health campaigns and leads bidirectional communication between the campaign planners and target populations (Valente, 2002), 2) a logo should be culturally compatible with clear meaning(s), 3) a logo must be practically applicable to activities to achieve the goals of the health campaign more effectively and, simultaneously, be attractive to target populations (Conroy & Channon, 1995). Based on these theoretical and practical foundations, this chapter presents four important and specific guidelines for designing health campaign logos: accuracy, cultural compatibility, comprehensibility, and narrativity, which are all necessary elements in designing health campaign logos.

Accuracy

It is not negotiable that a health campaign should deliver its message accurately. Accuracy of the message specifically means that the contents and images of health campaign materials should be specific and clearly understandable to the target populations without causing misunderstanding and misconception. In other words, there should be little communication noise between the message sender (a health campaign) and the receiver (target populations) as Shannon and Weaver's model (1949) and Eco's model (1976) of communication shows below in Figure 2.

Figure 2. Communication models

1) An Information-Communication Model (Shannon & Weaver, 1949)

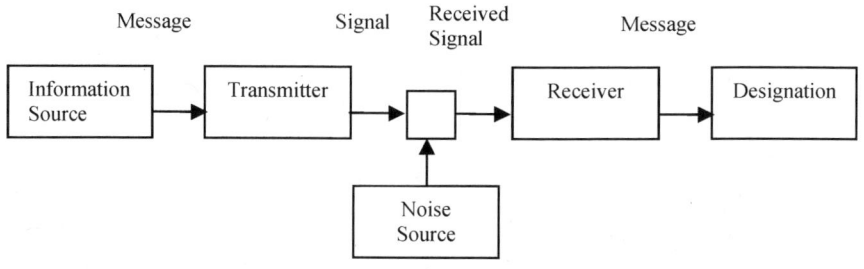

2) A Semiotic Model of Communication (Eco, 1976)

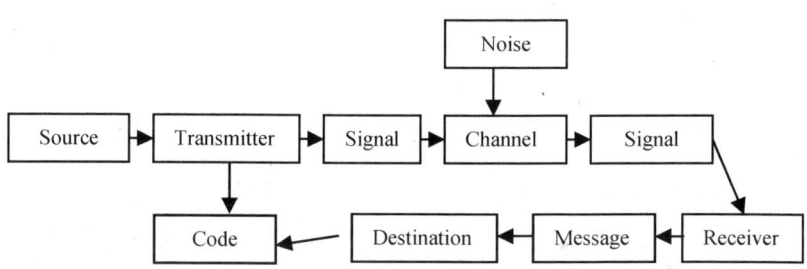

In Figure 2, the Shannon and Weaver model of information-communication has been known as a mathematical model of communication and applied to many technology and science fields. Communication scholars have also employed this model to explain how information is communicated between a sender and a receiver. In this model, communication noise results from uncertainty in understanding the meaning(s) of delivered information. In order to remove communication noise, Shannon and Weaver suggested that information should be designed and described in a more detailed and specific manner.

Similar to the Shannon and Weaver model, Eco (1976) provides a semiotic model of communication. The most noticeable similarity between the two models is that both models recognize the influence of communication noise in delivering information in the communication process. Based on this common feature, the main task to deliver information accurately is to reduce or remove communication noise. However, the semiotic communication model pays more attention to sharable code to prevent potential misunderstandings and enhance the effectiveness of information delivery. Applying this semiotic principle, a health campaign's intended messages and information should be encoded into a logo that considers how target populations decode the logo and understand its intended messages accurately with little communication noise. In this process, cultural relevance of a health campaign logo is a critical issue, which is discussed in the following section.

Cultural relevance

Cultural relevance is another key element when a logo is designed for a health campaign. It considers how an intended message makes sense to a target population. Needless to say, people in different cultures tend to have different ways of understanding as understanding is, in essence, a culturally and historically effected event (Gadamer, 2004). Therefore, health campaign professionals should pay much attention to how their target populations may understand a logo that is a means to deliver messages and information that a health campaign strives to implement in communication among target populations. This can be further specified with how well messages delivered by logos are tailored in the consideration of cultural difference and, similarly, how logos are culturally appropriate for the audiences to understand in their own cultures (Valente, 2002).

Cultural relevance is important not only to enhance accuracy in communicating health, but also to ensure credibility of the messages delivered by logos. Related to this, one of the principles in designing health campaigns is that target populations should perceive the message delivered by a health campaign as credible (Hovland et al., 1953). Again, people with different cultures have different belief systems, based upon different norms and values (Li, et al., 2012). Due to the complexity of culture, the pursuit of both accuracy and credibility seems to be a hard-to-achieve goal in designing a culturally relevant logo for health campaigns targeting people with different cultures. However, there are necessary principles for health campaign professionals to consider when they design or choose a logo for their health campaigns.

Regarding the cultural relevance of health campaign logos, it is also very important that health campaign professionals should have a culturally unbiased thought process in designing or choosing a logo for their health campaigns. In reality, it is highly possible, as shown in the example of the red ribbon logo, that health campaign professionals assume that the meaning of the sign they have chosen might be universal so that their target populations might also understand the sign as they do. According to MacDonald (1998), this type of health planners' perceptual bias in international health promotion efforts stems from the Western-centric perspective and economic imperialism. In addition, critical studies have also argued that Western economic imperialism in the past has been transformed into cultural imperialism (p. 35). This causes many mistakes in the design of health campaigns at present as well. In order to prevent mistakes caused by the health professionals' biased perspective, they should conduct sufficient research about their target populations' cultures by interviews, surveys, ethnography, as well as literature review before making a decision on their logos.

Comprehensibility

While cultural relevance is a more communal guideline, comprehensibility is a more individual and rational element. For designing a logo, comprehensibility refers to the degree that a logo can be rationally understood by an individual in a target population. In other words, comprehensibility relies on whether or not the information and messages delivered through a logo are logically designed, therefore, rationally acceptable by an individual. In that respect, designing a logo can be regarded as a sense-making process so that information and messages encoded into a logo make sense for target individuals to understand what it means. In business literature dealing with business logos, comprehensibility is closely related to subjective familiarity (Van der Lans, et al., 2009; Hendeson & Cote, 1998; Zajonc, 1968) which is a feeling of having seen a logo before. Related to subjective familiarity, comprehensibility can be often enhanced by the logo's compatibility with traditional symbols of a cultural group. In other words, the logos similar to previously well-known symbols are more comprehensive than a completely new one (Zajonc, 1968). This is why the theory of diffusion of innovations underlines compatibility as a perceived attribute of innovations that positively affect the innovation adoption (Rogers, 2003).

From the diffusion perspective, the degree of complexity of a logo is also related to the audiences' making sense of its meaning and adoption of the message delivered by the logo. Applying this tip, a simple logo increases its viewers' ability not only to understand what it is and what it means, but also to explain the logo to others, so that the logo is more easily communicated among target populations with less communication noise. This advantage of simplicity in the communication process further contributes to the target populations' ability to easily apply health messages attached to the logo to their lives, based upon their better understanding of health messages delivered by the logo. Semiotically, a simple logo can be interpreted by a simple decoding process that helps people understand the logo easily and accurately. This clear route for delivering and interpreting messages also removes the likelihood of information being lost or distorted.

Narrativity

The effectiveness of health communication depends much on the rapidity of diffusion of information and sustainability of information. Sustainability refers to a continuous process of target populations' engagement with health information delivered by a health campaign (Valente, 2002). This section introduces narratives as a means to pursue these double-tasks—the rapidity of diffusion and sustainability of information.

Garro and Mattingly (2000) explain, "Narrative is a fundamental human way of giving meaning to experience. In both telling and interpreting experiences, narrative mediates between an inner world of thought-feeling and an outer world of observable actions and states of affairs" (p. 1). According to Japp, Harter, and Beck (2005), narrativity has an inherently dialogic nature as a social communicative process because "personal narratives become the building blocks of public knowledge" (p. 3). More strategically within health contexts, shared narratives co-construct meanings of health through dialogic engagement among community members (Jamil & Dutta, 2012) and accelerate the diffusion of intended health messages among target populations (Rogers, 2003). In addition, if a narrative is interesting enough, the message out of the narrative remains in people's long-term memory as both narrative and edutainment theories have proved (Japp, 2005). From the semiotic perspective, a sign (logo) can be a seed to generate people's narratives telling stories related to the shape of the sign as well as the meaning behind it.

Due to the advantages of narrativity from both semiotics and the diffusion of innovations perspectives, narrativity is a core element in designing health campaign logos. Having all guidelines introduced previously, if a logo is designed in consideration of cultural relevance and simplicity so that target populations are able to understand it clearly, its encoded information is decoded accurately among target populations and also communicated among people by sharing their stories related to the logo itself and/or intended health messages attached to it. Once people start communicating with stories related to the logo, the diffusion of the messages is accelerated among target populations of health campaigns, and the health messages understood by storytelling remain in people's long-term memory. Based on this process, narrativity becomes a crucial communicative element for designing health logos as people engage in the ongoing communication. While applying the logo to their stories, narrativity of a logo not only brings a self-educational opportunity, but also enhances the likelihood of diffusing health information in more effective and entertaining ways. Due to this communicative nature, narrativity has been applied to many health communication programs using social marketing and entertainment-education strategies.

Conclusion

Logos are the most recognizable visual signs that represent health campaigns and simultaneously deliver health information to diverse target populations. Therefore, health campaign professionals should pay more attention to the role and effectiveness of logos when they design their health campaigns. Based on the theories of semiotics and the diffusion of innovations, this chapter presented four fundamental elements—accuracy, cultural relevance, comprehensibility, and narrativity—that help health campaign professionals design logos for their campaigns operated across different cultures. Figure 3 summarizes the guidelines for designing health campaign logos.

Figure 3. Designing health campaign logos with four guidelines

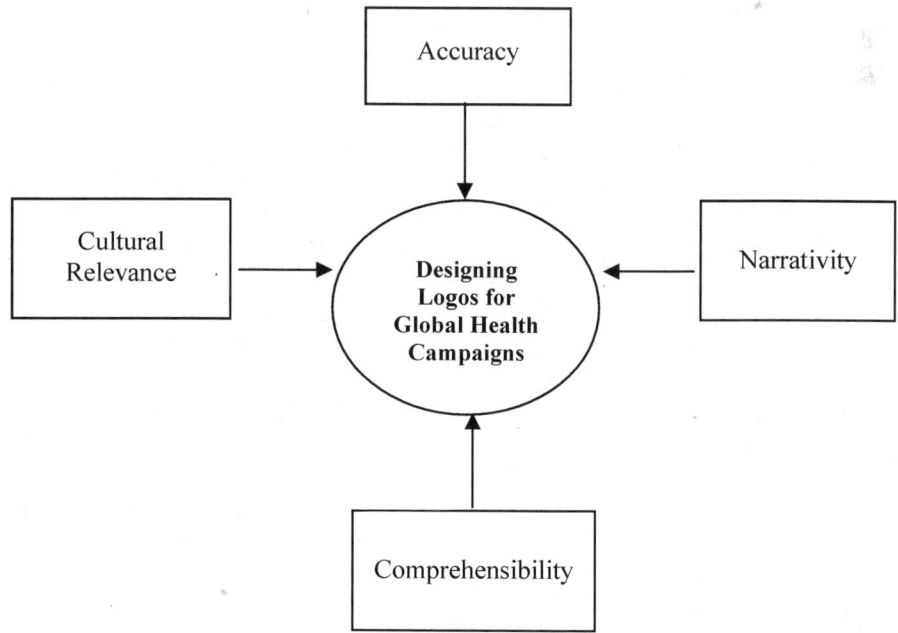

Recommended Readings

Airhihenbuwa, C. O. (1995). *Health and culture: Beyond the Western paradigm.* Thousand Oaks, CA: Sage Publications.
Beasley, R., & Danesi, M. (2002). *Persuasive signs: The semiotics of advertising.* Berlin: Mouton de Gruyter.
Eco, U. (1976). *A theory of semiotics.* Bloomington: Indiana University Press.
Henderson, P. W., & Cote, J. A. (1998). Guidelines for selecting or modifying logos. *Journal of Marketing, 62,* 14–30.
Peterson, R. A. (1979). Revitalizing the culture concept. *Annual Review of Sociology, 5,* 137–166.

Bibliography

Airhihenbuwa, C. O. (1995). *Health and culture: Beyond the Western paradigm.* Thousand Oaks, CA: Sage Publications.
American Family Traditions (2005). *Tie a yellow ribbon.* Retrieved March 20, 2013 from http://www.americanfamilytraditions.com/yellow_ribbon.htm
Babrow, A. S., & Mattson, M. (2003). Theorizing about health communication. In T.L. Thompson, A. M. Dorsey, K. I. Miller, & R. Parrott. (Eds.), *Handbook of Heath Communication* (pp. 35–61). Mahwah, NJ: Lawrence Erlbaum Associates.
Baldner, K. (1996). Subjectivity and the unity of the world. *The Philosophical Quarterly, 46,* 333–346.
Beasley, R., & Danesi, M. (2002). *Persuasive signs: The semiotics of advertising.* Berlin: Mouton de Gruyter.
Benbaji, Y., & Fisch, M. (2004). Through thick and thin: A new defense of cultural relativism. *The Southern Journal of Philosophy, XLII,* 1–24.
Berry, J. W. (1969). On cross-cultural comparability. *International Journal of Psychology, 1,* 207–229.
Conroy, M., & Shannon, W. (1995). Clinical guidelines: Their implementation in general practice. *British Journal of General Practice, 45,* 371–375.
Craig, R. T. (1999). Communication theory as a field. *Communication Theory, 9,* 119–161.
Culler, J. (1986). *Ferdinand de Saussure,* (rev. ed.). Ithaca, NY: Cornell University Press.
DeBar, L. L., Schneider, M., Ford, E. G., Hernandez, A. E., Showell, B., Drews, K. L., Moe, E. L., Gillis, B., Jessup, A. N., Stadler, D. D., & White, M. (2009). Social marketing-based communications to integrate and support the healthy study intervention. *International Journal of Obesity, 33(Sup. 4),* S52–S59.
Eco, U. (1976). *A theory of semiotics.* Bloomington: Indiana University Press.
Finan, N. (2002). Visual literacy in images used for medical education and health promotion. *Journal of Audiovisual Media in Medicine, 25,* 16–23.
Garro, L., & Mattingly, C. (2000). Narrative as construct and construction. In C. Mattingly & L. Garro. (Eds.). *Narrative and the Cultural Construction of Illness and Healing.* Berkeley: University of California Press.
Gadamer, H-G. (2004). *Truth and method* (2nd rev. ed.). New York: Continuum.

Harter, L., Japp, P., & Beck, C. S. (Eds.). (2005). *Narrative, health, and healing: Communication theory, research, and practice*. Mahwah, NJ: Erlbaum.

Henderson, P. W., & Cote, J. A. (1998). Guidelines for selecting or modifying logos. *Journal of Marketing, 62*, 14–30.

HIV-web, (2004). The history of the red ribbon. Retrieved October 9, 2006, from http://www.hiv.bg/about.hiv.bg.eng.htm

Hovland, C. I., Janis, I. L., & Kelly, H. H. (1953). *Communication and Persuasion*. New Haven, CT: Yale University Press.

Jamil, R., & Dutta, M. (2012). A culture-centered exploration of health: Constructions from rural Bangladesh. *Health Communication, 27*, 369–379.

Japp, P. M. (2005). Personal narratives and public dialogues. In L. M. Harter, P. M. Japp, & C. S. Beck. (Eds.), *Narratives, health, and healing: Communication theory, research, and practice* (pp. 53–59). Mahwah, NJ: Lawrence Erlbaum Associates.

Li, K., Seo, D-C., Torabi, M. R., Peng, C-Y. J., Kay, N. S., Kolbe, L. J. (2012). Social-ecological factors of leisure-time physical activity in black adults. *American Journal of Health Behavior, 36*, 797–810.

MacDonald, T. H. (1998). *Rethinking health promotion: A global approach*. London: Routledge.

Markus, H. R., & Kitayama, S. (1991). Culture and self: Implications for cognition, emotion, and motivation. *Psychological Review, 98*, 224–253.

Mick, D. G. (1986). Consumer research and semiotics: Exploring the morphology of signs, symbols, and significance. *Journal of Consumer Research, 13*, 196–213.

Mikulak, A. (2011). Mismatches between 'scientific' and 'non-scientific' ways of knowing and their contributions to public understanding of science. *Integrative Psychological & Behavioral Science, 45*, 201–215.

Peirce, C. S. (1958–66). *Collected papers*. In C. Hartshorne, P. Weiss, & A. W. Burks, (Eds.). Cambridge, MA: Harvard University Press.

Peterson, R. A. (1979). Revitalizing the culture concept. *Annual Review of Sociology, 5*, 137–166.

Putnam, H. (1990). *Realism with a human face*. Cambridge, MA: Harvard University Press.

Ransdell, J. (1977). Some leading ideas of Peirce's semiotic. *Semiotica, 19*, 157–178.

Rogers, E. M. (2003). *Diffusion of innovations* (5th ed.). New York: Free Press.

Shannon, C. E., & Weaver, W. (1949). *The mathematical theory of communication*. Urbana: University of Illinois Press.

Sofolahan, Y. A., & Airhihenbuwa, C. O. (2013). Cultural expectations and reproductive desires: Experiences of South African women living with HIV/AIDS. *Health Care for Women International, 34*, 263–280.

Solomon, J. (1988). *The signs of our time*. Los Angeles: Jeremy P. Tarcher.

Texas Department of State Health Services (2006). Red ribbon week: The story behind the symbol. Retrieved October 9, 2006, from: http://www.tcada.state.tx.us/redribbon/history.html

Trafimow, D., Triandis, H. C., & Goto, S. (1991). Some tests of the distinction between private self and collective self. *Journal of Personality and Social Psychology, 60*, 649–655.

Van der Lans, R., Cote, J. A., Cole, C. A., Leong, S. M., Smidts, A., Henderson, P. W., Bluemelhuber, C., Bottomley, P. A., Doyle, J. R., Fedorikhin, A., Moorthy, J., Ramaseshan, B., Schmitt, B. H. (2009). Cross-national logo evaluation analysis: An individual-level approach. *Marketing Science, 28*, 968–985.

Valente, T. W. (2002). *Evaluating health promotion programs*. New York: Oxford University Press.

Visual AIDS. (2004). History. Retrieved October 9, 2006, from http://www.thebody.com/visualaids/about.html

Yabrra, O., & Trafimow, D. (1998). How priming the private self or collective self affects the relative weights of attitudes and subjective norms. *Personality and Social Psychology Bulletin, 24*, 362–370.

Zajonc, R. B. (1968). Attitudinal effects of mere exposure. *Journal of Personality and Social Psychology, 9*, 27.

Health Advocacy and Activism

Chapter 16

Strategic Communication for Health Advocacy and Social Change

Gary L. Kreps, *George Mason University*

Introduction: Health Advocacy and the Health Care System

Health care consumers have a major stake in the quality of programs provided within the modern health care system. Yet consumers have had difficulty shaping health policies and practices due to a tremendous longstanding power imbalance within the modern health care system that accords far more authority to health care providers and administrators than to patients and family caregivers (Kreps, 2012; 1996). This traditional power imbalance limits consumer participation and influence within the modern health care system despite the fact that a large body of research demonstrates that increases in consumer participation in health care and health promotion efforts can significantly improve the quality of important health outcomes (Greenfield, Kaplan, & Ware, 1985; Kreps, 1988; Kreps, & Chapelsky Massimilla, 2002; Kreps & O'Hair, 1995).

Health advocacy groups and organizations have the potential to recalibrate the traditional imbalance of power in health care and health promotion efforts as a powerful social mechanism for promoting consumer-driven participation and change within the health care system (Kim, 2007). Health advocacy leaders can actively represent the voices, concerns, and needs of consumers within the health care system. Advocates have great opportunities to help make health care programs responsive and adaptive to consumer needs through the use of strategic health communication (Kreps, Kim, Sparks, Neuhauser, Daugherty, Canzona, Kim, & Jun, 2012). Strategic health advocacy communication can promote important influences on the development and refinement of health policies and practices. However, health advocates must learn how to communicate patients' perspectives and needs in compelling ways to key audiences using a variety of different communication channels and media to influence often entrenched health policies and practices (Kreps, 1996). This chapter describes the important communication activities that health advocates can perform to effectively represent the needs of consumers for reforming modern health care systems. The chapter also examines major communication challenges facing health advocates and suggests strategies for promoting effective health advocacy.

The Nature of Health Advocacy

Health advocacy typically occurs on multiple levels. The two most common levels for the delivery of health advocacy are the individual and the group levels. On the individual level health advocates work directly with specific patients to promote quality of care and informed decision making for these consumers, while on the group level advocacy groups and organizations represent the needs of many consumers confronting similar health challenges. Both of these levels of advocacy depend on effective and strategic health communication to be successful.

Individual level advocacy is delivered both informally and formally. At the informal level family members often serve as personal advocates for their own familial loved ones, particularly when these loved ones face serious health challenges or when the loved ones have difficulty representing their own health needs (perhaps due to reduced capacity related to their health conditions). Family advocates regularly support the health needs of children and elderly family members, but all health care consumers can benefit from effective personal health advocacy. There is tremendous potential for many people, particularly those who are well educated and those who are familiar with the health cares system, to serve as advocates for their friends, relatives, and others who are seeking health care services. Personal health advocacy can also help others adopt healthy behaviors and reduce significant health risks through education, support, and encouragement.

Individual level health advocacy is increasingly being delivered by formally trained care professionals, including health navigators, consumer advocates, patient educators, home health nurses, personal trainers, and social workers who can be assigned to work with specific consumers to help promote the best possible health outcomes for these consumers. Research has shown that these health advocates can dramatically enhance health consumer satisfaction, understanding, quality of care, and important health outcomes (Dohan & Schragg, 2005; Natale-Pereira, Enard, Nevarez, & Jones, 2011). Individual level health advocates provide invaluable support for health care consumers to insure these consumers receive the best care and advice to promote their health and well-being. These advocates depend on their strategic communication skills to gather relevant information concerning consumers' health concerns, interpreting health care recommendations and advice, and sharing this information clearly and compellingly with consumers.

There are also many different health advocacy groups and organizations that have been established to focus on promoting health and wellness for a large number of consumers experiencing specific similar health challenges, such as different cancers, heart disease, diabetes, and other health care issues. These advocacy organizations encourage focused research on specific health issues, influence legislation to promote consumer rights and responsive health care regulations, and help to refine health care delivery system programs, practices, and policies. Some of the larger and most well established health advocacy organizations have become familiar names such as the American Cancer Society, the Susan Komen Foundation, the Alzheimer's Association, and the American Heart Association. There are also numerous smaller (mom and pop) advocacy organizations and groups that are typically developed by consumers and/or their caregivers to address serious personal concerns they have had with the health care system based upon the care they (or their loved ones) have received. The leaders of both the large and small health advocacy groups/organizations depend on strategic health communication to achieve their goals. This chapter focuses primarily on the ways the leaders of health advocacy organizations can use strategic health communication to shape health policies and practices to support the needs of the health care consumers they represent.

There is a long history of health advocacy in the US that has powerfully influenced relevant health care research, as well as the development of important health policies and practices (Kim, 2007). For example, the American Cancer Society which was founded in 1913 as the American Society for the Control of Cancer by a group of prominent physicians and business leaders, has developed many influential programs to enhance the quality of cancer care and provide support to cancer patients. Prominent individuals have also had major influences on consumer advocacy by establishing influential health advocacy organizations. For example, Mary Woodward Lasker, who founded the Citizens Committee for the Conquest of Cancer when her husband Albert Lasker died from intestinal cancer in the early 1950s, was instrumental in promoting the introduction of the National Cancer Act of 1971 in the US that was signed into law by then President Richard Nixon. This landmark federal legislation initiated the national "War Against Cancer," which has spurred the development of important health organizations (such as the National Cancer Institute), the expenditure of billions of dollars of federal funding for important cancer research, the development of new cancer treatment strategies and medications, as well as the establishment of myriad new programs to support cancer prevention and control. However, it must be noted that it was not easy for individual advocates or their health advocacy organizations to accomplish such sweeping influences on public health policies. It took concerted strategic communication efforts, including the development of effective media relations programs, fundraising efforts, lobbying strategies, and the establishment of powerful public/private partnerships to achieve these important health promotion goals.

Advocacy, Communication, and Information in Health Care and Health Promotion

Communication is at the center of effective health care and health promotion, because communication provides consumers and providers with the relevant health information they need to get the best care and make their best health decisions (Kreps, 1988). Relevant and timely health information is a critical resource in health care and health promotion because it is the essential resource needed by practitioners who must guide strategic health behaviors, treatments, and decisions, as well as by consumers of health care who need to make important informed choices concerning the prevention of health risks, the promotion of their health, and the best health care treatments for them (Kreps, 1988). Health information includes the knowledge gleaned from health care interviews and laboratory tests used to diagnose health problems, the precedents developed through clinical research and practice used to determine the best available treatment strategies for specific health threats, the data gathered in checkups used to assess the efficacy of health care treatments, the input practitioners and consumers need to evaluate bioethical issues and weigh consequences in making complex health care decisions, the recognition of warning signs needed to detect imminent health risks, and the direct health behaviors that have been determined to help individuals avoid these risks (Kreps et al., 1998). Health care providers and consumers depend on their abilities to communicate effectively to generate, access, and exchange relevant health information for making important treatment decisions, for adjusting to changing health conditions, and for coordinating health-preserving activities. The process of communication also enables health promotion specialists to develop persuasive messages for dissemination over salient channels to provide target audiences with relevant health information to influence their health knowledge, attitudes, and behaviors. Health advocacy organizations have developed to help support these critically important health information needs.

Access to and effective use of relevant, accurate, and timely health information is critically important for guiding the important health-related decisions that consumers and providers must make across the continuum of care to promote health and well-being (Kreps, 2003; Kreps & Sivaram, 2010). This includes decisions about the prevention of health risks, health promotion behaviors, the detection and diagnosis of health problems, health care treatment strategies, and best practices for living with health threats (successful survivorship) (Kreps, 2003). Yet, health information is complex, with many different kinds of health risks, each with different causes, stages, symptoms, detection processes, and treatment strategies. Health care knowledge is rapidly evolving with advances in research and applications concerning etiology, prevention, detection, diagnosis, and treatment of health problems. It is extremely difficult for consumers, as well as many health care providers, to stay on top of all the health information they need to make their best health decisions. They need support to manage the complex and evolving health information environment.

A primary goal of health advocacy organizations is to help break through the complexity of health and health care by disseminating relevant, timely, accurate, and clear health information to consumers and providers to help guide informed health decision making. However, there are significant barriers to the dissemination of health information, especially for at-risk populations, due to limited access to health information, health literacy challenges, limited education levels, and the complexity of health research and health care processes (Kreps, 2012; 2006; Wen, Kreps, Zhu, & Miller, 2010). Health advocacy leaders must develop strategic communication programs for gathering relevant health information, interpreting that information, and presenting the information in meaningful ways to those who most need that information for guiding important health decisions.

Mediating the Complexity of the Modern Heath Care System

Health advocates must learn about the complex structures and processes that have been developed for delivering care and promoting health in the modern world. These health care structures are likely to operate quite differently from one location to another, particularly across different national health systems. Effective advocacy demands a detailed understanding of the different ways that health care delivery systems are organized and managed; the ways that health care services are financed; the ways that relevant treatments, medications, and technologies are developed, tested, and implemented; the ways that research programs are conducted to study health care and the promotion of health; as well as the ways that regulatory mechanisms and guidelines for governing the delivery of care are implemented.

This means that health advocates must be able to gather a great deal of complex information about health care systems and practices. They must learn about a wide range of different relevant health industries, including health care delivery systems, pharmaceutical companies, insurance organizations, and medical technology and supply industries. They need to learn about the many local, regional, and national government agencies that regulate heath care. They need to understand the ways that research programs are conducted to study health care tools, treatments, and processes. Moreover, they must learn the best ways to communicate with representatives of these different health care systems to promote cooperation and partnerships for refining health care practices and policies. In addition, health advocates need to understand the best ways to disseminate relevant information about the health care system to key audiences, particularly in reference to specific health consumers' needs and concerns. There is clearly a lot of information for health care advocates to gather and make sense of, as well as to strategically communicate to key audience to effectively advocate for meeting the health needs of consumers!

Coordinating the Efforts of Health Care Consumers and Volunteers

There is also a daunting administrative communication demand to developing effective and influential health advocacy organizations. Health advocacy group leaders cannot possibly accomplish the complex goals of influencing health care policies and practices to promote the goals of health care consumers all by themselves. They need to actively recruit followers who will become advocacy group members and volunteers to carry the group's messages and support group causes. Advocacy group leaders need to motivate, train, direct, and supervise these members to make sure they work effectively and cooperatively on behalf of the advocacy group/organization. Effective and adaptive leadership communication skills are needed to recruit, motivate, train, direct, and supervise personnel and volunteers (Kreps, Kim, Sparks, Neuhauser, Daugherty, Canzona, Kim, & Jun, 2012).

Advocacy group leaders also need to learn how to raise funds effectively to support health advocacy efforts. This is not an easy social influence process to accomplish! Fund raising is a complex strategic communication activity. Care must be taken to identify the most relevant audiences who are good potential sources for the donation of funds to specific health advocacy groups/organizations. Health advocacy group leaders must learn how to develop strategic development campaigns to motivate potential donors to provide financial support to advocacy organizations. These campaigns need to be strategically designed to capture the attention of key audiences of potential donors, elicit a strong sense of involvement with the advocacy organization among these audiences, and motivate commitment to provide needed financial support for health advocacy. This intricate communication process for eliciting financial support for health advocacy is complex and challenging. Moreover, there is tremendous competition between health advocacy groups for financial and material support. Health advocacy leadership demands strategic communication to navigate the complexities of raising funds to support advocacy organizations and the important activities of these organizations.

Working Cooperatively with Media Organizations for Health Advocacy

Popular media are primary tools for disseminating relevant health information concerning the health needs and issues affecting consumers. The right media coverage using the best media channels can be instrumental in helping advocacy organizations reach and influence key audiences. For example, advocacy organizations can use popular media to reach people who are concerned about the issues being championed by the organization to encourage these audience members to serve as potential members and volunteers. They need to reach potential donors to convince these audiences to provide financial and material support to the advocacy organization. They need to use the media to motivate public support for relevant legislation and policies. They also need media to encourage support from key public officials. However, it is not easy to control media messages and coverage. Strategic communication is needed to influence media cooperation with advocacy organizations.

The most direct way to control media coverage is for advocacy organization leaders to purchase media spots and advertising. Unfortunately, this can be very expensive, especially when paying for the use of the most dramatic and popular entertainment media, particularly television and film time, and to a lesser extent radio time. Another strategy for getting media coverage is for advocacy organization leaders to ask for it. For example, advocacy leaders often submit public service announcements to media outlets for free dissemination. Unfortunately, these public service announcements, even when accepted for presentation, rarely gain much exposure because they are typically programmed for inexpensive time periods. It is much more cost effective for health advocacy leaders to encourage free media coverage by earning it through the use of media advocacy (Wallack, Dorfman, Jernigan, & Themba, 1993).

Media advocacy is an intricate communication strategy for motivating mass media representatives to cover key stories that enhance the visibility and legitimacy of health advocacy organizations issues because the stories are attractive to these media representatives and promise to appeal to key audiences. In essence, advocacy leaders try to create news and encourage coverage of relevant and interesting stories. They can do this by building cooperative relationships with media representatives, staging newsworthy events, and linking advocacy group issues to breaking news or existing stories, as well as by providing editorial pieces and commentary on relevant issues.

Advocacy leaders can also encourage media advocacy coverage by preparing relevant stories, materials, and media kits for media representatives that make it easy for these representatives to cover the advocacy group stories (Houston Staples, 2009). They can provide succinct and persuasive summaries of advocacy organizations' positions of key public issues. They can distribute relevant fact sheets that provide compelling data and evidence in support of key issues they want covered. They can provide interesting press releases, with names and contact information of potential sources for the stories. They can also provide relevant background articles to media representatives, as well as providing clear and compelling background information about the advocacy organization.

By encouraging voluntary media coverage the health advocate hopes to encourage key support for the advocacy organization. The goal is to use free media coverage to influence and shape public debate, put pressure on policy makers, and encourage community support for the advocacy organization's key issues. Media coverage can help set the public agenda concerning health advocacy concerns by raising awareness about key issues, encouraging public discussion of these issues, and influencing private conversations about the issues to motivate support for social change (Wallack, Woodruff, Dorfman, & Diaz, 1999).

Building active collaborations with media representatives is critically important for motivating effective media coverage of health advocacy issues. There are several key questions that the health advocate needs to be able to answer. Who are the media representatives for the media outlets you want to cover your health advocacy issues? Are your messages right for the specific medium selected? Who are the audiences these media channels serve? What kinds of stories do these media outlets want to cover? What problems do you want addressed by the media? What are the ideal solutions to these problems? Who has the power to address these issues and must be mobilized to enact relevant social change? What messages would convince these key audiences to act on these issues? Do your messages have "news value" for the audiences the media outlets serve? How can you pitch your story to them? Can you help the media representatives do a good job? Are you responsive to media constraints (such as media time/space available for your story, the topics the media tends to cover, adjusting the level of complexity of ideas/language used to the appropriate level for the medium, the media outlets need for good visuals and/or sound bites, and the need for good personal testimony to humanize the story)? To utilize media channels effectively health advocacy leaders must be able to address these questions effectively. They must be able to develop strategic health communication responses to these questions so they can design compelling messages and encourage media support for disseminating these messages to key audiences.

Using Digital Media for Health Advocacy

An increasingly important channel for communicating health advocacy messages in the use of new, digital, e-health media (Whitten, Kreps, & Eastin, 2011). For example, the website has become a ubiquitous and pervasive part of the communication mix for health advocacy organizations (Gallant, Irizarry, & Kreps, 2007). The website is critical in helping to establish an identity for the advocacy organization and it also can serve as a primary portal for communication with key constituents if it is designed to be interactive. Unfortunately, too many health organization websites do not effectively utilize strategic interactive ehealth communication features and fail to maximize communication with key audiences (Kreps & Neuhauser, 2010). Many health websites fail to be particularly interactive, engaging, or dynamic (Gallant, Irizarry, Boone, & Kreps, 2011). To be effective, digital health programs must leverage the abilities of digital media to communicate vividly, interactively, and adaptively through the use of specialized mobile and interactive applications, video, tailored message systems, message boards, and social media (Kreps & Neuhauser, 2010). For example, the use of tailored information systems allows health advocacy organizations to adapt online communication to meet the unique needs, interests, orientations, and backgrounds of specific individuals, ensuring that online communication is personal and relevant for users (Kreps, 2000).

The website has morphed from being a mere repository of health information to being a portal to a range of exciting communication opportunities to connect, inform, and engage constituents of health advocacy groups. For example, health advocacy websites are often an entry point for access to online support groups, discussion boards, webinars, news feeds, and social media. Online support groups have become a staple health communication medium for many health advocacy organizations, enabling constituents who are confronting challenging health issues to connect with others confronting similar challenges to exchange ideas and to provide needed social support (Wen, McTavish, Kreps, Wise, & Gustafson, 2011). Evidence suggests that online support groups can be even more effective for supporting the needs of health care consumers than in-person support groups because they afford group members greater freedom to connect when they are in need, eliminate the need for travel to participate in the support group, and afford support group members a higher level of privacy and anonymity than in-person support groups (Whitten, Kreps, & Eastin, 2011). Online support groups have even begun to drive research about new therapies for challenging diseases (Frydman, 2009). Perhaps one of the greatest opportunities to health advocacy organizations is to leverage the use of digital media to promote collaborations, through the sharing of relevant information and the building of social action partnerships to promote change (Neuhauser & Kreps, 2010). As technology advances, there will be increasing opportunities to adopt new and powerful digital communication applications to promote the use of strategic communication to achieve the goals of health advocacy.

Case Study:
The GALA Program for Promoting Strategic Health Advocacy

To encourage the development of strategic communication programs by health advocacy organizations a new training and development organization has been established, the Global Advocacy Leadership Academy (GALA)

(Kreps, Kim, Sparks, Neuhauser, Daugherty, Canzona, Kim, & Jun, 2012). This case study will illustrate how the GALA program has integrated the multiple applications of strategic communication to enhance the effectiveness of health advocacy organizations. The GALA program has introduced new and relevant training, support, advising, and collaboration promoting programs to help health advocacy leaders build their knowledge base and learn how to communicate strategically with key representatives of different segments of the health care system. These health care system representatives that the advocates need to communicate with strategically include health researchers, educators, government and regulatory agency officials, health care delivery system personnel, health corporation leaders (from corporations such as pharmaceutical companies, insurance companies, medical equipment and device organizations, health informatics firms, supply organization, etc.), the media, as well as the leaders of other related advocacy and support organizations. Not only is the GALA program designed to teach leaders about these different relevant segments of the health care system, but the GALA program is designed to introduce health advocacy leaders to key representatives of these health sectors and help advocacy build cooperative relationships with these representatives (Kreps, Kim, Sparks, Neuhauser, Daugherty, Canzona, Kim, & Jun, 2012).

The GALA program is also designed to help educate advocacy leaders about the nature of health research, including how research is funded, who conducts the research, how research results are reported, how to make sense of health research findings, and how research is translated into relevant health care policies and practices. The GALA program will help advocacy leaders understand the intricacies of the modern health care system, including the design of health care delivery systems, the key roles performed by different professionals and support personnel working within the health care system, and the evolving policies governing health care delivery and reimbursement. The GALA program will also educate advocacy leaders about the development of government legislation for health care policies, programs, and research, corporate influences on the health care system, and the unique roles performed within the health care system by professional associations, regulatory agencies, educational institutions, support organizations, foundations, and other assorted non-profit, for-profit, and government agencies.

The GALA program is designed to help health advocacy leaders develop a wide range of necessary strategic health communication knowledge and skills to enable them to achieve important consumer goals. For example,

GALA can help health advocacy leaders learn how to support the information needs of the health care consumers they represent, providing these consumers with access to relevant, timely, and accurate health information. The GALA program is also designed to help advocacy organization leaders learn how to promote and advocate for increased funding for relevant health research needed to improve prevention, detection, treatment, and survivorship for the consumers they represent.

The GALA program has been designed to help leaders learn how to run effective advocacy organizations to serve the needs of their constituents and influence health practices. Strategies for recruiting, mobilizing, and serving the needs of organizational volunteers and personnel will be examined. Fund raising, investment, and fiscal management demands will be carefully examined. Strategies for using funds wisely for disseminating information, influencing legislation and policies, and planning and implementing influential health campaigns will also be examined.

The GALA program will help advocacy organization leaders learn how to disseminate relevant health information through a variety of media to raise awareness and educate health policy makers, health care administrators, providers, and consumers about the health issues of concern to their constituents. The GALA program will help advocacy organization leaders learn how to lobby legislators, regulators, and health care administrators to improve health care policies and practices. The health advocacy leaders will learn how to provide needed support and assistance to consumers confronting challenging health care problems, as well as to support the needs of their caregivers, family members, and loved ones. Perhaps most importantly, the GALA program is designed to promote local and global cooperation within the health care system to support health promotion, prevention, early detection, the best treatments, and successful survivorship for the health issues of concern to their constituents.

The Unique GALA Delivery Model

The GALA program is designed to provide advocacy leaders with relevant information and strategies for working effectively with key internal and external groups. For example, training programs will be conducted concerning development of effective relationships and collaborations with media representatives, government representatives, corporate leaders, researchers, and health care system representatives (Kreps, Kim, Sparks, Neuhauser, Daugherty, Canzona, Kim, & Jun, 2012). Moreover the GALA program will provide advocacy leaders with ongoing information support, consultation, updates on new opportunities/constraints, and continuing education to meet changing needs and refine advocacy knowledge and skills.

GALA programs will be delivered in several different complementary ways. Advocacy leaders will be invited to attend training programs conducted at a centralized site (George Mason University), where they will also be introduced to relevant government, corporate, and health care system representatives, researchers and scientists, legal, fiscal, and administration advisers, campaign planners and fundraising experts, as well as experienced and successful health advocacy organization leaders. In addition to centralized training programs, GALA program educators will travel to advocacy organizations in different parts of the world to provide on-site training programs. Arrangements will be made on demand to provide individual follow-up personal consultation with advocacy leaders to address specific emergent issues and concerns. Field experience opportunities will also be designed to guide advocates to participate in important meetings, conferences, and other relevant events, as well as to examine with GALA personnel the implications of these meetings. GALA is also proposing to link advocacy leaders and their constituents with an online information system (a collaboratory) to provide continuous support, on-line educational modules, repositories of health information documents, case studies, and media, as well as networking/collaboration opportunities for solving problems and developing new health advocacy initiatives.

The GALA training programs will model effective health advocacy leadership strategies. Leaders will learn how to establish and build effective advocacy organizations. They will learn how to recruit volunteers, organization members, and support staff. They will develop strategies for collaborating with other advocacy groups, locally, nationally, and internationally. They will develop skills for establishing working relationships with government representatives, corporate leaders, media representatives, educators, and researchers. They will also learn how to raise, manage, and invest funds for achieving advocacy goals.

The global nature of the GALA program is designed to promote international cooperation and collaboration for addressing advocacy issues, sharing resources, and implementing new policies and practices within the health care system. Advocacy leaders from different parts of the world who may be addressing similar issues will be linked to share information and resources for addressing these common issues. These leaders will be encouraged to build international collaborations for influencing global health practices and policies. The GALA program will combine support for leveraging research, theory, policies, and innovative applications to promote development of robust and adaptive advocacy programs to support the needs of health care consumers and their caregivers.

GALA Development Activities

To promote the growth and development of the GALA program, new strategies are being examined for seeking government and corporate support for GALA training and outreach programs. Survey data are being collected from key members of the advocacy, health care, government, and corporate communities to expand understanding about the unique training needs of advocacy organization leaders and the best strategies for meeting these training needs. GALA team members are identifying leading experts to work with the program to serve as mentors and trainers for aspiring advocacy leaders. New training modules, educational materials, and instructional guides are being designed and refined to use with the program. The GALA online collaboratory system is being designed and information is being collected to include in the collaboratory's online repository of documents, case studies, articles, research and funding opportunities, advocacy resources, and media programs. Information about the GALA program is being disseminated to key individuals and organizations around the globe to increase awareness and support for the new and exciting GALA health advocacy leadership activities.

Conclusion

Health advocacy organizations serve a vitally important role for representing the needs of health consumers within the modern health care system, refining public policies, and improving the quality of care and the promotion of health. However, effective health advocacy depends on the strategic use of health communication to gather relevant health information and to disseminate key information to important audiences in ways that will motivate cooperation and support for health advocacy issues. The Global Advocacy Leadership Academy (GALA) was described as an exciting new program for promoting the use of strategic health communication by health advocacy group leaders to achieve important health care and health promotion goals.

Recommended Readings

Kim, P. (2007). Public advocacy for cancer care. In H. D. O'Hair, G. L. Kreps, & L. Sparks. (Eds.). *The handbook of communication and cancer care.* (pp. 111–124). Cresskill, NJ: Hampton Press.

Kreps, G.L. (2012). Consumer control over and access to health information. *Annals of Family Medicine, 10(5).* To link to this article go to: http://www.annfammed.org/content/10/5/428.full/reply#annalsfm_el_25148

Kreps, G.L. (2006). Communication and racial inequities in health care. *American Behavioral Scientist, 49*(6), 760–774.

Kreps, G.L., Chen, Y-N. K., & Chan, J.M. (2011). Dialogue: Interdisciplinary and community-based approaches to health communication. *Communication and Society,* 17, 1–17

Kreps, G.L., Kim, P., Sparks, L., Neuhauser, L., Daugherty, C.G., Canzona, M.R., Kim, W., & Jun, J. (2012). Introducing the Global Advocacy Leadership Academy (GALA): Training health advocates around the world to champion the needs of health care consumers. In G.L. Kreps, & P. Dini, (Eds.), *Global health 2012: The first international conference on global health challenges* (pp. 97–100). Wilmington, DE: International Academy, Research, and Industry Association (IARIA).

Neuhauser, L., Schwab. M., Obarski, S. K., Syme, S. L., & Bieber, M. (1998). Community participation in health promotion: Evaluation of the California Wellness Guide. *Health Promotion International* 13(3).

References

Dohan, D., & Schrag, D. (2005). Using navigators to improve care of underserved patients: Current practices and approaches. *Cancer. 104(4):*848–855.

Frydman, G. (2009). Patient driven research: Rich opportunities and real risks. Journal of *Participatory Medicine,* 1, available at: http://www.jopm.org/evidence/reviews/2009/10/21/patient-driven-research-rich-opportunities-and-real-risks/

Gallant, L.M., Irizarry, C., Boone, G.M., & Kreps, G.L. (2011). Promoting participatory medicine with social media: New media applications on hospital websites that enhance health education and e-patients' voice. *Journal of Participatory Medicine,* 3. To link to this article go to: http://www.jopm.org/evidence/research/2011/10/31/promoting-participatory-medicine-with-social-media-new-media-applications-on-hospital-websites-that-enhance-health-education-and-e-patients-voices/.

Gallant, L.M., Irizarry, C., & Kreps, G.L. (2007). User-centric hospital websites: A case for trust and personalization. *e-Service Journal, 5:*2, 5–26.

Greenfield, S., Kaplan, S., & Ware, J. Jr. (1985). Expanding patient involvement in care: Effects on patient outcomes. *Annals of Internal Medicine, 102,* 520–528.

Houston Staples, A. (2009). Media advocacy: A powerful tool for policy change. *North Carolina Medical Journal, 70(2),* 175–178.

Kreps, G.L. (2012). Consumer control over and access to health information. *Annals of Family Medicine, 10(5).* To link to this article go to: http://www.annfammed.org/content/10/5/428.full/reply#annalsfm_el_25148

Kreps, G.L. (2006). Communication and racial inequities in health care. *American Behavioral Scientist, 49*(6), 760–774.

Kreps, G.L. (2003). The impact of communication on cancer risk, incidence, morbidity, mortality, and quality of life. *Health Communication, 15*(2), 161–169.

Kreps, G.L. (2000, November). The role of interactive technology in cancer communications interventions: Targeting key audience members by tailoring messages. Paper presented to the American Public Health Association annual conference, Boston.

Kreps, G.L. (1996). Communicating to promote justice in the modern health care system. *Journal of Health Communication, 1*, (1), 99–109.

Kreps, G.L. (1988). The pervasive role of information in health and health care: Implications for health communication policy. In *Communication yearbook 11*, ed. J.A. Anderson, 238–276. Newbury Park, CA: Sage.

Kreps, G.L., & Chapelsky Massimilla, D. (2002). Cancer communications research and health outcomes: Review and challenge. *Communication Studies, 53*(4), 318–336.

Kreps, G.L., Kim, P., Sparks, L., Neuhauser, L., Daugherty, C.G., Canzona, M.R., Kim, W., & Jun, J. (2012). Introducing the Global Advocacy Leadership Academy (GALA): Training health advocates around the world to champion the needs of health care consumers. In G.L. Kreps, & P. Dini, (Eds.), *Global health 2012: The first international conference on global health challenges* (pp. 97–100). Wilmington, DE: International Academy, Research, and Industry Association (IARIA).

Kreps, G.L., & Neuhauser, L. (2010). New directions in ehealth communication: Opportunities and challenges. *Patient Education and Counseling, 78*, 329–336.

Kreps, G. L., & O'Hair, D. (Eds.). (1995). *Communication and health outcomes*. Cresskill, NJ: Hampton Press.

Kreps, G.L., & Sivaram, R. (2010). The central role of strategic health communication in enhancing breast cancer outcomes across the continuum of care in limited-resource countries. *Cancer, 113*(S8), 2331–2337.

Natale-Pereira, A., Enard, K.R., Nevarez, L., & Jones, L.A. (2011). The role of patient navigators in eliminating health disparities. *Cancer. 117(15 Suppl),* 3543–3552.

Wallack, L., Woodruff, K., Dorfman, L., & Diaz, I. (1999). *News for a change: An advocate's guide to working with the media.* Thousand Oaks, CA: Sage Publications, Inc.

Wallack, L., Dorfman, L., Jernigan, D., & Themba, M. (1993). *Media advocacy and public health: Power for prevention.* Newbury Park, CA: Sage Publications, Inc.

Wen, K.-Y., Kreps, G.L., Zhu, F., & Miller, S. (2010). Consumers' perceptions about and use of the Internet for personal health records and health information exchange: Analysis of the 2007 Health Information National Trends Survey. *Journal of Medical Internet Research.* 12(4) e73, UR (4.41 impact factor). To link to this article go to: http://www.jmir.org/2010/4/e73/, doi:10.2196/jmir.1668

Wen, K.-Y., McTavish, F., Kreps, G.L., Wise, M., & Gustafson, D., (2011).From diagnosis to death: A narrative analysis of coping with breast cancer as seen through online discussion group messages. *Journal of Computer-Mediated Communication, 16 (2),* 331–361.

Whitten, P., Kreps, G.L., & Eastin, M. (Eds.) (2011). *E-Health: The advent of cancer online information services.* Cresskill, NJ: Hampton Press.

Chapter 17

Health Activism as Resistance: MOSOP as a Site of Culture-Centered Resistance in Niger Delta Region of Nigeria

Mohan J. Dutta, *National University of Singapore*
Agaptus Anaele, *Purdue University*

Introduction

One of the key elements in global health communication is the activist role of communication in drawing attention to global inequities and injustices, and in organizing through local, national, and global networks to challenge the unequal distribution of global health resources (Dutta, 2011). In this chapter, we introduce a culture-centered resistance site, the Movement for the Survival of Ogoni People (MOSOP) in the Niger Delta region of Nigeria. The history of MOSOP needs to be understood in the context of conflicts related to oil exploration and resistance in the broader Nigerian landscape. Nigeria is among the major crude oil producing countries of the world. The first oil well in Nigeria was identified in Oloibiri in the Niger Delta region in 1956, and subsequently several oil wells were located in the Niger Delta region that produces 90 per cent of Nigeria's oil (SPDC, 1995). The Niger Delta includes the following six states: Rivers, Delta, Edo, Calabar, Akwa Ibom, and Bayelsa. Unfortunately, the oil production in these states has not translated to better lives for the people, especially for the marginalized minority communities that have limited say in governance and the ways in which resources are distributed (Amnesty International, 2009). Instead, it has further impoverished communities where the oil wells are located due to environmental pollution and loss of farm lands, with large-scale contamination of property, crops and livestock, drinking water, and air (Pyagbara, 2007). Large-scale oil production in the region has resulted in a variety of adverse health effects resulting from exposure to oil, waste products from extraction and exploration, and extensive waste gas flaring (Gay, Shepherd, Thyden, &

Whitman, 2010; United Nations Environment Programme, 2011). The absence of basic facilities in the face of environmental pollution and the displacement of local indigenous populations from their forms of livelihood in the local communities have led to constant disagreement between oil corporations and the communities, embodied in local resistance in the oil region and resulting in large-scale violence, thus threatening community health (Gay et al., 2010; Pyagbara, 2007).

MOSOP gained global popularity in 1995, following the judicial execution of its founding leader Ken Saro-Wiwa by the Nigerian military leadership over his critique of the military, and the Anglo-Dutch Petroleum Company, Royal Dutch/Shell, for causing environmental degradation in Ogoni land. Saro-Wiwa was falsely framed for killing four Ogoni leaders, who later evidence suggested were actually killed by the military, allegedly working in collusion with Shell (Rowell & Lubbers, 2010). Saro-Wiwa's death attracted condemnation from human rights activists and civil societies around the globe, and the Ogoni movement emerged as a site of activism, co-creating a space for the articulation of local-global networks of resistance. We define the Ogoni resistance as an exemplar of culturally centered health activism because of the health consequences of displacement as well as the negative health outcomes of the seismic operations in the Niger Delta (Ogoni, 2011; Pyagbara, 2007). It is our hope that through examples such as the Ogoni Movement, the scope for considering health communication strategy in the global landscape is expanded to include resistance movements that seek to address the fundamental structural inequities underlying poor health outcomes in the global margins produced by unequal global policies (Dutta, 2011; Millen & Holtz, 2000; Millen, Irwin, & Kim, 2000; Pal & Dutta, 2008). Culturally centered health organizing attends to the local capacities of communities to participate in processes of change by challenging the inequities written into neoliberal global policies and by demanding opportunities for participation, recognition, and representation (Dutta, 2011). Against this background, our goal in the chapter is threefold: (a) present MOSOP as a site of resistance; (b) illustrate how structures respond to indigenous resistance against marginalization; and (c) document the outcomes of the interaction between MOSOP and the structures of organizing. We refer to structures in this essay to describe the state and oil corporations involved in seismic operations in the Niger Delta. Up to 1993, notable oil corporations in Ogoni land were Shell Petroleum Development Company (SPDC), Nigeria's National Petrochemical Company (NNPC), and Chevron. The local Ogoni protests and the disagreement between Shell and the communities over alleged non-compliance with international seismic operations forced SPDC to cease operations in Ogoni in 1993 (Amnesty International, 2009). Presently, Shell is in the process of ceding its oil wells in Ogoni to its joint venture partner, Nigerian National Petroleum Corporation (NNPC) (*Ogoni Star*, 2011).

Our interpretation of the interaction between MOSOP and the structures of organizing the oil industry in Nigeria is foregrounded in the culture-centered approach (CCA), a theoretical framework that seeks to understand the agency of indigenous communities in their resistance to top-down structures that marginalize them in decisions that impact their lives (Basu & Dutta, 2008, 2009; Dutta, 2011; Dutta-Bergman, 2004a, 2004b). Culturally centered organizing centralizes the local agency of communities, and foregrounds the voices of community members in disenfranchised contexts in the politics of social change (Pal & Dutta, 2008). The activities of MOSOP provide opportunities for listening to voices at the margins located in the global South that challenge top-down narratives that present neoliberal practices as panacea to social and development problems in a state that is heavily endowed with crude oil. Information gleaned from the MOSOP website is the primary data for this essay, documenting the practices of grassroots organizing in foregrounding the voices of community members at the margins (http://www.mosop.org/index.html). The MOSOP website is an important artifact of local activism, documenting the narratives co-constructed by MOSOP activists in their representation to a globally dispersed public, thus also serving as a resource for forging solidarities.

MOSOP Resistance in Ogoni Land

Ogoni land is an oil-rich area in Rivers State in the Niger Delta region of Nigeria, and has an estimated population of 500,000 persons (Amnesty International, 2009; MOSOP, 2011). The Ogonis depend primarily on subsistence farming and fishing. Therefore, the occupation of their farm lands by oil corporations and associated environmental degradation pose dangerous threat to their health and sources of livelihood, adversely affecting the land, agriculture, and farming (Amnesty International, 2009). Gas flaring, the burning of the gas separated during oil extraction as waste, destroys plants and wildlife by poisoning the atmosphere, causing acid rain (Amnesty International, 2009; UNEP, 2011; UNHCR, 1995). Frequent oil spills into the land destroy the land and oil spills into the rivers kill the aquatic organisms, while pipelines built across farm lands render the farm lands unusable, therefore rendering community members jobless and without food resources (Amnesty International, 2009; Pyagbara, 2007). Seismic surveys and construction of oil industry infrastructures have displaced large areas of land used for farming and fisheries, created obstructions in flows of water resulting in unbalanced asphyxiation and desiccation, and caused saltwater to flow into freshwater ecosystems, damaging both fisheries as well as local drinking water systems (Amnesty International, 2009). The absence of pipe-borne water, poor electricity supply, paved roads, and fully equipped hospitals are indications that oil corporations and the Nigerian state fail to adequately share the resources accruing from Ogoni with the communities where the oil is drilled from, with the absence of community participation in the ownership and distribution of resources (Amnesty International, 2009).

MOSOP is an ethnic activist group that challenges the imperial activities of global oil corporations that explore crude oil from the oil fields in Ogoni communities. MOSOP is a reaction to many years of oil exploration and mining in the region endowed with abundant crude oil and mineral resources, exemplifying a new form of colonialism that extracted wealth from communities through collusion between TNCs and local elites and without the participation of local community members. MOSOP was formed as a collective voice that speaks against the marginalization of Ogonis on their land, articulated through the everyday experiences of the Ogoni people with the adverse effects of the oil wells, oil spills, and gas flaring. The members of MOSOP are drawn from different organizations, and include women, youth, churches, teachers, students, and other professionals. The organizational website notes that "MOSOP stands for the Ogoni people's right to choose the use of our land and its resources. We have survived being marginalized and occupied by the state into the new era of Nigeria's fragile and imperfect democracy" (MOSOP, 2012. The statement added, "MOSOP strives for a future where all 'stakeholders' in the Ogonis' human and natural wealth can experience peace and prosperity as equal partners."

Evident in the statement is the marginalization suffered by the Ogonis in the hands of oil corporations and Nigerian government. The statement particularly draws attention to the oppression of the Ogonis during the 10-year military rule in Nigeria, a period that was characterized by human rights abuses, forceful detention of activists, and other forms of oppression. During this period, the right of the Ogoni to participate in decisions about the utilization of their lands was usurped by the government and the oil corporations, continuing the legacy of colonialism experienced by the Ogoni people. Therefore, the voices of resistance represented on the MOSOP website narrate the sovereignty of the Ogoni people and their right to have a say in the uses of their land and resources. The struggle for representation and recognition is fundamental to the struggle of the Ogoni people for social justice (MOSOP, 2012).

The exploration activities in Ogoni land are characterized by corrupt practices by oil corporations and government representatives that marginalize community members by excluding them from exploratory agreements on their farm lands, and when employment promises are made to the communities, they are not fulfilled. MOSOP draws attention to these unjust practices. Often the rhetoric of employment provision is used by the corporations and their agents as a tactic to co-opt the communities in generating support for the agendas of the corporations. Furthermore, when the employment promises are fulfilled, community members are hired as unskilled workers, such as drivers, cooks, cleaners, and the corporations in turn use these numbers to justify their project of development in the communities. The oil operations on Ogoni land produce a variety of health and environmental effects (UNEP, 2011). In addition to the deforestation of farm lands belonging to the community due to gas flaring, the Ogonis are also exposed to respiratory and other health complications as a result of the activities of the oil corporations (Amnesty International, 2009; MOSOP, 2012).

MOSOP stands in resistance to the violations of the fundamental human rights of the Ogoni people, and was founded in 1990 by Ken Saro-Wiwa, who was executed by Nigeria's military leadership in 1995 over alleged incitement of youth against the state and oil corporations (MOSOP, 1995). Through a collective voice, MOSOP resists the activities of oil corporations and seeks ways of regaining its rights from the government and the corporations. For more than two decades (1990 to date), MOSOP has been continuing to challenge environmental pollution of its farm lands by oil corporation that explore oil from Ogoniland, an area that houses over 30 oil wells that has generated over $30 billion in oil revenue for the Nigerian state in the past two decades (UNHCR, 1995).

Following its inauguration in 1990, MOSOP demanded from the Nigerian State and Shell Petroleum Corporation (SPDC) the right to participate in decisions about oil exploration on their lands. Additionally, they claimed that oil corporations in Ogoni should conduct environmental impact assessment and adhere to internationally stipulated seismic operations. Their demands were contained in the Ogoni Bill of Rights, a document that remains a reference point in the history of MOSOP. Specifically, the Bill of Rights requested SPDC to conduct environmental impact assessments of its activities on their land with the ultimate goal of ensuring best practices in seismic operations (MOSOP, 1994). In this Chapter, through the example of the MOSOP resistance movement, we elucidate the strategies of global health activism directed at challenging the unequal structures of global policies that generate a wide variety of negative health effects.

Resistive Strategies and Tactics

MOSOP adopts different strategies to resist marginalization of the Ogonis from the operations of oil corporations on Ogoni land. These include peaceful demonstrations, publication of a newspaper, *Ogoni Star*, petitions, and disruption of oil production activities. We provide an outline of some of these strategies in the following sections, seeking to draw attention to the role of communication as an agent of change in the backdrop of global health.

Demonstrations and voices

In the face of their marginalization, Ogonis organized through community meetings, performances, and demonstrations, coming together through the sharing of stories, songs, speeches, and poems. Meetings emerged as spaces of resistance, where the everyday accounts of community members served as the organizing framework for joining community members in networks of local resistance. Several forms of protest of the Ogonis draw upon the notion that the freedom to non-violently express resistance is an internationally recognized human right. Demonstrations, open representations of protests in public spaces, are seen as a resistance tactic used by activist groups to compel structures to effect changes in policy decisions and has recorded success at different sites of resistance. Notable forms of demonstration include peaceful marches against unfavorable policies, display of placards, performances, chanting of slogans, and hunger strikes (Dutta, 2011). In some instances, peaceful demonstrations turn violent especially when state security agents use force to compel activist groups to withdraw from protest against unfavorable policies, and the Ogoni narrative draws attention to various forms of State-sponsored violence. The Ogoni website represents an image of Ken Saro-Wiwa at the first Ogoni Day demonstration held in 1993:

Ken Saro-Wiwa at the first *Ogoni Day* held on 4 January 1993, which drew an unprecedented crowd of more than 300,000 Ogoni people. It is a special day on which our people celebrate their victory over the evil forces of marginalization, unconscionable military brutality against defenseless and law-abiding citizens, untold oppression, economic deprivation, environmental despoliation, and criminal neglect by the Nigerian state and their corporate agents including Shell.

The demonstration emerges as a site for documenting the marginalization of the Ogoni protestors, narrating the stories of police brutality and oppression, and drawing attention to the economic exploitation of the Ogoni people. The images of Ogoni Day celebrations are presented in the *Ogoni Star*, depicting protest marches, meetings, speeches, songs, and dances (http://www.mosop.org/02_Ogoni_Star_17_31_January_2011_Special_Edition.pdf).

MOSOP has collectively resisted top-down oppression in Ogoni through peaceful demonstrations. Some of these peaceful demonstrations resulted in the killing of Ogoni indigenes by governmental security forces, which use force to either guard corporation's oil stations, or to prevent the community from disrupting oil production at the oil wells. For instance, in 1992, MOSOP issued an ultimatum to the oil corporations (Shell, Chevron, and the Nigerian National Petroleum Corporation) to pay $10 billion accumulated royalties to its communities and to stop further pollution of its farm lands. MOSOP also demanded mutual agreement with the community on further drilling on its land, and threatened to embark on the disruption of oil operations should the corporations fail to honor their demands.

In response to the demands raised by MOSOP at the protest marches and demonstrations, Nigeria's federal government banned all public gatherings against oil production activities, and put forth a decree that such gatherings shall be considered as treason. The government move did not deter MOSOP. During the commemoration of the United Nations Year of Indigenous People in 1993, MOSOP mobilized over 300,000 persons to inaugurate the Ogoni Day, an event that raised public awareness about the suffering of the Ogonis due to the seismic operations on its land. The event snowballed into a demonstration that led to the beating of a Shell Petroleum Development Company staff by the community members, and the incident attracted state security forces. Consequently, the incident led to violence between SPDC and the community, and claimed the lives of over 1,000 Ogonis, arrest and detention of MOSOP members, and destruction of properties belonging to the Ogonis. Furthermore, the demonstration led to a four-year military occupation of Ogoniland (MOSOP, 1995).

Consequently, the founder of MOSOP, Saro-Wiwa and eight members of the group were arrested and detained by the state security agencies in 1994, and executed in November 1995 on the grounds that they incited the youth against the government and were involved in the killing of moderate Ogoni leaders. Several international observers condemned his execution and described it as judicial murder. According to MOSOP, the state used military forces to quell community resistance against oil corporations, and such military interventions were characterized by flagrant abuse of human rights, rape, indiscriminate shootings, extortion, and extra-judicial executions that contravened Nigeria's Constitution to protect the rights of its citizens (UNCHR, 1995).

Worth noting is that these events occurred during the era of military rule in Nigeria. Although the situation is not totally different, it is important that human rights and freedom of speech is receiving fair attention in Ogoni land. For instance, on August 3, 2012, MOSOP declared political autonomy from the Nigerian state. In his declarative statement, present leader of MOSOP, Goodluck Diigbo, said: "we are acting with legitimacy to reclaim all of our rights without exception" (MOSOP, 2012). Speaking on MOSOP's newly established radio station, *Voice of Ogoni*, he said, "By this declaration of political autonomy, we the Ogoni people are determined to enforce the United Nations Declaration of Rights of Individual People without fear or retreat" (MOSOP, 2012). Further, he noted that the self-government would allow MOSOP to collectively review the controversial UNEP Ogoni land oil assessment report. Whether the cession from the Nigerian State is successful remains to be seen, however, the lesson is a fair level of freedom of expression in the civilian rule. Historically, such attempts would have led to arrest, detention and jungle trials of the leaders of MOSOP.

Songs of protest

Songs have been a traditional part of Ogoni culture, serving as communicative expressions of the local culture and the stories of the local culture. As forms of resistance, songs interrogate the literacy-driven organizing logic of the State, instead finding meaningful resistance in the voices, performances, and solidarity of the people who have been marginalized from the processes of State formation. In the backdrop of the continued marginalization of

Ogoni people, songs emerge as communication channels for identifying the effects of oil pollution and for framing the oppressive effects of oil extraction in Ogoniland. Through songs, the community of Ogoni people came together to articulate their struggles and to share the story of their everyday oppressions in the hands of the hegemonic state, voicing the exploitation of Ogonis and rendering visible the various forms of oppression that remain hidden amid the hegemonic narratives of the State-TNC apparatus.

At nearly every protest gathering, songs are sung as performances that overtly challenge the oppressions of the State. Songs counter-organize oppositional narratives of development, documenting first-hand the lived experiences of community members living with the effects of the oil spills, contaminated land, and displacement from everyday forms of livelihood. The more than 3000 or so separate oil spills in the region that are experienced by the Ogoni are narrated through their songs. Consider for instance the following song (Ratical, 2012):

"The flames of Shell are flames of Hell,
We bask below their light,
Nought for us to serve the blight,
Of cursed neglect and cursed Shell."

The over 3000 oil spills have been poorly managed. The depiction of the flames of Shell as the flames of hell works to document the plight of the Ogoni people. Through songs, community members share their experiences with the oil spills and the neglect of the oil company in cleaning up the spills. The songs also juxtapose the structural violence embodied in the profiteering from the oil industry in the backdrop of the everyday experiences of Ogoni people who have lost their land and their forms of livelihood.

The sense of collective efficacy of the Ogoni struggle develops in the backdrop of these oppressive forms of exploitation. The song *"Aaken, aaken, Ogoni aaken"* (Arise, arise, Ogoni Arise) sung at almost every Ogoni gathering and protest march asserts Ogoni cultural identity in the face of the mainstream politics of erasure. The collective expression of Ogoni cultural identity stands in resistance to the structural exploitation of the Ogoni people, and asserts its political agency in claiming Ogoni representation. An Ogoni song reiterates "Be proud, be proud, Ogoni people be proud, We shall no longer allow the world to cheat us" (Nigeria Dialogue, 2011). The sense of pride as a people is the basis for the expression of an Ogoni consciousness, voiced in the resistance to the continued oppression of Ogonis. Songs emerged as performative sites for sharing evidence and offering grassroots information on the felt effects of the oil spills in the everyday lives of Ogonis.

Mass Media Strategy

Building networks with activist groups globally and drawing attention through global media were strategies that were effectively used by Saro-Wiwa. In televised interviews, not only did Saro-Wiwa document the plight of the Ogoni people, but he also presented visual evidence of the oil spills and gas flares in Ogoniland. Recently, MOSOP launched a television station, *Voice of* Ogoni. The newly established station was the medium through which it announced its political autonomy from the Nigerian state. Also, from 2009 to 2011, MOSOP published *Ogoni Star*, every fortnight. The newspaper was its official channel to raise awareness about the marginalization and human rights abuses on its land. It also used the paper as a medium to challenge and counter claims by the state and oil corporations. The following are some headlines on the newspapers: "MOSOP faults shell on project claims" (*Ogoni Star,* 2011). In the report, MOSOP faulted Shell's claim in national media that it spent N5.3 billion in recent years on development projects in Ogoni. Here is another headline in *Ogoni Star* "Motorists, Commuters Groan on Eleme Road" (*Ogoni Star*, 2011). The report chronicles the absence of paved roads in Eleme, one of the communities in Ogoni, and presents the harrowing experiences of commuters due to the occupation of the deplorable roads by petroleum tankers that are conveying petroleum products from the refineries located in the area. Again, here is another headline: "NNPC to begin production on Shell's Ogoni Wells. FG yet to discuss with Ogoni MOSOP" (*Ogoni Star*, 2011). The report highlights the government's plan to resume oil mining in the oil wells that belong to SPDC without dialogue with the community.

SPDC abandoned its 30 oil wells in 1993 following repeated disagreement with the community over its failure to adhere to internationally stipulated seismic operations. Through these publications, MOSOP draws attention to the marginalization techniques of the government and oil corporations involved in seismic operations in the Ogoni lands. For instance, Nigeria National Petroleum Corporation (NNPC) is Shell's joint partner, and represents Nigeria's arm of oil exploring company. Drawing attention to the linkage between NNPC and Shell emerges as a tactic for depicting the old transnational sources of power operating in Ogoni land.

Bill of Rights and Petitions

The Ogoni Bill of Rights, created by the Ogoni people through large-scale community participation, community meetings, and community-wide organizing processes, emerges as the voice of recognition and representation of the Ogonis. The Bill of Rights articulates the environmental and health consequences of the mining operations, witnessed through the everyday experiences of the Ogoni people. Here is an excerpt from the Bill of Rights (http://www.mosop.org/ogoni_bill_of_rights.html):

> Ogoni has suffered and continues to suffer the degrading effects of oil exploration and exploitation: lands, streams and creeks are totally and continually polluted; the atmosphere is forever charged with hydrocarbons, carbon monoxide and carbon dioxide; many villages experience the infernal quaking of the wrath of gas flares which have been burning 24 hours a day for 33 years; acid rain, oil spillages and blowouts are common. The result of such unchecked environmental pollution and degradation are that (i) The Ogoni can no longer farm successfully. Once the food basket of the eastern Niger Delta, the Ogoni now buy food (when they can afford it); (ii) Fish, once a common source of protein, is now rare. Owing to the constant and continual pollution of our streams and creeks, fish can only be caught in deeper and offshore waters for which the Ogoni are not equipped. (iii) All wildlife is dead. (iv). The ecology is changing fast. The mangrove tree, the aerial roots of which normally provide a natural and welcome habitat for many a sea food—crabs, periwinkles, mudskippers, cockles, mussels, shrimps and all—is now being gradually replaced by unknown and otherwise useless palms. (v) The health hazards generated by an atmosphere charged with hydrocarbon vapour, carbon monoxide and carbon dioxide are innumerable.

The Bill of Rights documents the effects of oil exploration. The Bill draws upon scientific evidence to document the effects on the environment that is charged with hydrocarbons, carbon monoxide, and carbon dioxide, complementing the scientific evidence with the lived everyday experiences of Ogonis. The effects of oil exploration are evidenced in the acid rain, oil spillages and blowouts experienced by the villages in the area. The impact on the lives of Ogoni people is documented in terms of food shortage, the destruction of Ogoni agriculture, and the rendering of the Ogoni people as market dependent for sources of food. The gradual loss of fish and seafood as a result of the oil-drilling operations is narrated, and the health consequences are articulated in the frame. The Bill narrates the erasure of Ogoni lives, the depletion of Ogoni resources, and the death of Ogoni culture as a result of the environmental pollution and resulting food insecurity. The death of the Ogoni people is juxtaposed in the backdrop of the greed of British and American oil companies. The deprivation of the Ogoni people is framed in relationship to the greed of oil companies and the encroachment of Ogoni land.

MOSOP also uses petitions as a communicative strategy to resist oppression and marginalization by the oil corporations and by the state. On March 7, 2010, the group resisted the state's attempt to relocate the military cantonment from the Port Harcourt, the state capital to Ogoni land. The Rivers State government had proposed the idea of relocating the military cantonment located in Port Harcourt, the state capital to Ogoni land. In pushing its agenda forward, the government used the rhetoric of development and employment opportunities that will result from the relocation of the military base to justify its decision. In its collective objection to the idea, the group articulated concerns regarding the shortage of land for farming and industrial development, articulated in the backdrop of the high population density in the region and the already ongoing development projects that have caused displacement.

Worth noting here is the claim of the Ogoni people to their land. Resisting displacement, the Ogonis note that they have offered enough and in return have been further oppressed. It is in this backdrop of the narratives of oppression that the voices of resistance draw attention to the need to stand in opposition to the persistent suppression. Further noting its rejection of the idea of development that is based on the displacement and massacre of Ogoni people, the group observes that establishing a military cantonment in Ogoni will not create job opportunities for the people and instead create further suppression. Pointing to the high percentage of unemployed graduates in Ogoni, the group voices the need for infrastructural facilities and projects rather than further militarization.

Once again, the narrative of resistance symbolically ruptures the monolithic narrative of development that utilizes the promise of jobs to carry out top-down interventions. The voices of the Ogoni participants note that establishing the military cantonment will not create jobs and will instead create further oppression. The one-side story of job creation is set in the backdrop of Ogoni voices that question the logics of the story. References to the oppressive role of the military in the region are shared as entry points for pointing to the possible violence and threats to health posed by the proposal to set up the military cantonment.

Petitions emerge as voices of change. Through the petitions, the Ogoni people seek out recognition and representing, offering alternative narratives that interrogate the grand narrative of development. Noting the material and physical aggression suffered by the Ogoni's due to oil exploration and mining, the group points out that militarization is a tactical strategy to encroach on Ogoni landed property. Once again, the interrogation of the military presence in the region draws attention to the oppressive practices of the government, depicting the military presence as a precursor to bringing back Shell. This point is further noted in the following excerpt:

> We cannot help but note that this plot to reinforce an already over militarized Ogoni territory may not be unconnected with an attempt to return Shell to the area by a governor who has consistently lamented non resumption of oil production in Ogoni and who has been putting pressure on our leaders to allow Shell back. We will resist this plot to the last man in Ogoni. We urge the Rivers State Government to immediately halt the plan to relocate a military barracks to Ogoni. We will not accept this obvious act of callous insensitivity to the plight of the Ogoni people despite all we have suffered in the hands of the military since we started demanding a fair share of our oil resources in 1990.

The militarization of Ogoni land is seen as a strategy for expanding the Shell operations in the region. Evident from the statement is the level of marginalization and neglect suffered by indigenes of an area that has witnessed 40 years of seismic operations on its land. The narratives also attend to the development paradox, depicting how a region endowed with natural resources has the highest unemployment rate in the country. It is not clear if the petition contributed to the hold on the relocation plan of the military base by the state, but the broader policy climate reflected discussions of the Ogoni protests.

MOSOP embodies resilience in important ways. Despite the use of force by the oil corporations and the Nigeria state, MOSOP remain a formidable force against oppression and marginalization of its rights, continuing to emerge as a voice of protest and drawing attention to the threats to human health that are posed by the oil occupations in the region. Regardless of the judicial execution of its founding leader in controversial circumstance in (1995), the group continues to challenge the operations of oil corporations on its land. Presently, it maintains a heavy online presence by publishing a newspaper, *Ogoni Star* every fortnight. The newspaper is a channel through which MOSOP challenges oppressive policies on its land, emerging as a voice that stands in defiance.

The voices of resistance in Ogoni land provide a site for documenting the complicity between transnational corporations, the state, and the elite classes in the marginalization of the community carried out through neoliberal development programs. The resistance literature shows the nexus between translational corporations and the state in forcefully implementing the agenda of the former in communities, and simultaneously attends to the creative ways in which communities organize to resist the concentration of resources in the hands of transnational hegemony (Dutta, 2012).There are visible markers of such collaboration in Ogoni land. See for instance how MOSOP articulated the collaboration among the oil corporations and the state against the Ogonis in the following excerpt: "MOSOP still requires local as well as international support in dealing with a ground swell of an unholy alliance between the political class and transnational oil corporations" (MOSOP 1994, p.1). In the excerpt, MOSOP draws public attention to the complicit role of the elite classes in carrying out the oppression of its community members.

Social change through solidarity and structural transformations

One of the earliest outcomes of MOSOP organizing was the withdrawal of Shell from Ogoni land. The killing of Saro-Wiwa catalyzed widespread global protests, co-creating spaces for transnational local-global networks of solidarity and organizing global resistance against the Shell-military nexus in Nigeria. The horizontal networks of solidarity within Nigeria fostered local organizing against oil spills across various sites. In March 2012, 11,000 members of the Bodo fishing community in Niger delta initiated a case against Shell in London's High Court, demanding compensation for two oil spills that occurred in 2008 (Bawden, 2012). Transnational solidarity networks fostered the involvement of global organizations such as Amnesty International, United Nations Environmental Program, and Human Rights Watch, resulting in multiple fact-finding missions, grassroots information gathering, and research-driven networks. Solidarity networks fostering local global connections created avenues for litigation in courts in the global North where the TNCs could be held accountable. For instance, organizations such as the Center for Constitutional Rights and EarthRights International worked with the families of Saro-Wiwa and murdered activists from Ogoniland to charge Shell in the Federal District

Court in New York for its complicity in the murder of the activists (Center for Constitutional Rights, 2009). The case was settled, providing $15.5 million to the plaintiffs for the injuries suffered due to the death of their family members and creating The Kiisi Trust for various development activities in Ogoni. Following the return of democratically elected government in 1999, the agitations of MOSOP are more widely accepted, and both the state and oil corporations are slowly paying attention to the lack of essential facilities in the area that has lost its farm lands and sources of livelihood due to several years of seismic operations. SPDC is beginning to pay attention to the need to conduct environmental impact assessment on Ogoni land and the need for cleanup of the spills that occur on the farm lands. The activities in Ogoni also had a multiplier effect in that it triggered pockets of youth resistance in the Ijaw area, where Riverine communities are facing similar threats due to seismic operations on their lands.

Notable groups such as the Niger Delta Militants resorted to obstruction and seizure of oil platforms belonging to oil corporations, thus disrupting oil production in the oil wells located in their communities. The activities of the Niger Delta Militants in turn resulted in heavy military campaign in the region. Given the difficulty in sustaining oil production in a hostile environment, the activities of the militia compelled the federal government to engage the groups in a negotiation over environmental degradation, community rights and resource allocation, the core agendas of MOSOP. Drawing upon the activities of MOSOP, it is apparent that resistance and collective action catalyze social change and policy reform. Importantly, it could branch off as an olive tree with branches going to different directions as seen in the MOSOP scenario, where its activities triggered similar activities in Ogoni and different communities in the Niger Delta, thus serving as an entry point for catalyzing local-global resistance networks.

Conclusion: Grassroots Strategies of Change

The Ogoni resistance movement exemplifies health activism because of its direct emphasis on addressing issues of health that result from oil operations and explorations, documenting the relationships between environmental pollution and health outcomes. In the backdrop of large-scale liberalization across the globe that has resulted in the increasing concentration of resources in the hands of the resource rich, the opportunities of the marginalized to participate in decisions that severely impact their health have been limited. This is evident in the development of large-scale mining and oil exploration operations across the globe without attending to the communities and the people that experience the health consequences of these operations. In many instances, mining and oil exploration projects have been carried out through deception, manipulation and the use of violence, without consulting the communities that are severely impacted by these operations. Ranging from displacements to toxic reactions to food insecurity to death that result from top-down development projects carried on in the name of development, the health effects of mining and oil exploration operations are documented, witnessed, and addressed through grassroots resistance movements that foreground local voices as agents of change. Localized forms of resistance in disenfranchised communities emerge on the landscape of global politics by challenging the basic assumptions of development, and by simultaneously documenting the negative health effects of development projects through their localized experiences. Voices of resistance emerging from the global South resist liberal democratic understandings of dialogue underpinning neoliberal governance, noting the hypocrisies and paradoxes embodied in dialogic calls issued by the TNC and the Nigerian government.

Health communication as health activism, as depicted in the example of Ogoni resistance against the oil operations on Ogoni land, develops as a strategy for addressing structural inequities and power imbalances through the presence of marginalized voices. In the global context, with the increasing inequalities between the haves and have-nots, health activism emerges as a communicative site for challenging inequitable structures that remain the sites of poor health outcomes. Of particular relevance for health communicators are the (a) gathering of information resources that serve as evidence in documenting structural violence, and (b) the framing of health and environmental justice issues from the standpoint of communities at the margins that are erased from dominant discursive spaces. Additional health communication scholarship needs to examine the various communicative strategies that are deployed across globally dispersed sites of local action against environmental and material threats to health posed by development projects pushed under the narrative of economic growth. The fundamental organizing of local, national and global networks driven by local voices offers a framework for understanding the ways in which communities at the margins that are erased from dominant discursive spaces go about securing spaces of recognition and representation.

The Ogoni movement depicts the struggles of the margins to seek avenues for participation and representation. As depicted through the case study we have shared in this Chapter, the struggle of the margins is first and foremost for recognition and representation in those discursive spaces where decisions are made regarding their lives. These struggles for representation then emerge into the mainstream discursive spaces through the voices of the margins. Through a variety of communication channels such as demonstrations, protest marches, petitions, dissemination through mass media, the Ogoni movement carries forth its message of resistance to uneven development in Ogoni land. The articulation of the health effects and environmental effects emerges as the entry point for the politics of change. The everyday experiences of community members with poor health outcomes are narrated in the backdrop of the state-oil company narrative. It is through the foregrounding of the local as a site of knowledge production that MOSOP challenges the expert narratives of the state-TNC nexus.

Recommended Readings

Dutta, M. J. (2012). *Voices of resistance*. West Lafayette, IN: Purdue University Press.
Kim, J. Y., Millen, J. V., Irwin, A., Gershman, J. (Eds.). (2000). *Dying for growth: Global inequality and the health of the poor*. Monroe, ME: Common Courage Press.

References

Amnesty International. (2009). *Petroleum, pollution, and poverty in the Niger Delta*. London, UK: Amnesty International.
Basu, A., & Dutta, M. (2008). Participatory change in a campaign led by sex workers: Connecting resistance to action-oriented agency. *Qualitative Health Research, 18*, 106[en]119.
Basu, A., & Dutta, M. (2009). Sex workers and HIV/AIDS: Analyzing participatory culture-centered health communication strategies. *Human Communication Research, 35*, 86[en]114.
Bawden, T. (May 12, 2012). Africa's oil theft crisis. *The Independent*. Retrieved from http://www.independent.co.uk/news/business/analysis-and-features/africas-oil-theft-crisis-7737955.html on January 20, 2012.
Center for Constitutional Rights. (2009). Backgrounder: Wiwa v. Royal Dutch Shell and Wiwa v. Anderson—Oil giant goes on trial for complicity in human rights abuses. Retrieved from wiwavshell.org on January 20, 2013.
Chambers, R. (1983). *Rural development: Putting the last first*. Essex, England: Longman.
Dutta, M. J. (2011). *Communicating social change: Structure, culture, agency*. New York: Routledge.

Dutta-Bergman, M. J. (2004a). The unheard voices of Santalis: Communicating about health from the margins of India. *Communication Theory, 14,* 237–263.

Dutta-Bergman, M. (2004b). Poverty, structural barriers and health: A Santali narrative of health communication. *Qualitative Health Research, 14,* 1–16.

Gay, J., Shepherd, O., Thyden, M., & Whitman, M. (2010). *The health effects of oil contamination: A compilation of research.* Worcester Polytechnic Institute.

Melkote, S., & Steeves, L. (2001). *Communication for development in the Third World.* New Delhi: Sage.

Millen, J., & Holtz, T. (2000). Dying for growth, Part I: Transnational corporations and the health of the poor. In J. Y. Kim, J. V. Millen, A. Irwin, & J. Gershman (Eds.), *Dying for growth: Global inequality and the health of the poor* (pp. 177–223). Monroe, ME: Common Courage Press.

Millen, J., Irwin, A., & Kim, J. (2000). Introduction: What is growing? Who is dying? In J. Y. Kim, J. V. Millen, A. Irwin, & J. Gershman (Eds.), *Dying for growth: Global inequality and the health of the poor* (pp. 3–10). Monroe, ME: Common Courage Press.

MOSOP. (2012). Objectives and aims. Retrieved from www.mosop.org,p.1 on January 19, 2013.

Nigeria Dialogue. (September 13, 2011). *Shell and the Ogoni narrative.* Retrieved from www.nigeriadialogue.com on January 19, 2013.

Ogoni Star. (2011). *Ogoni Star,* 12. Retrieved from http://www.mosop.org/02_Ogoni_Star_17_31_January_2011_Special_Edition.pdf on October 20, 2012.

Pal, M., & Dutta, M. (2008b). Theorizing resistance in a global context: Processes, strategies and tactics in communication scholarship. *Communication Yearbook, 32,* 41–87.

Pyagbara, L. S. (2007). International expert group meeting on indigenous peoples and protection of the environment. Department of Economic and Social Affairs, United Nations.

Ratical. (2012). Factsheet of the Ogoni struggle. Retrieved from www.ratical.org on January 19, 2013.

Rowell, A., & Lubbers, E. (December 5, 2010). Ken Saro-Wiwa was framed, secret evidence shows. *The Independent.* Retrieved from http://www.independent.co.uk/news/world/africa/ken-sarowiwa-was-framed-secret-evidence-shows-2151577.html on January 20, 2013.

United Nations Environment Programme. (2011). Environmental assessment of Ogoniland. Retrieved from http://www.unep.org/nigeria/ on January 20, 2013.

UNHCR. (1995). Human Rights Watch, *The Ogoni Crisis: A Case-Study of Military Repression in Southeastern Nigeria,* 1 July 1995, available at: http://www.unhcr.org/refworld/docid/3ae6a7d8c.html [accessed 20 January 2013]

Valuing Data

Chapter 18

National Health Communication Surveillance Systems

Bradford W. Hesse, David E. Nelson, Richard P. Moser,
Kelly D. Blake, & Wen-ying Sylvia Chou,
National Cancer Institute
Lila J Finney Rutten, *Mayo Clinic*
Ellen Burke Beckjord, *University of Pittsburgh*

> *"Public health surveillance is the foundation for decision making in public health and empowers decision makers to lead and manage more effectively by providing timely, useful evidence."*
>
> —Thacker, Qualters, & Lee, 2012

Introduction

In articulating a vision for public health surveillance in the 21st century, program directors from the U.S. Centers for Disease Control and Prevention (CDC) offer a definition of what public health surveillance has evolved to mean: "the systematic, ongoing collection, management, analysis, and interpretation of data followed by the dissemination of these data to public health programs to stimulate…action" (Thacker, et al., 2012). Although the practice of public health surveillance has origins in monitoring for infectious disease, it has expanded to include data from a variety of sources assessing a variety of outcomes. Whatever these new sources may add, the basic premise remains the same: to create an empirically based system for gathering the intelligence needed to protect and improve the public's health. The Surgeon General of the U.S. from 1998–2002 proclaimed that: "In public health, we can't do anything without surveillance; that's where public health begins" (Satcher, 2009). For many, the CDC directors argued, "it is the cornerstone of public health activity" (Thacker, et al., 2012). In this chapter, we explain how the public health surveillance system can be extended to monitor changes in the communication environment by providing an example of a national communication surveillance system launched in the United States.

A Historical Evolution of National Surveillance Systems

One of the first examples of a classic public surveillance exercise can be traced back to the use of city maps in London to track the incidence of disease outbreaks of cholera in 1854. Physician John Snow (the "father of modern epidemiology") used hand-drawn maps to mark the incidence of cholera deaths in hopes of finding a pattern underlying the outbreak of cholera and identify potential patterns of transmission within the Soho district of London. In studying the maps, and conducting interviews with residents, Snow traced the origin of the outbreak to a contaminated pump on Broad Street. He concluded from this analysis that the cholera germ was not being transmitted through "bad air," which was the prevailing theory at the time, but that it was being transferred through polluted water from the pump. The exercise not only changed the way city leaders would prevent future outbreaks, but it also revolutionized scientific theory relevant to disease transmission.

Over time, the use of surveillance systems to monitor the health of communities became an important part of providing for the common welfare of communities and countries. Disease registries began to diffuse as a staple among public health advocates, as did the use of routine surveillance of the food, drug, and water supplies. In the mid-1800s, a community report by the Massachusetts Sanitary Commission in the U.S. led to arguments for standardized nomenclature for diseases and their antecedents, thus ensuring consistency of information derived from disparate sources could be combined together, along with a proposal to collect health data along with basic sociodemographic characteristics as part of a decennial census. Consistent with the zeitgeist surrounding that proposal, governments from around the world began setting aside resources to monitor the health of their respective populations routinely though national surveys, systematic examinations of data from medical records, routine environmental inspections, analyses of blood and tissue samples, and through an examination of contextual determinants (Hall, Correa, Yoon, & Braden, 2012).

Although many of these surveillance efforts were producing actionable data at the local level, their use across international boundaries would be limited without an attempt to reach agreement on the indicators needed to monitor disease etiologies and transmission vectors (Louis, 2012). In 1893, a French physician by the name of Jacques Bertillon released the *Bertillon Classification of Causes of Death*, which became the starting point for international consensus on the classification of disease and health issues

(American Public Health Association, 1899). Throughout the latter part of the 20th century, the World Health Organization (WHO) continued to make the case for using a standard classification of disease and to begin collecting surveillance data in a comparable way across countries. To that end, the organization has maintained a whole family of classifications that it has used to promote common reporting on disease, disability, health, and health interventions. In particular, the tenth edition of the International Classification of Disease, commonly referred to as ICD-10, was put in place in 1992 and underlies the common reporting of disease and mortality statistics from the organization's 194 member states. The newest iteration of the classification system is being modified to synchronize with SNOMED, the emerging standard for maintaining health information within electronic health record systems (www.who.int/classifications/icd).

Extending Surveillance to Include Behavior and Communication

To take advantage of alerting state governments to disease breaks, and to help researchers and practitioners understand preventable risk, leaders at the Centers for Disease Control and Prevention in the U.S. launched the Behavioral Risk Factor Surveillance System (BRFSS) in 1984 (Gentry, et al., 1985). Its purpose was to collect the data needed to assess the U.S. population's behavior related to preventing serious disease, especially chronic disease, before it would occur, thus, saving costs in advanced medical care and enhancing the welfare and quality of life of citizens. Each of the 50 states, the District of Columbia, and the territories of Guam, Puerto Rico, and the U.S. Virgin Islands began conducting the survey on a routine basis. Common questions integrated into the core of the surveillance system have made it possible to assess trends in behavioral risk at the national level, while items integrated from the local jurisdictions have made it possible to collect information of interest to state planners (Mokdad, 2009). By focusing on behavior, BRFSS has given public health planners a mechanism of insight into the behavioral and environmental influences that, if left unchecked, could lead to serious health problems in the future.

One of the more influential facets of the overall public health environment has to do with the influence that the information environment exerts on health-related behaviors (Hesse, 2010; Kreps, 2010; Viswanath, 2005). Communication influences have been implicated directly or indirectly in the rise of tobacco-related deaths internationally (National Cancer Institute,

2008), to the rise of an "obesity epidemic" in the U.S. (Fitzgibbon, et al., 2007), to increases in vaccine-preventable disease (Lewandowsky, Ecker, Seifert, Schwarz, & Cook, 2012), to errors and utilization rates within medical systems (Mazor, et al., 2012), and to rises in public confusion over scientific recommendations (Bubela, et al., 2012). Rapid changes in the information environment, due in a large part to international diffusion of the Internet and global media channels, can promote public access to valuable health information, as well as public confusion (Berland, et al., 2001). To understand the influence of the communication environment on individual behavior over time, experts assembled in a 1998 symposium convened by the U.S. National Cancer Institute (NCI) recommended launching a surveillance system focused on communication. In response to that recommendation, NCI launched the Health Information National Trends Survey (HINTS) in 2001 (Nelson, et al., 2004).

Theoretical Framework

The HINTS surveillance system was initiated as a biennial survey through the Behavioral Research Program at the National Cancer Institute as a complementary effort to existing national surveillance systems. By design, the system was created with linkages to other national systems through common data elements, in addition to important unique components. Some of the common data elements included self-reports of health risk factors such as tobacco use, diet and exercise, alcohol use, vaccination (HPV), cancer screening, healthcare utilization, and experiences with chronic disease as assessed routinely by BRFSS, the National Health Interview Survey (NHIS), the National Health and Nutrition Examination Survey (NHANES), the Consumer Assessment of Healthcare Providers and Systems (CAHPS), and the California Health Interview Survey (CHIS). Some of the key demographic distinctions were drawn from surveys conducted by the National Census Bureau to be consistent with federal reporting requirements to allow for standardized reporting of outcomes. Because the survey was intended to match self-reports of health experiences with responses to the communication environment and the Internet specifically, care was taken to include items used by the University of Pennsylvania's *Annenberg National Health Communication Survey* and the Pew Research Center's *Internet and American Life Project*. Constructs unique to HINTS, and routinely assessed in the survey, include trust in health information sources, experiences with health information seeking, use of media for health information seeking, communication with clinicians and other healthcare professionals, health-related use of the Internet and emerging communication technologies.

In addition to the surveillance aim, the HINTS program was founded with the objective of providing a data resource for conducting behavioral and communication research. As such, key constructs in HINTS and item development were informed by theories of health communication, media usage, risk information processing, diffusion of innovations and behavior change (Croyle & Lerman, 1999; Fischhoff, Bostrom, & Quadrel, 1993; Glanz, Lewis, & Rimer, 1997; Rogers, 1995; Weinstein, 1993). Another feature of the HINTS program is that it was created to be part of the translational bridge between basic laboratory science, where much of the psychological research on message development and socially influenced cognition was conducted, and the broad national environment in which "real world" cancer control activities occurred. This aspect of the framework took its inspiration from the Canadian Cancer Control system. In Canada, national cancer control efforts were balanced between investments in basic science, intervention research, application delivery, and surveillance efforts. The U.S. NCI has embraced that framework in the programmatic activities it has adopted in cancer control and prevention (Hiatt & Rimer, 1999).

Following that framework, the HINTS surveillance system was developed as a complementary surveillance channel—to work in tandem with disease registries and other surveillance channels—in offering researchers, intervention developers, application developers and policy makers a framework through which to track population-wide influence. This system's level surveillance framework, as illustrated in Figure 1, reflects a national push to link data streams for the purpose of "connecting the dots" between research, clinical practice, and public health. It is enabled especially by advances in health information technology (Savel & Foldy, 2012) and analytic technology (Rolka, et al., 2012). Predictions are that those advances should also enable improved global health surveillance (Louis, 2012).

Figure 1. A framework for reducing disease burden based on complementary investments in fundamental research, intervention research, program delivery, and surveillance research (Hiatt & Rimer, 1999)

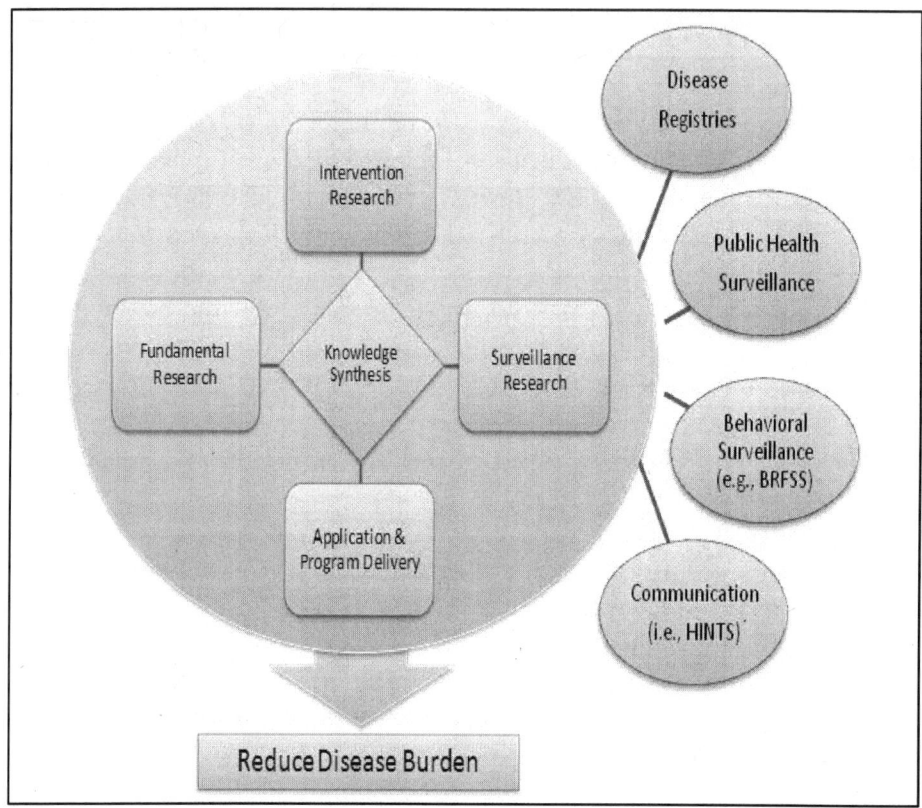

Designing, Implementing, Evaluating, and Disseminating Results of a Surveillance System

In implementing the HINTS program, we followed many of the best practice guidelines established by the American Association of Public Opinion Researchers (AAPOR), the Council of American Survey Research Organizations (CASRO), and academic survey research professionals to develop reliable and statistically valid point estimates to use for national surveillance purposes.

Designing the System

The main purpose for developing a surveillance system of any kind is to collect data in a scientifically accurate and precise way, while managing the demands of resources and budget, in order to produce actionable information for public benefit (Thacker, et al., 2012). The HINTS system is designed to be a survey of self-reported attitudes, knowledge, and behaviors from the general U.S. population of non-institutionalized adults aged 18 years and older. Surveys use sampling methods to obtain data from a randomly selected subset of a pre-defined segment of the overall population, called a sample frame. Sampling theory suggests that if accurate measurements are drawn in a truly random fashion from a larger population, then the mean of those measurements will begin to approximate the overall mean of the underlying population within specifiable degrees of confidence (Groves, 2009). Survey administrators thus seek to minimize the deviation of all the obtained measures of central tendency from true measures in the underlying population and total survey error across *coverage, sampling, nonresponse, and measurement* (Dillman, Smyth, & Christian, 2009).

Coverage errors occur when not all members of the overall population are given an equal, nonzero probability of being included in the sample. Door-to-door, or area-probability-sampling, techniques often provide the best guarantee of coverage; however, these techniques can be very expensive. When the HINTS system was launched in 2001, it used a list-assisted, Random Digit Dial telephone technique. With this technique, lists of valid telephone numbers are purchased from an external vendor and then a computer-assisted sampling program is used to dial numbers from those lists at random. Recently, the number households with landline telephones began to decline (Blumberg & Luke, 2008), as did phone survey response rates (Keeter, Kennedy, Dimock, Best, & Craighill, 2006) since many individuals, especially those who were young and mobile, elected to maintain cellular telephone service in lieu of their landlines. Like other federal surveillance systems, the HINTS program retooled its approach in 2007 to experiment with a dual-frame RDD and postal survey. Comparisons of results suggested that the newly available postal frame offered better coverage of noninstitutionalized adults than the telephone survey and in 2011 the system was converted to a postal frame in its entirety.

Sampling error refers to the degree to which the precision of estimates is limited because not everyone in the sampling frame had an equal opportunity to be represented in the obtained sample. The HINTS management team experimented with several techniques to be sure that each adult member of the household had equal chances of being selected for inclusion. The method of respondent selection that proved to be the most effective was referred to as the "Next Birthday Method" wherein recipients of the telephone call or the mailed package were instructed to select that adult member of the house whose birthday was coming up next (Rizzo, Park, Hesse, & Willis, 2004).

Nonresponse error refers to the unequal representation of members within a sampling frame due to differences in willingness to respond across subgroups. The HINTS management team made a concerted effort to minimize nonresponse bias: telephone operations were conducted both during the day and during the evening across all U.S. time zones to improve the probability of response; advance materials were sent to the home in advance of the telephone call to elicit a sense of civic opportunity; and two dollar bills were included with the materials to attract attention ($2 bills are rare in the U.S.) and to serve as a token of expressed appreciation.

Finally, measurement error refers to the degree to which respondents' interpretations of questions match the measurement objectives of survey designers in a reliable way across the sample. To address clarity of survey items, formatting and content issues, the HINTS team used cognitive interviewing techniques in which paid participants were brought into a laboratory and asked to verbalize their thinking when interpreting the questions and formulating responses. After the cognitive interviews were conducted, and the survey was finalized, a fully implemented field test of the procedures was conducted to shore up the reliability of procedures and address any remaining content issues. The HINTS instrument was also translated into Spanish, and cognitive interviewing was done in Spanish for the translated version to ensure cultural competence of the survey items.

Implementing the System

To date, there have been four full administrations of HINTS. Contracts for the first three (HINTS 1–3) were awarded biennially. The fourth contract (HINTS 4) was awarded to cover a four-year period, and represented a change in protocol. The first year of the fourth contract was to be set aside for the development of an "over-inclusive" item pool to submit for government clearance with the stipulations set aside by United States Code (U.S.C.) § 3501 to §3521. Once approval was obtained, the survey administrators were asked to begin an iterative sequence of administration across four cycles of data collection. Each cycle would draw strategically from the over-inclusive item pool, with some items repeated across all or half of the cycles administered for trending purposes. Within each survey administration, the process for development follows a fairly consistent plan (see Table 1). For the HINTS 4 administration, a special Web 2.0 platform was constructed for soliciting nominations of items from the general user community in addition to soliciting items from content experts in more customary ways (Moser, Beckjord, Finney Rutten, Blake, & Hesse, 2012).

Table 1. Implementation steps for completing single cycle of HINTS data collection.

Step	Description	Product
1. Solicit item pool	Worked with subject matter experts to identify relevant measurement goals, items, and harmonized data elements.	Pool of testable survey items for clearance and subsequent refinement.
2. Formulate sampling plan	Worked with survey statisticians to finalize strategies for optimizing coverage, reducing sampling error, improving validity of measurements, and protecting response rates.	Sampling plan available as a technical document on the HINTS website.
3. Obtain clearances	Clearance procedures in the U.S. included requests for an expedited Internal Review Board (IRB) and approval from the Office of Management and Budget (OMB).	Official clearance with OMB number to print on all respondent materials.
4. Develop procedures	Survey administrators developed survey management system, computer-assisted telephone interview, and paper forms.	All materials prepared for survey administration.
5. Test & evaluate	All items were submitted to a concurrent protocol analysis (i.e., think aloud procedure) within the cognitive laboratory. Pilot study was used to test and refine procedures.	Finalized content and operational protocols.
6. Administer survey	Surveys were administered over approximately a four-month period. Quality control procedures and frequent reporting ensured that the sample was released in a judicious, effective way and methods adhered to protocol.	Initial data set from all respondents.
7. Data cleaning and weighting	Data specialists removed redundancies, coded for missing or uninterpretable values, checked internal consistency, completed format libraries, and added statistical weights for accurate variance estimation.	Final, deidentified data set delivered to program managers.
8. Data release	Final data files and all technical documentation were made available to HINTS community through website; an electronic codebook was used to portray population estimates to general public in real time.	Public release data sets and accompanying technical material.

Evaluation

Evaluation was built into the fabric of the HINTS program from its inception. During each phase of instrument construction, versions of the instrument were brought into a survey laboratory for successive rounds of cognitive testing. Cognitive testing is a procedure used by survey designers to evaluate the manner in which respondents interpret and respond to the wording and format of questions in the instrument. The HINTS formative evaluation team used a concurrent protocol analysis procedure in which representative participants were presented with questions from the draft instrument and then asked to verbalize their thought processes when interpreting and responding to questions. Approximately nine participants were brought into the laboratory independently for each of three cycles for a total of approximately 27 hours of recorded interviews (3 cycles X 9 participants X 1 hour). Testing procedures followed best practice as articulated by Sudman, Bradburn, and Schwarz (Sudman, Bradburn, & Schwarz, 1996).

Once the survey was readied for the field, a trial pilot test was conducted to test all of the administrative procedures in real world conditions. Pilot studies typically aimed for a sample size of about 150 respondents. Sampling procedures for the pilot tests were set to oversample telephone exchanges (in the first three administrations) or postal areas (in the third and fourth administrations) in which high numbers of multilingual respondents lived. This ensured that the administration procedures would run smoothly in even the most challenging of coverage areas. Results for the pilot test were used to adjust final procedures and to calibrate selection algorithms in the Random Digit Dial surveys.

In years 5 and 7 of the survey, two separate program evaluations were conducted by independent contractors to assess the reach and effectiveness of the program from the perspective of prospective stakeholders and beneficiaries. The evaluation contractors reviewed the program's web presence with recommendations for improving usability; they evaluated the network of knowledge products being generated by the HINTS community; and the conducted interviews during relevant conferences with interested users. Revisions were made to the program's dissemination efforts based on the independent evaluators' recommendations.

Summaries of the evaluation activities can be found on the HINTS website at http://hints.cancer.gov.

Dissemination

The HINTS dissemination plan focused on two primary audiences: data users and results. Data users included communication scientists, public health analysts, graduate students, and other research professionals who would be interested in taking the raw data from the HINTS surveys and converting them for peer-reviewed publications. Results users, in contrast, included public health planners, policy makers, journalists, and other information intermediaries who could help turn the results of scientific findings into public health action.

To support data users, the HINTS website was developed to provide direct access to deidentified, self-documented copies of the data in SAS®, SPSS®, and STATA® formats. Replicate weighting vectors were included to improve accuracy of population estimates. The website was also used to keep track of scientists' ongoing publications and to support collaborative work in similar topic areas. To support results users, the HINTS website offered an easy-to-use catalogue of each questions. Catalogue entries included weighted population estimates for item responses, sample values, question text, notes, skip patterns, and source information. In addition, the program produced a series of easy-to-comprehend synopses—called HINTS Briefs—to summarize salient points from the scientific literature for use in public health planning. The HINTS Briefs were made available in both English and Spanish, and have been published quarterly.

Case Studies

Using HINTS Domestically

Over the decade in which the HINTS program was founded, there have been several instances in which the surveillance system interacted with results from the basic science community and with other monitoring programs to inform public health planning. One such instance included the development and diffusion of vaccines to prevent cervical cancer from human papillomavirus (HPV) infections. Surveillance data, such as data from the disease registries depicted on the right side of Figure 1, have suggested that roughly half of sexually active adults will contract HPV unless precautions are taken to prevent infection. Throughout the later part of the 1980s and the 1990s medical researchers at Georgetown University, the University of Rochester, University of Queensland in Australia, and the U.S. National Cancer Institute took that population signal as evidence for a need to create a better preventive measure, and began working on a vaccine that would elicit an antibody reaction to certain strains of the virus before infection occurred. In 2006, the US Food and Drug Administration approved a quadrivalent vaccine (i.e., a vaccine that was effective in preventing four different strains of HPV) for public marketing. In other words, surveillance data drove a need for basic, fundamental discovery to prevent HPV infection through the development of a vaccine; while intervention trials led to program delivery through the legislative safety mechanisms employed through the Food and Drug Administration. By 2006, two of the HPV vaccines, Gardasil and Cervarix, were ready for market and health communication researchers began looking for a surveillance system to track population level awareness.

Understanding that a marketing campaign for the HPV vaccine was imminent led the HINTS management team to include items on HPV awareness, knowledge, and usage within the 2005 administration. From those data, researchers learned that only about 38% of women in the U.S. had ever heard of HPV and from among those only about half knew that the virus could lead to cancer (Tiro, Meissner, Kobrin, & Chollette, 2007). Factors associated with HPV awareness were of the unequal diffusion of health information among populations within the U.S as documented by previous HINTS studies (Viswanath, et al., 2006); that is, those who knew the most about HPV were younger, well-educated, non-Hispanic whites.

By including the same HPV items used in previous iterations for trending purposes, HINTS researchers were able to track an increase in awareness of HPV from approximately 38% of the population in 2005 (Tiro, et al., 2007) to 68% in 2008 (Kontos, Emmons, Puleo, & Viswanath, 2012) as well as increases in knowledge about the links between the virus and cervical cancer (Kobetz, et al., 2010; Kontos, et al., 2012). Many of the same researchers were able to explore further associations between diffusion of HPV awareness and sociodemographic characteristics. Ongoing analyses of the HINTS data on HPV vaccine use have been underway to understand the complex cognitive and attitudinal relationships between awareness and subsequent behavior (Fang, Coups, & Heckman, 2010), and have begun to trigger new, fundamental behavioral research to understand the nature of vaccine hesitancy. In 2012, the HINTS data featured prominently in policy discussions initiated by the U.S. President's Cancer Panel focused on bolstering national vaccine usage rates.

There are many other examples of how the HINTS program has been used to monitor changes in the domestic communication environment. Studies of technology diffusion within the national landscape are serving to inform policy discussions related to the adoption of patient-provider email, personal health records, and electronic health records (Beckjord, et al., 2007; Hesse, et al., 2010). Studies of new media utilization from HINTS data are informing the use of social media strategies for health purposes and are providing physicians and health system administrators with data on the sources of first access and trust in medical information for personal use (Beckjord, et al., 2007; Chou, Hunt, Beckjord, Moser, & Hesse, 2009; Finney Rutten, et al., 2012; Hesse, et al., 2005). In 2011, HINTS was selected to provide national-level indicators on the U.S.'s Healthy People 2020 goals in the area of Health Communication and Informatics (DHHS, 2012).

Using HINTS Globally

A defining hallmark of the new information environment is its global reach (Friedman, 2007). Increasingly, economies from all around the world are benefiting from, and contributing to, a global network of information resources supported by diffusion of Internet technologies, mobile telephone technologies, and satellite communications. The HINTS program is serving the global community by offering a comparative framework and a set of common measures for evaluating communication planning in different environments internationally. For example, an administration of HINTS on the Caribbean island of Puerto Rico illustrated how the diffusion of mobile telephones may have leapfrogged other communication technologies in providing citizens with access to health information. In 2012, the National Cancer Institute began working with representatives from the Ministry of Health in the Peoples' Republic of China to conduct an ambitious survey of 100,000 Chinese citizens using the HINTS framework (Kreps, et al., 2012). Results of the survey should contribute to the global knowledge base on how health information is interpreted and acted upon in different regions and from different cultures.

By expanding our understanding of the health information environment internationally, we hope that future collaborations of partners and populations will inform communication planning around the world. The timing is especially critical, we believe, because estimates from the World Health Organization and the United Nations place the encroachment of non-communicable disease as the greatest challenge to face the international community in the century to come. For example, estimates from the World Health Organization suggest that deaths from tobacco consumption worldwide, if left unchecked, will take the lives of 8 million people annually by 2030 (World Health Organization, 2008). An examination of corporate planning documents suggests that when confronted with a shrinking domestic market, tobacco companies took their advertising campaigns into international markets (National Cancer Institute, 2008). Surveillance tools such as HINTS should help the global community work together in counteracting the influence of these international threats to health by shining a scientific light on the information environment in which all citizens live.

Recommended Readings

Dillman, D. A., Smyth, J. D., Christian, L. M. *Internet, mail, and mixed-mode surveys: the tailored design method.* 3rd ed. Hoboken, NJ: Wiley & Sons; 2009.

Finney Rutten, L. J., Hesse, B. W., Moser, R. P., Kreps, G. L. *Building the Evidence Base in Cancer Communication.* Cresskill, NJ: Hampton Press; 2010.

Groves RM. *Survey methodology.* 2nd ed. Hoboken, NJ: Wiley; 2009.

Hesse, B.W. (Guest Editor). (2005) The Health Information National Trends Survey (HINTS): Research from the baseline. *Journal of Health Communication, 10, Supp 1.* New York: Taylor and Francis.

Rutten, L. F., Hesse, B.W., Moser, R. P., & Blake, K. (Guest Eds.). (2010). Partners in Progress: Informing the Practice and Science of Health Communication through National Surveillance. *Journal of Health Communication, 15, Supp 3.* New York: Taylor and Francis.

Online Tools and Resources

American Association for Public Opinion Research: www.aapor.org
The Health Information National Trends Survey (HINTS): http://hints.cancer.gov
The World Health Organization: www.who.int

References

American Public Health Association. (1899). *The Bertillon classification of causes of death.* Lansing, MI: R. Smith Print. Co.

Beckjord, E. B., Finney Rutten, L. J., Squiers, L., Arora, N. K., Volckmann, L., Moser, R. P., et al. (2007). Use of the internet to communicate with health care providers in the United States: Estimates from the 2003 and 2005 Health Information National Trends Surveys (HINTS). *J Med Internet Res, 9*(3), e20.

Berland, G. K., Elliott, M. N., Morales, L. S., Algazy, J. I., Kravitz, R. L., Broder, M. S., et al. (2001). Health information on the Internet: Accessibility, quality, and readability in English and Spanish. *JAMA, 285*(20), 2612–2621.

Blumberg, S. J., & Luke, J. V. (2008). *Wireless substitution: Early release of estimates from the National Health Interview Survey, July–December 2007.*: National Center for Health Statistics. .

Bubela, T., Nisbet, M. C., Borchelt, R., Brunger, F., Critchley, C., Einsiedel, E., et al. (2012). Science Communication Reconsidered. *Nature Biotechnology, 27*(6), 514–518.

Chou, W. Y., Hunt, Y. M., Beckjord, E. B., Moser, R. P., & Hesse, B. W. (2009). Social media use in the United States: Implications for health communication. *J Med Internet Res, 11*(4), e48.

Croyle, R. T., & Lerman, C. (1999). Risk communication in genetic testing for cancer susceptibility. *J Natl Cancer Inst Monogr*(25), 59–66.

DHHS. (2012). Healthy People 2020 Objectives. Retrieved September 25, from http://www.healthypeople.gov/2020/topicsobjectives2020/objectiveslist.aspx?topicId=18

Dillman, D. A., Smyth, J. D., & Christian, L. M. (2009). *Internet, mail, and mixed-mode surveys : the tailored design method* (3rd ed.). Hoboken, N.J.: Wiley & Sons.

Fang, C. Y., Coups, E. J., & Heckman, C. J. (2010). Behavioral correlates of HPV vaccine acceptability in the 2007 Health Information National Trends Survey (HINTS). *Cancer Epidemiol Biomarkers Prev, 19*(2), 319–326.

Finney Rutten, L. J., Hesse, B. W., Moser, R. P., Ortiz Martinez, A. P., Kornfeld, J., Vanderpool, R. C., et al. (2012). Socioeconomic and geographic disparities in health information seeking and internet use in Puerto Rico. *J Med Internet Res, 14*(4), e104.

Fischhoff, B., Bostrom, A., & Quadrel, M. J. (1993). Risk perception and communication. *Annu Rev Public Health, 14*, 183–203.

Fitzgibbon, M., Gans, K. M., Evans, W. D., Viswanath, K., Johnson-Taylor, W. L., Krebs-Smith, S. M., et al. (2007). Communicating healthy eating: Lessons learned and future directions. *J Nutr Educ Behav, 39*(2 Suppl), S63–71.

Friedman, T. L. (2007). *The world is flat : A brief history of the twenty-first century* (Rev. pbk. ed.). New York: Picador.

Gentry, E. M., Kalsbeek, W. D., Hogelin, G. C., Jones, J. T., Gaines, K. L., & Forman, M. R. (1985). The behavioral risk factor surveys: II. Design, methods, and estimates from combined state data. *American Journal of Preventive Medicine, 1*(6), 9–14.

Glanz, K., Lewis, F. M., & Rimer, B. K. (1997). *Health behavior and health education.* San Francisco: John Wiley & Sons, Inc.

Groves, R. M. (2009). *Survey methodology* (2nd ed.). Hoboken, N.J.: Wiley.

Hall, H. I., Correa, A., Yoon, P. W., & Braden, C. R. (2012). Lexicon, definitions, and conceptual framework for public health surveillance. *MMWR Surveill Summ, 61*(Supplement), 10–14.

Hesse, B. W. (2010). Health communication in a world gone flat: Programmatic overview of HINTS. In L. J. Finney Rutten, B. W. Hesse, R. P. Moser & G. L. Kreps (Eds.), *Building the evidence base in cancer communication.* Cresskill, NJ: Hampton Press.

Hesse, B. W., Hansen, D., Finholt, T., Munson, S., Kellogg, W., & Thomas, J. C. (2010). Social participation in health 2.0. *IEEE Computer, 43*(11), 45–52.

Hesse, B. W., Nelson, D. E., Kreps, G. L., Croyle, R. T., Arora, N. K., Rimer, B. K., et al. (2005). Trust and sources of health information: The impact of the Internet and its implications for health care providers: Findings from the first Health Information National Trends Survey. *Arch Intern Med, 165*(22), 2618–2624.

Hiatt, R. A., & Rimer, B. K. (1999). A new strategy for cancer control research. *Cancer Epidemiol Biomarkers Prev, 8*(11), 957–964.

Keeter, S., Kennedy, C., Dimock, M., Best, J., & Craighill, P. (2006). Gauging the impact of growing nonresponse on estimates from a national RDD telephone survey. *Public Opinion Quarterly, 70*(5), 759–779.

Kobetz, E., Kornfeld, J., Vanderpool, R. C., Finney Rutten, L. J., Parekh, N., O'Bryan, G., et al. (2010). Knowledge of HPV among United States Hispanic women: Opportunities and challenges for cancer prevention. *J Health Commun, 15 Suppl 3*, 22–29.

Kontos, E. Z., Emmons, K. M., Puleo, E., & Viswanath, K. (2012). Contribution of communication inequalities to disparities in human papillomavirus vaccine awareness and knowledge. *Am J Public Health, 102*(10), 1911–1920.

Kreps, G. L. (2010). *Health communication*. Los Angeles: SAGE.

Kreps, G. L., Yu, G., Zhao, X., Chou, W. Y., Zihao, X., Meijie, S., et al. (2012). *Extending the US Health Information National Trends Survey to China and Beyond: Promoting Global Access to Consumer Health Information Needs and Practices.* Paper presented at the Global Health 2012, Venice, Italy.

Lewandowsky, S., Ecker, U. K. H., Seifert, C. M., Schwarz, N., & Cook, J. (2012). Misinformation and its correction: Continued influence and successful debiasing. *Psychological Science in the Public Interest, 13*(3), 106–131.

Louis, M. (2012). Global health surveillance. *MMWR Surveill Summ, 61*(Supplement: July 27, 2012).

Mazor, K. M., Roblin, D. W., Greene, S. M., Lemay, C. A., Firneno, C. L., Calvi, J., et al. (2012). Toward patient-centered cancer care: Patient perceptions of problematic events, impact, and response. *J Clin Oncol, 30*(15), 1784–1790.

Mokdad, A. H. (2009). The Behavioral Risk Factors Surveillance System: Past, present, and future. *Annu Rev Public Health, 30*, 43–54.

Moser, R. P., Beckjord, E. B., Finney Rutten, L. J., Blake, K., & Hesse, B. W. (2012). Using collaborative web technology to construct the health information national trends survey (HINTS). *Journal of Health Communication, 17*, 990–1000.

National Cancer Institute. (2008). *The role of the media in promoting and reducing tobacco use. Tobacco Control Monograph No. 19* (No. NIH Pub. No. 07-6242). Bethesda, MD: U.S. Department of Health and Human Services, National Institutes of Health, National Cancer Institute.

Nelson, D. E., Kreps, G. L., Hesse, B. W., Croyle, R. T., Willis, G., Arora, N. K., et al. (2004). The Health Information National Trends Survey (HINTS): Development, design, and dissemination. *J Health Commun, 9*(5), 443–460; discussion 481–444.

Rizzo, L., Park, I., Hesse, B., & Willis, G. (2004). *Effect of incentives on survey response and survey quality: A designed experiment within the HINTS I RDD sample.* Paper presented at the Annual meeting of the American Association of Public Opinion Research, Phoenix, AZ.

Rogers, E. M. (1995). Lessons for guidelines from the diffusion of innovations. *The Joint Commission Journal on Quality Improvement, 21*(7), 324–328.

Rolka, H., Walker, D. W., English, R., Katzoff, M. J., Scogin, G., & Neuhaus, E. (2012). Analytical challenges for emerging public health surveillance. *MMWR Surveill Summ, 61*, 35–40.

Satcher, S. B. (2009). *Keynote Address: CDC's Vision for Public Health Surveillance.*

Savel, T. G., & Foldy, S. (2012). The role of public health informatics in enhancing public health surveillance. *MMWR Surveill Summ, 61*, 20–24.

Sudman, S., Bradburn, N. M., & Schwarz, N. (1996). *Thinking about answers: the application of cognitive processes to survey methodology* (1st ed.). San Francisco: Jossey-Bass Publishers.

Thacker, S. B., Qualters, J. R., & Lee, L. M. (2012). Public health surveillance in the United States: Evolution and challenges. *MMWR Surveill Summ, 61*, 3–9.

Tiro, J. A., Meissner, H. I., Kobrin, S., & Chollette, V. (2007). What do women in the U.S. know about human papillomavirus and cervical cancer? *Cancer Epidemiol Biomarkers Prev, 16*(2), 288–294.

Viswanath, K. (2005). Science and society: The communications revolution and cancer control. *Nat Rev Cancer, 5*(10), 828–835.

Viswanath, K., Breen, N., Meissner, H., Moser, R. P., Hesse, B. W., Steele, W. R., et al. (2006). Cancer knowledge and disparities in the information age. *J Health Commun, 11 Suppl 1*, 1–17.

Weinstein, N. D. (1993). Testing four competing theories of health-protective behavior. *Health Psychol, 12*(4), 324–333.

World Health Organization. (2008). *WHO Report on the Global Tobacco Epidemic, 2009.* Geneva: World Health Organization.

Chapter 19

Cultural Beacons in Health Communication: Leveraging Overlooked Indicators and Grassroots Wisdoms[1]

Laurel J. Felt, *University of Southern California*
Lucía Durá & Arvind Singhal, *The University of Texas at El Paso*

Said the Eye one day,
"I see beyond these valleys a mountain veiled with blue mist. Is it not beautiful?"
The Ear listened, and after listening intently awhile, said,
"But where is any mountain? I do not hear it."
Then the Hand spoke and said,
"I am trying in vain to feel it or touch it, and I can find no mountain."
And the Nose said,
"There is no mountain, I cannot smell it."
Then the Eye turned the other way, and they all began to talk together about the Eye's strange delusion.
And they said, "Something must be the matter with the Eye."

—Kahlil Gibran[2]

What do we see, hear, touch, and feel? What do we not see, not hear, not touch, and not feel? These two queries–both their intellectual substance and their riddle-esque style–capture key challenges around designing, implementing, and evaluating health communication interventions. Consider a team of health practitioners and researchers collaborating to design a nutrition program in a community, and administering a pre-intervention needs assessment survey that asks: *What is the general wellness of the community? Who is malnourished and who is thriving? Which citizens perform Nutrition Strategies X, Y, and Z?* Post-intervention, the team might re-distribute the survey, seeking answers to the same questions in order to gauge the effect of the intervention.

---

1 This article draws upon research conducted by the present authors in Uganda, India, Perú, and Sénégal.
2 From *The Madman: His Parables and Poems*, first published in 1918.

This pre-post data can begin to illuminate the intervention's effects. However, the team will only learn about the predetermined survey constructs—i.e., the survey will deliver a limited knowledge product. Further, the respondents' answers will be codified in pre-determined response categories—i.e., the data collected is bounded by the narrow knowledge-generating framework. Like each body part enumerated in Gibran's parable, this survey instrument can detect and process only a certain type of information. By definition, the survey instrument cannot discover or process any other type of information.

We call on health communicators to purposely and mindfully gather information that is traditionally overlooked and omitted, for such can yield surprising and invaluable insights. What if the hypothetical nutrition team had subjected its corpus to the following critical questions: Whose experiences do these data reflect, and whose voices are absent? What data is collected, and what is not? What data characteristics lend credibility to local wisdom, and what characteristics prompt its dismissal? In this scenario and for all health communicators, the answers to these questions begin to guide the discovery of overlooked indicators and grassroots wisdoms.

We call these overlooked indicators and grassroots wisdoms *cultural beacons* (CBs) (Durá, Felt & Singhal, 2012). This chapter will explore the nature of CBs as well as offer tools for putting CBs into practice. Specifically, it will examine CBs' theoretical underpinnings, provide case studies in which CBs emerged, recommend strategies for designing, implementing, and evaluating interventions that integrate CBs, and recommend more sources of practical information for enriching and extending our practice. Our purpose is to take seriously the essence of Gibran's tale and to not miss, or discredit, what's really out there.

Theoretical Frame for Cultural Beacons

Much like a beam from a lighthouse, cultural beacons can guide outsiders, helping them to negotiate unexpected features of a landscape as well as establish moorings upon a solid base. (Durá, Felt, & Singhal, 2013)

In our exploratory work on cultural beacons, we termed overlooked indicators and local wisdoms *cultural scorecards*: culturally embedded, user-defined measures for understanding communicative meaning(s), components, and sites of change (Singhal & Durá, 2009; Singhal, Durá, & Felt, 2011). The term was later changed to *cultural beacons* (Durá, Felt, &

Singhal, 2013). This latter designation acknowledges the capacity of on-the-ground insights to illuminate (as beacons do) unique features of people and places. Here, we call upon health communicators to more mindfully consider cultural beacons (CBs) for three key reasons: (1) traditional data-gathering does not wholly capture program-related transformations (Smith, 1999; Shiva, 2005; Dutta & Pal, 2010); (2) non-traditional, non-textual, and participatory forms of knowledge-generation can yield overlooked data; and (3) local wisdoms, enshrined in grassroots epistemologies, can enrich program design and evaluation.

Traditional Data-Gathering Delimits Understanding

Let us return to the nutrition example where a pre-post survey asks: What is the community's general wellness now? Who are malnourished or thriving, respectively? Who now performs Nutritional Strategies X, Y, and Z? Such a survey instrument is unequipped to capture certain program-related transformations. For instance, it does not measure the quantity of nutritional supplements sold at the local store, nor does it ask for observed changes, such as the extent to which common lands show signs of scavenging. Although this instrument might allow space for "any additional comment," its design does not prioritize unexpected outcomes, such as heavy rainfall, abundant fodder, and improved livestock wellness.

By design, tools like surveys, and protocols for in-depth interviews and focus groups, circumscribe range and depth of self-expression (especially with taboo topics), context (time and place of assessment), and sample size. Investigator agendas are almost always ranked above the participants' and thus participants' lived realities are often absent from data corpuses. Not surprisingly, program evaluation literature that has focused on traditional indicators of participant knowledge, attitude, and behavior change has been found wanting in gauging program effectiveness (e.g., Saegert, Benitez, Eizenberg, Hsieh, & Lamb, 2004; Ebrahim, 2005).

To change our mindsets about datasets is difficult for both participants and researchers. We tend to re-enact established operating procedures, or follow our learned scripts. To justify our scripts, we label them as "tried and true" or as "effective," "efficient," or "generalizable." Although scripts are necessary and often deliver satisfactory results, they become dangerous when fossilized as dogma. Kenneth Burke (1954) described this phenomenon of losing the ability to think beyond one's training as *trained incapacities* (p. 7).

Trained incapacities curtail not only what we can see, hear, or execute but also delimit what we cannot see, cannot hear, or cannot do.

Participatory, Non-Textual Data-Gathering Enhances Understanding

In the Western tradition of conducting research, information not codified in print has been repressed, disqualified, and/or dismissed. This perspective, in which unlettered knowledge is considered illegitimate, has been described as "textocentric" (Conquergood, 2002; Singhal & Rattine-Flaherty, 2006). We argue that indigenous, informal, and *non-textocentric* data gathering can deeply enhance understanding of interventional effectiveness. What are these non-textual, participatory forms of knowledge generation? Artistic, musical, oral, and visual performances represent formats for the traditionally silent to raise their proverbial voices (e.g., Boal, 1979; Fals-Borda & Rahman, 1991; Singhal, Harter, Chitnis, & Sharma, 2007). Participatory visualization techniques (e.g., participatory photography and sketching) accompanied by oral narratives are low-cost, audience-centered methodologies to assess participants' perceptions and interpretations of a social change intervention (Singhal & Devi, 2003; Singhal & Rattine-Flaherty, 2006). The Most Significant Change (MSC) technique also solicits participants' experiences of program-produced change, enabling the articulation of unexpected outcomes, appreciation of diverse participation, and facilitation of organizational learning (Dart & Davies, 2003; Davies & Dart, 2005). Additional participatory methodologies include (but are not limited to) participatory appraisal and asset mapping.

How do non-textual, participatory data add value to what one obtains from traditional data gathering methods? In terms of knowledge *product*, cultural beacons (CBs) add value by considering grassroots "meanings that are masked, camouflaged, indirect, embedded, or hidden in context" (Conquergood, 2002, p. 146). CBs are *culturally embedded*—that is, so specific to a culture that they often seem "invisible" to outsiders. They are *user-defined*—that is, the participants recognize the value/ascribe significance to these data themselves. Thus, in terms of knowledge *process*, participatory, non-textocentric methods inherently reveal the world of respondents, sharing clues as to "what counts" in their cultural contexts. CBs also can reinforce validity by inductively informing how we measure, what we measure, and with whose indicators we measure.

Local Wisdom and Grassroots Epistemologies Need to Be Understood

Robert Chambers, a leading scholar of participation, power, and social change, maintains that participatory research methodologies (PMs) illuminate on-the-ground realities for outsiders. Chambers (2010) points to the importance of local wisdom in this story from Bangladesh:

"...A team led by a consultant used an array of PRA [participatory rural appraisal] tools, a listening study, and drama to generate value statements from members of the movement. The over 8,000 resulting key statements from groups and committees were 'peppered with perspectives which had never occurred to staff'" (p. 38).

Similarly, public health scholar Meredith Minkler (2000) affirms the value of local wisdom. The community members' feedback "at first seemed to make little sense from an epidemiological perspective. Yet, as residents described the logic behind their sorting, it soon became clear that their analyses were based on a sophisticated knowledge of the communities in which they lived" (p. 194).

Participatory methodologies invoke grassroots wisdoms to surface. Usually PMs are deployed within the context of participatory action research (PAR), a dialogic and collaborative process that invites participants and practitioners to co-construct research design and contribute to ongoing data collection. Minkler (2000) lauds PAR as "an empowering process through which participants can increase control over their lives by nurturing community strengths and problem-solving abilities" (p. 193). In terms of benefits, PAR also can "sensitize both the community and the providers about the feelings and constraints of the other side," ensuring that the dialogue does not become adversarial (Singh & Shah, n.d., p. 6). Educational researchers Marilyn Cochran-Smith and Susan L. Lytle (2009) also interrogate epistemological frameworks, characterizing knowledge as fluid, dynamic, and constructed; as such, any search for "truth" must include joint construction of local knowledge, questioning of common assumptions, and scrutiny of whose perspectives are left out (p. 2).

To illustrate the processes through which local knowledge can be co-constructed between researchers and the respondents, we turn to two case studies that are rich with cultural beacons: One from Uganda; the other from India.

Cultural Beacons Revealed in the Field[3]

The general purpose of both the Uganda and the India projects was to create a more healthy community in a geographically circumscribed area. The insights reported here come from both formal, structured (participatory) evaluation activities, and also from informal observations and interrogations that were noted in our field journals and photographically.

Mats, Home Goods, G-nuts and Birds in Uganda[4]

As the Lord's Resistance Army (LRA) civil conflict showed signs of ebbing in northern Uganda in 2007 and 2008, thousands of abductees were rescued or managed to escape captivity. Five thousand of the estimated 26,000 returnees were female (Okot, Lamunu, & Oketch, 2011). While in captivity they were forced to act as porters and cooks, often as soldiers (compelling them to commit atrocities themselves), and almost universally as sex slaves. As a result, "home" communities tended to reject these "LRA-tainted" women, many of whom returned pregnant or with their captor-sired children in tow. Two of the present authors collected data to evaluate a Save the Children project that aimed to reintegrate these stigmatized returned abductees within their communities. In a participatory sketching activity with returned abductees to gauge post-intervention change, it was noted that several respondents drew a homestead, an adjacent tree, and a mat beneath this tree. In a casual conversation about this observed pattern, a local project coordinator explained to us that for the Acholi people of northern Uganda, a mat beneath a homestead-adjacent tree means, "You are welcome. Please come, sit, and share a cup of tea in the shade." This mat is a culturally embedded, user-defined indicator of individuals' capacity for hospitality and leisure. It implies psychosocial healing, material well-being, and evidence of feeling that one belongs to the community, i.e., triumph over social stigma. The repetitive drawing of the mat under a tree signifies that the respondents felt they had achieved a certain level of reintegration within their communities.

More CBs denoting social reintegration appeared unexpectedly. Several project participants invited us into their homesteads. Without fail, each hostess urged us to sit on plastic patio chairs and proudly pointed to her array of possessions—a radio set, hand-held mirrors, large sacks of g-nuts (peanuts), and plastic water bottles of a liter or more filled with shea smearing oil. We

---

3   This section draws upon and builds on our previous work (Durá, Felt, & Singhal, 2012; Singhal, Durá, & Felt, 2011; Singhal & Durá 2010).
4   This section draws upon Singhal and Durá (2008).

asked each woman we visited how she felt about her position in the community. A typical response was, "Before, I couldn't look at my face in the mirror, but now I am proud." Many would say, "I like putting smearing oil on my face. I like to look nice" (Singhal & Durá, 2008, p. 66). Thus, we came to understand that the mirrors and smearing oil were CBs; they represented a sense of self-worth and belonging, as well as a commitment to hygiene and personal grooming. We later learned about the significance of the chairs. Having chairs and a table confers social status. It shows that one has the means and the pride to treat guests with honor, sparing them from sitting or eating on the dirt floor. As for the radio, participants explained that this made them feel connected to the outside world. Such a commitment to information and connection, especially when the world beyond their walls had treated them so brutally, suggests the women's healing—the radio was a CB too.

An off-the-cuff field conversation provided a third occasion to discover two CBs. As we walked for several kilometers in the Acholi bush, we noticed whole g-nut shells scattered along the road. Staff member Jimmy explained that g-nuts on the ground are a sign of abundance. Before, people were so hungry that if ever there were a g-nut on the ground, it would be eaten immediately. Now, he said, you also see birds in the campsites. Before, birds didn't come because there were no spare food scraps for them to eat (Singhal & Durá, 2008). Jimmy's words reveal the g-nuts and campsite birds as CBs that represent abundance. Their presence shows, in no uncertain terms, that residents now have enough to eat

These CBs in Uganda are bright spots of devastated communities that are moving toward health and healing. They indicate growing psychological and material well-being as the previously stigmatized now exhibit signs of self-worth, dignity, and belonging. Even the trodden earth shows hints of community abundance.

Birthdays, Boyfriends and Bicycles in India[5]

In the Indian state of Bihar, an entertainment-education radio serial called *Taru* commanded the airwaves from 2002 to 2003. *Taru* was a media and community-based intervention to create healthy communities in rural India. *Taru*'s purpose was to promote gender equality, reproductive health, caste and communal harmony, and community development. One of the present authors led the program evaluation of the *Taru* project. Participants in the *Taru* project

---

5 This section draws upon Singhal (2010).

were asked to photograph and narrate visible signs of change in their communities after active program viewing. In an in-depth interview, one respondent described the first ever celebration of a birthday party for a young girl, attributing it as an effect of *Taru*. While many boys in rural Bihar celebrate their birthdays, such is not the case for girls—a sign of girls' unequal status. Thus, this girl's party, inspired by the soap opera's modeling of a young girl's birthday, was a CB. It demonstrated a courageous change of long-standing tradition; the party's significance was further vetted by the discovery that several other young girls celebrated their birthdays in the following months.

Figure 1. Vandana posing for a picture next to her platonic male friend

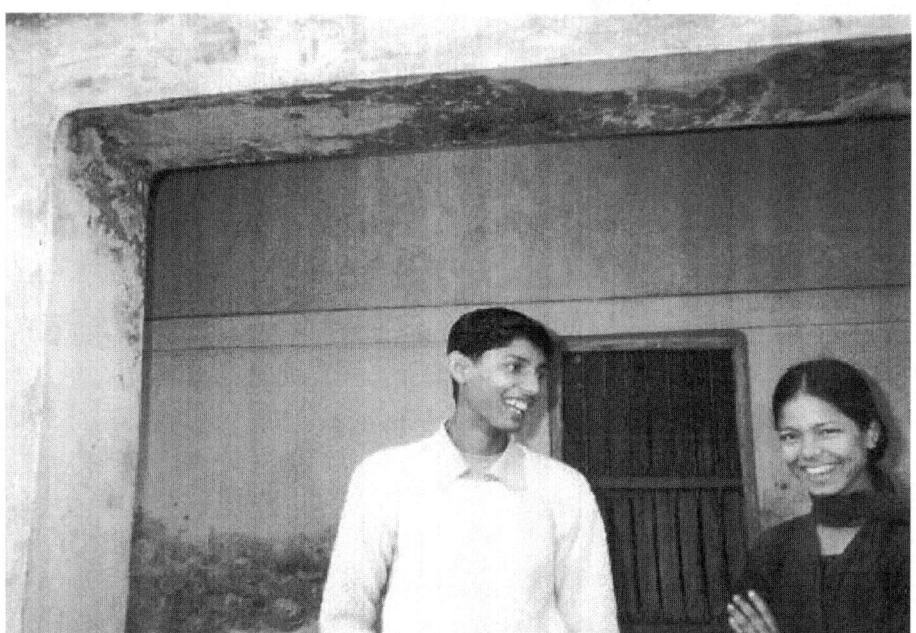

A 17-year-old girl named Vandana explained two CBs embedded in a photograph of herself. First, Vandana was wearing jeans in the picture. Since conservative villagers deem jeans inappropriate, her fashion challenges historically accepted gender roles and tradition—a goal of the *Taru* project. That Vandana felt strong enough to take such a stand suggests an improved sense of confidence. Second, the jeans-clad Vandana was standing beside a boy—perhaps the first time in Kamtaul Village history that a young woman invited a platonic male friend to stand beside her in a picture. So, this companionship choice is also a CB indicating empowerment.

Another CB emerged from a snapshot (see Figure 2) of two girls walking with a bicycle.

Figure 2. Girls using a bicycle in Bihar, India

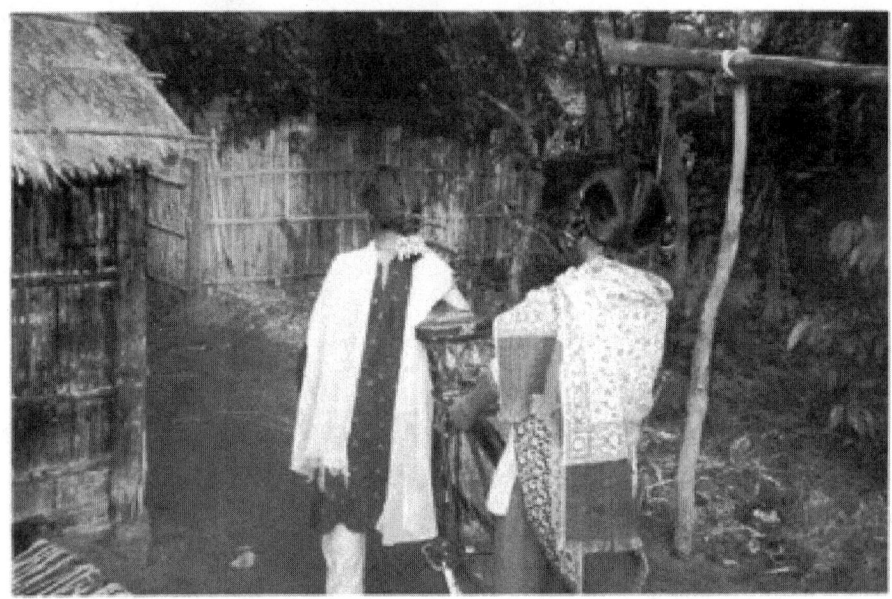

To explain the significance of this image, a local male resident stated: "These girls are trying to learn to ride a bike. After listening to *Taru*, girls are changing. By listening to radio these girls learn of new ideas and act on them" (Singhal, 2010, p. 16). This is two CBs in one: not only does it suggest female empowerment, but it also points to radio's ability to impact cultural norms.

Our field experiences in Uganda and India suggest to us that cultural beacons can appear in at least three forms:

1. *Material possessions whose ownership indicates functional or cultural well-being (e.g., a mat, a radio, mirrors, smearing oils, chairs);*
2. *Natural resources whose presence or state indicates social conditions (e.g., g-nuts on the ground, birds at campsites);*
3. *Social behaviors whose performance indicates change for individuals or collectives (e.g., celebrating girls' birthdays, wearing jeans, riding bicycles).*

Implications for Designing Health Communication Projects

From the Uganda and India illustrations of cultural beacons, it is clear that CBs are grassroots, locally relevant indicators that tend to be invisible to outsiders and embedded within local culture. So, how can one design, discover, and evaluate health communication projects to more readily reveal cultural beacons? In so doing, how can health communicators expand their understanding of local wisdoms and grassroots epistemologies?

Designing with Cultural Beacons in Mind

How can health communication projects be designed so that cultural beacons may more readily surface? Designing for CBs requires "untraining" fossilized scripts related to research design and data collection, sharpening observation and listening skills, and nurturing relationships between and among multiple stakeholders. In light of Gibran's parable, those looking for CBs should be prepared to listen with their eyes and see with their ears. What concrete actions might be taken to "watch" and "listen" for CBs?

Incorporate Participatory Practices. To design for CBs, health communication projects may consider incorporating some form of participatory action research (PAR). PAR values co-constructed knowledge building through collaboration, and relies upon an iterative cycle of planning, action, and reflection over time (Aringay, 2008). Embracing PAR can enable the conditions for CBs to emerge. Our work in Uganda demonstrated how participatory methodologies, such as sketching and narration, off-the-cuff conversations with the participants and local project staff (e.g., Why the plastic chairs?), clarification from participants (e.g., g-nuts indicate community abundance), and reflection upon what this all meant shaped our ensuing work.

Embrace "Unusual Suspects." Before designing a health communication project, the universe of stakeholders must be identified. Who stands to gain or lose from this project? Whose input is crucial to the project's success? It also helps to plan for "unusual suspects": those who, traditionally, have not been considered crucial to the project's success but who might yield unexpected insights. For instance, let us return to the photo of two young girls in rural Bihar trying to help each other in riding a bicycle. The picture and narration came from 22-year-old Mukesh, a male resident of Abirpur village, who connected the dots. Here were two young girls who were listening to *Taru,* learning about gender equality, and who began to do things, i.e., ride a bicycle—behaviors attributed to men. Mukesh represents an "unusual suspect" because, in order to ascertain the empowerment of young girls, researchers usually survey young girls, their parents, or their peers exclusively. Rarely would young men in the community be asked for local signifiers of girls' empowerment. To increase the odds of noticing CBs through unusual suspects, health communicators may ask: *What am I not seeing or hearing? Who else do I need to speak with?*

Nurture Relationships. The cornerstones of healthy relationships between researchers, respondents, and project staff are respect, trust, and productive communication. This emerges from *mutual demystification*—that is, parties knowing one another and being known. Sharing meals, extending courtesies, and dialoguing about non-task issues help in building relationships. In our work in Uganda, we invested about 30 to 40 percent of our time doing so. This sense of familiarity and, importantly, trust allowed us to approach colleagues such as Jimmy and ask about the g-nuts on the ground, or the plastic chairs for visitors. The benefit of familiarity and trust cuts both ways; because project participants trusted us, they invited us to their homesteads after formal data collection had concluded. We noted our observations in field journals and, appreciating these data's richness, requested permission from the participants to report. Again, due to trust, they consented. The success of projects—and the health of communities, for that matter—hinges upon partners' relationships (Kim & Ball-Rokeach, 2006). Such is true for discovering cultural beacons, as well.

Share Vision(s) and Ownership. Now that you know *of* all the stakeholders in the project, you can be sure that you're inviting everyone you should to participate in the collaborative vision-sharing. And, because now you *know* all of the stakeholders in the project, the odds of them sharing frank, comprehensive, and productive insights are quite good.

Whether you use needs assessment, asset-mapping, SWOT (strengths, weaknesses, opportunities, threats) analysis, or another methodology to establish consensus as to the project's goals and scope, arriving at goals together will lay the groundwork for shared ownership of project processes. Jointly develop a program and research plan that enfranchises diverse individuals in multiple activities (e.g., data collection, training) across the project's scope and sequence. Co-construct multiple means of both gathering participants' insights and translating this rich data.

Open Space for the Unexpected. In our experience, many CBs revealed themselves during off-the-cuff conversations and unplanned follow-up questions. The implication: be curious and purposely schedule flexible time to capitalize on emergent opportunities, e.g., accept invitations to visit participant homes so you can ask about what they do with the shea smearing oil, or walk (instead of drive) from one homestead to another so you can notice g-nuts on the ground, and so on.

A simple design check-list is provided below.

Cultural Beacons Design Checklist

√	DESIGN TASK
	With diverse colleagues, identify all stakeholders and unusual suspects. Ask, Who else needs to be here?
	Do not miss an opportunity to build relationships with field staff and respondents. Engage in mutual demystification.
	Be curious. Ask questions. Be open to wonder and surprise.

Discovering CBs: "Invisible" and Embedded Indicators

How can stakeholders in health communication projects more readily discover cultural beacons? Participatory, non-textocentric methodologies invite locals to share culturally embedded, user-defined insights. Participatory sketching / photography, coupled with the artists' narration of these images, led to our recognition of CBs on multiple occasions. In order to "discover" that these were CBs and held special meaning or importance, we looked for the frequency with which these images appeared across various participants. For instance, a sketch of the mat under a tree appeared with repeated frequency to indicate a cultural pattern.

More importantly, when any part of an image was not explained, we asked a follow-up question; since CBs' significance is always "invisible" to outsiders, locals' clarification is the only way to uncover the precious within the seemingly banal.

A simple discovery check-list is provided below.

Cultural Beacons Discovery Checklist

√	DISCOVERY TASK
	Act in ways that will facilitate CBs' discovery: visit locals in their cultural context(s), use participatory, non-textocentric methodologies
	Scrutinize likely CB sites: material possessions, natural resources, social behaviors

Evaluating Cultural Beacons

How can health communication projects evaluate the robustness of cultural beacons?

To evaluate a CB, first ascertain whether an artifact meets the two criteria of a CB. Is it (1) culturally embedded—that is, so specific to a culture that it may seem "invisible" to outsiders; and (2) user-defined—that is, the participants recognize the value/ascribe significance to these data themselves? If these qualifications are met, then the reliability and validity of the CB can be further explored through various strategies: triangulation, quantitative validation, scaling considerations, and measures of organizational learning.

Triangulation. Suppose a participant of a hand-washing campaign sketched a restroom wastebasket, then explained its significance: prior to the intervention, no one had wastebaskets in their restrooms because they didn't need to throw away paper towels (either because they weren't washing their hands at all or because they weren't drying their hands on this sanitary, disposable vector). The participant's account turns restroom wastebaskets into a CB. But to what extent does this CB, if it was mentioned only once, represent community conditions?

Triangulating, or using multiple measures to capture data on a single construct, could reveal whether a phenomenon (in this case, increased paper towel waste due to sanitary hand-washing practice) suggested by a CB (the restroom wastebasket) is occurring widely. External measures, such as vendors' records of wastebaskets, paper towels, and soap sold, or observed changes, such as the extent to which these wastebaskets are filled with paper towels, also could support the CB. If these measures are substantially and significantly correlated with the CB-derived data, then the CB acquires significance.

Quantitative Checks. The above hand-washing example offers ways to examine the program-related impacts of CBs in quantitative terms, e.g., repeated sales of paper towels and soap, frequency of emptying of wastebaskets, and such. Performance of private behaviors can be corroborated by means other than self-report. In so doing, the researchers may expand their depth and breadth of a particular effect and be motivated to pursue more data metrics.

Scaling Considerations. Identifying CBs can expand our notion of what it means to scale. Scaling, or increasing access to "solutions," should not be seen only along a vertical axis. Since participants may take skills/ experiences/innovations from one project and apply it to another lateral concern, scaling also can be understood horizontally. For instance, participants in the hand-washing intervention may apply what they learned about germs to change their habits around preparing food, treating wounds, or disposing waste. They also might leverage their participation in less direct ways, such as by applying their self-efficacy as learners to other learning contexts. This hyper-local approach may be a more productive and sustainable way to scale than widely disseminating a single-issue intervention.

Organizational Learning. Finally, CBs can enrich organizational learning and serve diverse stakeholders. Because CBs have the potential to more fully illuminate program impact, organizations can better ascertain the relative efficiencies of their efforts and the ripple effects engendered. For example, the organization behind the hand-washing campaign could use related CBs to estimate campaign embrace and local economic impact, as well as contextualize the community's decrease in hospital visits since the campaign began. Moreover, processes associated with participation can significantly benefit participants, delivering opportunities for developing skills, relationships, and self-efficacy in important areas. The utility and longevity of such assets contributes to the value and sustainability of an intervention.

A simple evaluation check-list is provided below.

Cultural Beacons Evaluation Checklist

√	EVALUATION TASK
	Test whether a CB meets the two-fold threshold for qualification
	Use multiple measures to triangulate
	Corroborate beyond self-report, e.g., with external measures or observed changes
	Investigate horizontal scaling impacts related to the phenomenon represented by the CB (optional)
	Evaluate how CBs impact organizational and individual learning

Conclusion

In this chapter, we proposed strategies for the design, implementation, and evaluation of overlooked indicators and grassroots wisdoms, which we call cultural beacons. Our research is anchored by the theoretical observations that traditional data-gathering methods are insufficient for capturing all program-related changes, and "other" ways of knowing yield legitimate data that can enrich programmatic efforts and formal reports. We illustrate these theoretical observations through two case studies from Uganda and India, comprising almost a dozen examples of CBs.

The exploration of cultural beacons in general and the tools we have presented in this chapter are by no means exhaustive, nor are they meant to be prescriptive. Rather, they are meant to be beacons themselves: guiding practice and, in the spirit of action research, informed by practice as well. In the Appendix we suggest readings and resources for continued exploration and enrichment. Further work with CBs should necessarily follow, including an attention to research ethics. Thoughtful consideration must be given to Institutional Review Board (IRB)-approved activities, participants' informed consent, and researcher-participant norms.

To honor IRB-approved plans as well as open space for detecting CBs, research designs should include flexible contexts for data gathering, such as key informant interviews, participant-observation, and ethnographic documentation. When it seems as though a specific mode for CB detection might fall outside previously approved research plans, investigators should petition the IRB to make modifications so this opportunity is not lost.

Data cannot be gathered without participants' informed consent. In the case of g-nuts on the ground, a staff member acted as a key informant—Jimmy provided data. When we realized the richness of his insight, we reminded Jimmy of his rights and requested his participation in the research. Because of the rapport we had established with Jimmy, we believed that he freely chose to engage; however, because of Jimmy's professional role, we needed to ensure that he did not feel coerced. A special informed consent protocol might be useful in cases like these, and merits further exploration. To design for CBs, it is probably useful to define the research population in the original IRB submission as community members and stakeholders.

Norms in terms of researcher-participant interactions also might require reevaluation. In order to protect researchers' "objectivity," their engagement with project participants is usually confined to formal data collection activities. But such spaces limit opportunities for building trust and meaningfully learning about the local context on participants' terms, in their spaces. Rather than understanding validity as a function of distance, it might be more productive to understand it as a function of comprehension. The better we comprehend a community and its residents, the more valid are our reports of program-related outcomes. Our understanding of how to approach health communication interventions and research with CBs in mind is young and, from our collaborative efforts with diverse stakeholders, will continue to grow.

Acknowledgements

We thank our various collaborators, respondents, and colleagues who helped us with our respective projects in Uganda, India, Perú, and Sénégal. We began to explore the notion of cultural scorecards about nine years ago, and broached them in a very preliminary form with Spanish readers (Singhal & Durá, 2010). Since then we have expanded our ideas both theoretically and methodologically.

We especially thank Drs. Mohan Dutta, Earl Babbie, and D. Lawrence Kincaid who read our manuscripts at different points in time and provided invaluable suggestions for refinement and improvement. Dr. Kincaid was the one who broached with us the importance of computing reliability and validity estimates for cultural beacons.

Recommended Readings

Dutta, M., & Pal, M. (2010). Dialog theory in marginalized settings: A subaltern studies approach. *Communication Theory, 20*, 363–386.
Chambers, R. (2010). Paradigms, poverty, and adaptive pluralism. *Institute of Development Studies, 2010* (344), 1–57.
Greiner, K., & Singhal, A. (2009). Communication and invitational social change. *Journal of Development Communication, 20*(2), 31–44.
Zoller, H.M. (2000). "A place you haven't visited before": Creating the conditions for community dialogue. Dialogue [Special issue]. *The Southern Communication Journal, 65* (2 & 3), 191–207.

Additional Resources

The 4 Cs of Participation Inventory (Reilly, Jenkins, Felt, & Vartabedian, 2012, p. 18) was developed for educators to identify their learning contexts' participation opportunities. Its greater objective is to facilitate learning in a culture where "…members believe their contributions matter, and feel some degree of social connection with one another" (Jenkins, Purushotma, Clinton, Weigel, & Robison, 2006, p. 3). Because this sense of self-efficacy and community describes a participatory action research (PAR) project, the tool may help PAR practitioners to reflect upon and address participants' enfranchisement.

- How do we provide mechanisms to **CREATE**?
- How do we support opportunities for media to **CIRCULATE** across platforms, disciplines and ages?
- How do we help learners to **COLLABORATE** and build upon others' knowledge?
- How do we encourage learners to **CONNECT** with counterparts and establish productive networks?

References

Aringay, E. (2008). *Action Research*. Retrieved from http://labsome.rmit.edu.au/liki/index.php/Action_research

Boal, A. (1979). *The theatre of the oppressed*. New York: Urizen Books.

Burke, K. (1954/1984). *Permanence and change*. Berkeley: University of California Press.

Chambers, R. (2010). Paradigms, poverty, and adaptive pluralism. *Institute of Development Studies, 2010* (344), 1–57.

Cochran-Smith, M. & Lytle, S.L. (2009). *Inquiry as stance: Practitioner research for the next generation*. New York: Teachers College Press.

Conquergood, D. (2002). Performance studies: Interventions and radical research. *The Drama Review: A Journal of Performance Studies, 46* (2), 145–156.

Dart, J., & Davies, R. (2003). A dialogical, story-based evaluation tool: The Most Significant Change Technique. *American Journal of Evaluation*, 24 (2), 137–155.

Davies, R., & Dart, J. (2005). The 'Most Significant Change' (MSC) Technique. United Kingdom: CARE International. Retrieved from: www.mande.co.uk/docs/MSCGuide.pdf

Durá, L., Felt, L.J., & Singhal, A. (2013). *Cultural beacons: Grassroots indicators of change*. Paper presented at 63rd Annual International Communication Association Conference, London, UK.

Dutta, M., & Pal, M. (2010). Dialog theory in marginalized settings: A subaltern studies approach. *Communication Theory, 20*, 363–386.

Ebrahim, A. (2005). Accountability myopia: Losing sight of organizational learning. *Nonprofit and Voluntary Sector Quarterly, 34* (1), 56–87.

Fals-Borda, O., & Rahman, M.A. (1991). *Action and knowledge: Breaking the monopoly with participatory action-research*. New York: The Apex Press.

Glasser, B.G., & Strauss, A.L. (1967). *The discovery of grounded theory: Strategies for qualitative research*. Chicago: Aldine Publishing Company.

Grabill, J. (2007). Sustaining community-based work: Community-based research and community building. In P. Takayoshi & P. Sullivan (Eds.), *Labor, writing technologies, and the shaping of composition in the academy* (pp. 325–339). Cresskill, NJ: Hampton Press.

Grabill, J. (2001). *Community literacy programs and the politics of change*. Albany: State University of New York Press.

Greiner, K., & Singhal, A. (2010). Inviting—not requiring—social change. *MAZI: The Communication for Social Change Report*. 20. Retrieved from http://www.communicationforsocialchange.org/mazi-articles.php?id=408

Greiner, K., & Singhal, A. (2009). Communication and invitational social change. *Journal of Development Communication*. 20: 2.

Jenkins, H., Purushotma, R., Clinton, K., Weigel, M., & Robison, A. J. (2006). *Confronting the challenges of participatory culture: Media education for the 21st century*. Chicago: The John D. and Catherine T. MacArthur Foundation.

Kim, Y. C., & Ball-Rokeach, S. (2006). Community storytelling network, neighborhood context, and civic engagement: A multilevel approach. *Human Communication Research, 32*, 411–439.

Minkler, M. (2000). Using participatory action research to build healthy communities. *Public Health Reports, 115,* 191–197.
Okot, A., Lamunu, G., & Oketch, B. (2011). Female abductees suffer reintegration pain. *Report news, International Justice, ICC Institute for War & Peace Reporting.* ACR Issue 305. Retrieved from http://iwpr.net/report-news/female-abductees-suffer-reintegration-pain-0
Parks, W., Gray-Felder, D., Hunt, J., & Byrne, A. (2005). *Who measures change? An introduction to participatory monitoring and evaluation of communication for social change.* South Orange, NJ: Communication for Social Change Consortium.
Reilly, E., Jenkins, H., Felt, L.J., & Vartabedian, V. (2012). *Shall we PLAY?* Los Angeles: Annenberg Innovation Lab at the University of Southern California.
Saegert, S., Benitez, L., Eisenberg, E., Hsieh, T.S., & Lamb, M. (2004). Participatory evaluation: How it can enhance effectiveness and credibility of nonprofit work. *The Nonprofit Quarterly, 11*(1): 54–60.
Shiva, V. (2005). *Earth democracy: Justice, sustainability, and peace.* Cambridge, MA: South End Press.
Simmons, W.M. (2007). *Participation and power: Civic discourse in environmental policy decisions.* New York: SUNY.
Singhal, A. (2010). Riding high on Taru fever: Entertainment-education broadcasts, ground mobilization, and service delivery in rural India. *Entertainment-Education and Social Change Wisdom Series, 1* (1), 1–19. Netherlands: Oxfam-Novib.
Singhal, A., & Devi, K. (2003). Visual voices in participatory communication. *Communicator, 37,* 1–15.
Singhal, A., & Durá, L. (2010). Tarjetas de valoracion cultural: Un llamado para desarrollar sentidos participativos de moniteero y evaluacion. *Folios, 23*(January–June): 161–180.
Singhal, A., & Durá, L. (2009). *Protecting children from exploitation and trafficking: Using the positive deviance approach in Uganda and Indonesia.* Washington DC: Save the Children.
Singhal, A., Durá, L., & Felt, L.J. (2011). *What counts? For whom? Valuing cultural scorecards.* Paper presented at 97th Annual National Communication Association Conference. New Orleans, LA.
Singhal, A., Harter, L., Chitnis, K., & Sharma, D. (2007). Participatory photography as theory, method, and praxis: Analyzing an entertainment-education project in India. *Critical Arts, 21* (1), 212–227.
Singhal, A., & Rattine-Flaherty, E. (2006). Pencils and photos as tools of communicative research and praxis: Analyzing Minga Peru's quest for social justice in the Amazon. *Gazette, 68* (4), 313–330.
Smith, L. (1999). *Decolonizing methodologies: Research and indigenous peoples.* London: Zed Books.
Wilkins, K. (2008). *Questioning the politics of numbers: How to read and critique research.* Austin, TX: Unpublished manuscript.
Zoller, H.M. (2000). "A place you haven't visited before": Creating the conditions for community dialogue. Dialogue [Special issue]. *The Southern Communication Journal, 65* (2), 191–207.

Chapter 20

Evaluating Health Communication Interventions

Gary L. Kreps, *George Mason University*

Introduction: Health Communication and the Need for Evaluation Research

Health communication programs have become an essential and ubiquitous part of the delivery of health care and the promotion of public health in the modern world. These programs provide basic health information, warnings about health risks, guidelines for delivering self-care, education about diseases and therapies, feedback about changing health conditions, updates about medical test results, strategies for breaking negative health habits and adopting healthy behaviors, and support for making complex health decisions. Common health communication programs include the use of simple posters, instructional handouts, and pamphlets, professional counseling and health education interactions in medical offices and clinics, as well as the introduction of intricate health information websites, public service announcements, on-line patient and caregiver support groups, tailored health information systems, webinar-based tutorials, entertainment education programs, tele-health home monitoring and interaction systems, interactive patient-centered health records, patient computer portals, mobile health applications, and even (my favorite) the use of intelligent interactive human agents (avatars and robots) to provide counseling and health education to consumers (Neuhauser & Kreps, 2003; Neuhauser & Kreps, 2010).

While the use of health communication programs has proliferated, we are not always well informed about the influences these programs are having on the different audiences they are designed for. Typically these health communication programs are designed with lofty intentions to help people, but with limited data to guide their development, implementation, refinement, and institutionalization. Often these health communication programs can evoke differential responses from diverse audiences, unintended influences, and even negative (iatrogenic) effects on health outcomes. It is critically important to conduct regular, ongoing, and strategic evaluations of health communication intervention programs to assess their effectiveness in achieving primary program goals. Ideally, rigorously gathered evaluation data should guide the development of health communication program, refinement of these programs, and strategic planning for future health communication efforts (Green & Glasgow, 2006).

The Goals of Evaluation Research

Evaluation research programs are essential for helping to increase understanding about how well health communication intervention programs work (Rootman, Goodstadt, McQueen, Potvin, Springett, & Ziglio, 2001). Failure to engage in careful and concerted evaluation research is likely to doom the success of health communication interventions (Kreps, 2002). Such research can answer important questions about the specific influences health communication programs are having on different audiences, who (if anyone) is paying attention to these communication programs, and what is being learned from these programs. It is critically important to learn if the communication programs are having any unintended influences, including boomerang and iatrogenic (negative) effects (Cho & Salmon, 2007; Rinegold, 2002). Too often communication intervention programs have been found to lead to negative influences on target audiences, such as with the National Youth Anti-drug Media Campaign, which actually increased interest in using illegal drugs by at-risk youth (Hornik, Jacobsohn, Orwin, Piesse, & Kalton, 2008). Moreover, evaluation research can help explain why some health communication programs appear to work and what parts of these programs work the best.

Evaluation research also can help health communication program developers take stock of their programs answering key questions about the goals and purposes of these programs. For example, good evaluation data can help clarify what interventionists want to accomplish with specific health communication progams, which audiences they want to reach and influence with these programs, and what they want members of these audiences to do in response to the health communication programs. Based upon this information derived through evaluation research they can establish measurable goals and outcomes for the health communication programs. They can establish a baseline for current activity in these areas to track over time. They can identify relevant theories and intervention strategies to guide their development and implementation of health communication interventions. They can also make sure that the programs are sensitive to unique audience needs, cultural orientations, literacy levels, and expectations (Neuhauser & Paul, 2011, US Department of Health and Human Services, 2010).

The Need for Evaluation Data

The ultimate goal for evaluation research is to guide improvements in health communication programs to enhance their abilities to promote health. Good evaluation data are like turning on the lights in a dark room. "Now I can see!" It is very difficult to design complex health communication interventions to work just right initially. Good data will identify problems with these health communication interventions and suggest directions for improving and refining these programs. Evaluation data can help identify best strategies for designing interventions to meet the unique needs of different audiences. It is unrealistic to think that any one health communication intervention strategy will work equally well with all relevant audiences. Moreover, during the process of collecting evaluation data from key representatives of audiences the interventions are designed for, health communication experts can begin to build collaborative relationships with these representatives to invite them to assist with "user-centered design" of health communication programs and to engage in community participative research and intervention program development (Neuhauser, 2001; Neuhauser & Kreps, 2011; Neuhauser, Schwab, Obarski, Syme, & Bieber, 1998).

Good evaluation research can examine the costs and benefits of intervention programs to determine whether the outcomes received from these interventions are worth the time and expense invested in them. If the evaluation data gathered clearly suggest the benefits of the interventions are greater than their costs, these data can be used to justify larger long-term investments in these programs that can lead to sustaining and institutionalizing the best programs within communities. Carefully gathered evaluation data speak loudly and can help researchers advocate for needed support to expand programs for health promotion (Green & Glasgow, 2006).

The Nature of Evaluation Research

Evaluation research is disciplined inquiry that involves studying health communication intervention programs in a careful, planned, and rigorous manner to understand program influences and potential challenges to achieving program goals (Kreps, 2002). Carefully planned and well-conducted evaluation research can produce valid results for guiding program development, implementation, refinement, and sustainability. The best evaluation research typically involves the use of multiple research methods, including survey, textual analytic, experimental, and ethnographic methods

Good evaluation data provides health communication program planners with critically important information about:

- Level of demand for health communication programs and the issues they cover
- Environmental constraints and specifications for the implementation of communication programs
- Specific design flaws and limitations of communication programs
- User assessments of the efficiency and effectiveness of communication programs
- The appropriate fit for these programs with specific audiences and contexts
- Strategies for adapting communication programs to fit the unique demands of users

Validity of Evaluation Research

It is important to develop the best (most valid) evaluation research designs and methods to inform health communication program design and refinements. Poorly conducted research (with low levels of validity) is worse than no research at all (since false information is worse than no information). Invalid evaluation research will mislead communication planners about the needs for and directions of changes to communication programs. Evaluation researchers should carefully plan their studies to produce findings that can be trusted and generalized. Evaluation of research findings should always take into consideration the limitations of the research before applying the findings to health communication programs.

There are two primary forms of validity of concern to evaluation researchers, internal validity and external validity. Internal validity concerns the accuracy of conclusions drawn from evaluation research. Is the study conducted in such a way that it leads to accurate findings about the communication programs being studied? External validity concerns the generalizability of the findings from evaluation research studies. Can the conclusions from the study be applied to other people, programs, places, and/or times? The primary concern about internal validity is that poorly conducted research (with low levels of internal validity) would result in false and misleading evaluation results. To promote internal validity evaluation researchers should take care to increase the rigor over the ways the research is conducted to insure that variables are operationalized to promote measurement validity and reliability, to make sure that research participant responses are not biased by their experiences with the research, their biases, history, selection, or any demand effects from the research, as well as to make sure that their own personal attributes, goals, and observational biases as researchers do not influence research findings. To promote external validity in evaluation research researchers must take care to ensure that the sampling strategies they use are as representative as possible to the populations they want to generalize findings to, that the research methods have ecological validity, are realistic to real life settings they want to generalize findings to, and that studies can be replicated with different subjects and settings to validate the generalizability of results.

Formative and Summative Evaluation Research

Formative evaluation is an essential process in the development and refinement of health communication intervention programs. Formative research is used to test the adequacy of current programs, providing relevant data for improving the programs. Formative evaluation assesses the need for communication intervention programs through a process of needs analysis. What is the nature of the health problems that need to be addressed by communication interventions? How complex and intractable are these problems? Formative research also helps to identify and segment the key audiences that need to be reached to address the specific health problems. By examining key components of the issues to be addressed, the audiences to be reached, and the key components of the intervention programs developed, evaluation researchers can identify any shortfalls in these communication programs and provide clear directions for the development of improvements to these programs.

To conduct formative research intervention programs are carefully assessed to determine their suitability for addressing the specific health issues they were designed for. Tests are conducted to determine the adequacy of message strategies used and the communication channels deployed to disseminate health messages. Field tests are conducted to determine how well the intervention programs have been implemented in key settings. User responses to programs are tracked over time, especially after refinements are made to the programs. Programs are tested to determine how acceptable and usable they are for key audience representatives. These tests often generate user recommendations for refining program features that can be implemented to improve intervention programs.

Summative evaluation research is used to measure overall intervention program influences and outcomes. Summative research documents the positive and negative influences of health communication intervention programs. These data provide important measures of the utility of health communication intervention programs for health care and health promotion (Nutbeam, 1998). Summative data should examine overall patterns of program use, user satisfaction with programs, message exposure and retention from the programs, changes in key outcome variables (such as learning, relevant health behaviors, health services utilization, and health status) related to the intervention, as well as economic analyses of program costs and benefits (cost-benefit analysis). Summative research also identifies strategies for sustaining the best intervention program. Strong summative evaluation data can be very influential in securing support for program sustainability and institutionalization.

Formative and summative evaluation research should not be viewed as separate and unrelated intervention research processes. Rather, they can be viewed as different parts of an evaluation research continuum. While formative research looks at key parts of health communication interventions, providing a microscopic analysis of individual components and influences of the programs, summative research looks at the big picture of the overall influences of health communication intervention programs. Formative and summative evaluation research should ideally work together in evaluating health communication intervention programs. In fact, formative research findings should inform summative research conclusions, providing key pieces of the data needed to assess overall program influence and effectiveness. Results from formative research efforts should be mined and combined to compile summative research conclusions.

Audience Analysis Research

Audience analysis is a critically important part of evaluation research. It is a necessary prerequisite to creating and refining health communication programs that are responsive to the concerns, needs, perspectives, and communication styles of targeted (intended) audiences of people that communicators want to reach with health messages. Intervention programs that are designed based on rigorous audience analysis data are likely to be seen by key audience members as personally relevant, be attended to, comprehended, carefully considered, and accepted because these programs are developed with audience members' concerns and expectations in mind.

Needs analyses are initial applications of audience analysis research that gather data from potential program users to establish levels of program demand and opportunities to design unique intervention programs to fit audiences' specific health needs. Needs analysis should identify relevant performance gaps between ideal and actual health outcomes that might necessitate development of targeted health communication interventions. Needs analysis should also identify whether there is sufficient demand for new communication program interventions for promoting health.

After needs analyses are conducted, it is time to get to know the unique factors of the individuals health communication interventionists want to reach. Key audience analysis data that should be collected include demographics (age, gender, race, ethnicity, education, income, etc.), current and past related health behaviors, communication characteristics (such as media use patterns, media preferences, literacy levels, and language preferences), audience members' knowledge, attitudes, values, and emotions related to the intervention topics, their cultural habits and preferences, effective motivational factors, and potential barriers to accepting information and changing health behaviors. These data should let evaluation researchers know about the perceptions of program users about the intervention, identifying any concerns and limitations to these interventions, and developing evidence-based strategies from the data gathered to refine and improve the programs to better meet audience needs and expectations.

All health communication intervention programs should be based upon clear evidence of what works and what is not working very well. There is a wealth of important data, often lying dormant, in every health care/promotion setting that indicates what has and what has not worked in the past to achieve health promotion goals. Audience analysis data should identify important user expectations and predispositions that can guide program design, implementation, and ultimately program acceptance and utilization. The more revealing the audience analysis data gathered are, the better these data can be used to design and refine effective health communication intervention programs.

There are two general strategies for collecting audience analysis data. The evaluation researcher can review existing data about key audiences, such as federal, state, and local health statistics, extant research literature about targeted audiences, or conduct secondary analysis of previously collected dated from targeted audiences. (This strategy can save the researcher time and money, but is dependent upon the quality of the available data sets). The second strategy is to collect new audience analysis data, such as conducting personal interview, conducting focus group discussions, administering surveys, or analyzing audience documents (such as letters, photographs, Facebook posts, or online discussions). Often evaluation researchers will use a combination of analyzing existing audience data and collecting their own new audience analysis data to learn about the unique features of targeted audience members.

There are a number of key considerations for effectively collecting and using audience analysis data. Audience analysis data should always guide program development. It is hard to believe that health communication intervention programs are developed without audience analysis data. Furthermore, audience analysis data should assess differences between different audiences to help program planners segment target audiences and develop appropriate and effective interventions that meet the needs of unique groups. Interviews, focus group discussions, surveys, and textual analyses are all good sources of audience analysis data. It is a good idea to use a combination of these data gathering strategies for collecting audience analyses. Interviews and focus group discussions are particularly useful for identifying topics and questions for designing survey instruments. These methods are also very good for elaborating on findings from surveys, providing greater depth of audience analysis data. Surveys are particularly good for examining audience characteristics, especially when they are conducted with representative samples. Interviews and focus group discussions are particularly good for generating new ideas for program development and refinement from key audience representatives.

Evidence-Based Intervention Efforts

The best intervention programs are based upon strong evaluation data. Strong evaluation data should provide clear evidence about what has and has not worked in the past to promote health. These data should help demonstrate the need for change and intervention within the health care system. These data should help identify the kinds of health communication intervention programs that will best fit the needs of specific audiences and fit within the constraints of specific social contexts and environments. The data should clearly demonstrate the utility of proposed interventions, the most promising intervention strategies, and test the effectiveness of health communication intervention programs in action (Kreps, 2002).

There are rich natural data sources that should be identified during audience analysis research efforts that can provide strong evidence for developing and designing health communication intervention programs. These data sources can also assess the relative success of intervention programs. For example, the evaluation researcher can identify "natural" (normally collected) records of key events (such as medical records, attendance records, purchase records, error rates, and usage levels) that can provide interesting trend data to track relevant audience activities before and after implementation of health communication intervention programs (Webb, Campbell, Schwartz, & Sechrist, 1972). Natural data collected before implementation of health communication intervention programs can provide a clear baseline measure from which to track system changes that can, at least in part, be related to intervention programs. (Care must be taken to recognize multiple influences on system performance due to uncontrolled events, secular trends, and extraneous variance, so as not to overstate (or understate) the influence of health communication interventions. Control measures in similar contexts where the communication interventions have not been implemented can provide important points of comparison for clarifying the influences of health communication intervention programs on health outcomes.

It is a good evaluation strategy to implement user response mechanisms (such as user feedback programs, help requests, and suggestion systems) into health communication intervention programs (Kreps, 2002). These response mechanisms can both be passive (providing invisible data collected automatically by tracking and recording use of communication programs, such as the use of tracking cookies on computer programs) and active feedback systems that require users to provide feedback, comments, and suggestions. Passive usage data is easy to collect, but often provides limited and sometimes misleading information about the quality of communication programs, especially when used in isolation of other sources of performance evaluation data. For example, common passive measures of computer-based communication program use are hit rates on websites or total time on websites. These measures might indicate the popularity of program use, or they could also indicate errors in reaching the site or problems with navigating the site. On the other hand, active response data can suffer from validity issues concerning self-report data, particularly if the responses are not anonymous and are shared with other users. It is a good idea to use passive and active response data together, as well as in tandem with other user data, to clarify user responses to health communication interventions.

Prior to implementation of health communication intervention programs, as well as after programs have been implemented, it is important to conduct usability tests of these programs and the technologies used to deliver the programs (Neuhauser & Paul, 2011; Nielsen, 2000). Usability tests assess program users' evaluations of their experiences accessing and navigating communication programs, including the ease, comfort, efficiency, speed, and effectiveness of use, as well as track users' perceptions about, abilities to operate the programs, achieve their health goals with the programs, and their suggestions for improving the programs (Kreps, 2002). Can users accomplish the goals the health communication intervention programs were designed to help them accomplish? How easily can new users learn how to use a specific communication program? Which users are likely to be most and least successful with using a specific communication program? Usability data will help answer these questions and suggest strategies for refining health communication programs.

Methodological Issues in Evaluation Research

There are a number of factors that often limit the effectiveness of evaluation research efforts. For example, a major limitation in the way that evaluation research is often conducted is the over-use of cross-sectional data. Cross-sectional data are collected at a single point in time. How do we know whether that one point in time is representative of the use of the communication program? It is important to determine how health communication programs are accepted and utilized over time. There are often peaks and valleys in program use that cannot be captured with cross-sectional data. Users have to learn how to access and navigate communication programs, get used to these programs, experiment with them, and it may also take some time for users to benefit from the programs. Gathering cross-sectional data is likely to miss key moments and evolutionary trends in the use and application of health communication programs, missing both potential strengths and weaknesses of these programs.

Another common problem in the ways that evaluation research is conducted involves over-reliance on self-report data. Self-report data is information requested from respondents, typically through the use of survey tools such as interviews, focus group discussions, and questionnaires. In too many cases self-report data has become the default research tool for gathering evaluation data. While self-reports often provide interesting data, they can also be biased, especially in organizational contexts (such as health care centers and clinics) where there may be sociopolitical pressures that influence responses. Respondents often try to provide the "right" answer to questions to please researchers. Sometimes respondents answer questions in ways that make them look good, such as answers to questions concerning health behaviors like their levels of alcohol consumption, illegal drug use, tobacco use, exercise behaviors, and dietary choices. Sometimes respondents give the most expedient answer to survey questions to get through with the survey quickly, sometimes referred to as response-set. Due to these threats to the validity of self-report data caution must be taken in interpreting these results. It is also a good idea to gather additional, more objective data, from records, observations, and textual analyses to check the accuracy of self-report responses.

Too often evaluation researchers focus on tangential variables (variables that are not directly relevant to evaluating health communication programs). There is a tendency for researchers to use existing research tools and standardized scales that they are familiar with and have already been validated, but may not measure variables of direct relevance to the programs being evaluated. Sometimes this is referred to as the "law of the hammer," where researchers are apt to use a familiar tool even if it is not the right tool for the job (Kreps, 2002). The measurement of tangential variables inevitably will provide weak and equivocal evaluation data. Care must be taken to identify or develop measures that will clearly operationalize variables that are central to the goals of the health communication intervention program being evaluated.

A final common methodological problem with evaluation research to be addressed here that has already been alluded to in the discussion of passive and active response mechanisms earlier in this chapter, is the over-reliance on shallow data in evaluation studies. A common example of shallow data is the number of web hits. It is difficult to determine what the number of hits means when evaluating a communication program. Does a lot of hits mean it is a good program? Who is accessing the website? What are they doing at the site? Are they able to use the information on the website to achieve the health promotion goals? It is unclear. Conclusions made based on shallow data are often unwarranted. Additional information is typically needed to determine how users perceive and apply information from health communication programs. Effective evaluation research programs must be designed to provide needed depth of information about use and satisfaction with communication programs if the data are to be useful in assessing program effectiveness and guiding program refinements.

Data Reduction and Information Overload

Clarity in the ways that evaluation research data are reported is essential in enabling the application of these data for program assessments and improvements. Too often evaluation data are reported in complex and equivocal ways that limit understanding and application. This only increases information overload rather than increasing understanding. Statistical presentations of evaluation research results are often complex and confusing for lay audiences, especially those who have low levels of numeracy. Who are the data being reported to? Other researchers? Policy makers? Funders and investors? Health care providers? Consumers and family caregivers? Reports of evaluation research must be prepared to meet the literacy level and vested interests of the audiences for these data.

To get the most out of evaluation research results, researchers have to translate findings in clear and compelling ways. Strategic use of tables, charts, diagrams, and examples can help bring evaluation data to life. It is incumbent on the evaluation researcher to clearly identify the implications, applications, and limitations of evaluation research for key audiences.

Best Practices for Conducting Evaluation Research

The following suggestions are designed to help evaluation researchers enhance the effectiveness of their evaluations of health communication intervention programs:

Use of longitudinal research designs will help capture variations in program use and help to provide a clear picture of health communication program strengths and weaknesses (Kreps, 2011). It is important to gather evaluation data at multiple points in time to capture the evolution of program adoption and utilization. This means conducting surveys, observations, and textual analyses at different intervals, as well as to use pre-post experimental designs that compare outcome measures at different points of time beyond the baseline measures. It is always best, if possible, to establish baseline measures prior to the implementation of the health communication intervention program.

The use of multi-methodological research designs will provide evaluation researchers with a full assessment of health communication intervention programs (Kreps, 2011). Multi-methodological research designs combine different methods to provide different kinds of evaluation data. Typically one method can augment weaknesses if data collection for another method and the different sources of data can provide reality checks for the accuracy of data collected. This is particularly useful in validating the accuracy of data collected via self-report measures.

Combining quantitative and qualitative data can enrich evaluation research efforts. While quantitative data can be powerfully analyzed statistically and appears to carry strong scientific weight and objectivity, it often fails to provide great depth of information and explanation about why users react to programs the ways they do. Alternatively, qualitative data, while sometimes appearing rather impressionistic, typically provides great depth of information. When reported in narrative form, qualitative data can be most compelling. The combination (triangulation) of quantitative and qualitative data gives evaluation research both precision and depth of analysis.

The use of unobtrusive measures can provide evaluation researchers with interesting and non-reactive data about health communication program utilization and influences (Kreps, 2011). Unobtrusive measures do not depend on user self-reports about communication programs. By observing naturally occurring data, such as examinations of archival records and passive user-response mechanisms, researcher can gather revealing data about consumer behavior that is not influenced by self-editing and socio-political constraints. Unobtrusive data can also be used to check the accuracy of self-report data, increasing confidence in survey results.

It is important to build in careful operationalizations and measurements of key economic and health outcome variables in evaluation research of health communication intervention programs. By measuring relevant health outcome variables evaluation researchers can assess the influences of health communication programs on important health consequences, such as user knowledge, attitudes, values, intentions, behaviors, and health states, including levels of morbidity and mortality. Economic analysis of the costs and benefits of health interventions can clearly illustrate the relative value of these programs. Measurement of important economic and health outcomes is especially relevant for summative evaluation research to assess the relative contributions of health communication programs on health promotion.

It is imperative for evaluation researchers to use strong evaluation data to demonstrate progress and guide future health communication intervention efforts. Good evaluation research efforts should provide clear information about the contributions of health communication intervention programs on the accomplishment of important health promotion goals and outcomes (Nutbeam, 1998). By carefully tracking progress, evaluation researchers can identify the achievements and shortfalls of health communication intervention programs, and help to guide the development of refined programs for enhancing health promotion in the future.

Building Evaluation Research into Every Communication Program

Evaluation research should be an indispensable part of the development and refinement of every health communication intervention program (Rootman et al., 2001). Evaluation researchers should identify available sources of audience analysis data. What do we already know about key audiences? Are there natural sources of information about key events that can inform evaluation efforts, such as medical billing records, public records, or message transcripts)? Program developers should build in user-response mechanisms into every health communication intervention program to provide feedback about program use. Researchers should seek existing or establish baseline measures of key audience attributes and behaviors to use as benchmarks for later comparisons after use of health communication programs. Usability tests should be conducted regularly to determine the effectiveness of communication programs for different groups of users. Researchers should work closely with key representatives from targeted audiences to conduct user-centered design and community participative evaluation research (Neuhauser, Constantine, Constantine, Sokal-Gutierrez, Obarski, Clayton, Desai, Sumner, & Syme, 2007). Data from evaluation research should be applied to refining and improving all health communication programs.

Suggested Readings

Kreps, G.L. (2002). Evaluating new health information technologies: Expanding the frontiers of health care delivery and health promotion. *Studies in Health Technology and Informatics, 80,* 205–212.

Kreps, G.L. (2011). Methodological diversity and integration in health communication inquiry. *Patient Education and Counseling, 82,* 285–291.

Neuhauser, L. (2001). Participatory design for better interactive health communication: A statewide model in the USA. *Electronic Journal of Communication* 11, nos. 3&4.

Neuhauser, L., & Kreps, G.L. (2011). Participatory design and artificial intelligence: Strategies to improve health communication for diverse audiences. In N. Green, S. Rubinelli, & D. Scott. (Eds.). *Artificial Intelligence and Health Communication* (pp. 49–52). Cambridge, MA: AAAI Press.

Neuhauser, L., Schwab, M., Obarski, S. K., Syme, S. L., & Bieber, M. (1998). Community participation in health promotion: Evaluation of the California Wellness Guide. *Health Promotion International* 13(3).

Nutbeam, D. (1998). Evaluating health promotion—progress, problems, and solutions. *Health Promotion International, 13*, 27–44.

Rootman, I., Goodstadt, M., McQueen, D., Potvin, L., Springett, J., & Ziglio, E. (Eds.). (2001). *Evaluation in health promotion: Principles and perspectives*. WHO (EURO), Copenhagen.

References

Cho, H., & Salmon, C.T. (2007). Unintended effects of health communication campaigns. *Journal of Communication, 57(2)*, 293–317.

Green, L. W., & Glasgow, R. E. (2006). Evaluating the relevance, generalization, and applicability of research: Issues in external validation and translation methodology. *Evaluation and the Health Professions, 29*(1), 126–153.

Hornik, R., Jacobsohm L., Orwin, R., Piesse, A., & Klton, G. (2008). Effects of the National Youth Anti-Drug media campaign on youths. *American Journal of Public Health, 98(12)*, 2229–2236.

Kreps, G.L. (2002). Evaluating new health information technologies: Expanding the frontiers of health care delivery and health promotion. *Studies in Health Technology and Informatics, 80,* 205–212.

Kreps, G.L. (2011). Methodological diversity and integration in health communication inquiry. *Patient Education and Counseling, 82,* 285–291.

Neuhauser, L. (2001). Participatory design for better interactive health communication: A statewide model in the USA. *Electronic Journal of Communication* 11, nos. 3&4.

Neuhauser, L., Constantine, W. L., Constantine, N. A., Sokal-Gutierrez, K., Obarski, S. K., Clayton, L., Desai, M., Sumner, G., Syme, S. L. (2007). Promoting prenatal and early childhood health: Evaluation of a statewide materials-based intervention for parents. *American Journal of Public Health,* 97(10): 813–819.

Neuhauser, L., & Kreps, G. (2003). Rethinking communication in the e-health era. *Journal of Health Psychology, 8,* 7–22.

Neuhauser, L., & Kreps, G. (2010). Ehealth communication and behavior change: Promise and performance. *Journal of Social Semiotics,* 20:1, 9–27.

Neuhauser, L., & Kreps, G.L. (2011). Participatory design and artificial intelligence: Strategies to improve health communication for diverse audiences. In N. Green, S. Rubinelli, & D. Scott. (Eds.). *Artificial Intelligence and Health Communication* (pp. 49–52). Cambridge, MA: AAAI Press. http://www.aaai.org/ocs/index.php/SSS/SSS11/paper/viewFile/2475/2857

Neuhauser, L., & Paul, K. (2011). Readability, comprehension and usability. In: *Communicating Risks and Benefits: An Evidence-Based User's Guide*. Silver Spring, MD: U.S. Department of Health and Human Services. Bethesda MD: Food and Drug Administration.

Neuhauser, L., Schwab, M., Obarski, S. K., Syme, S. L., & Bieber, M. (1998). Community participation in health promotion: Evaluation of the California Wellness Guide. *Health Promotion International,* 13(3).

Nielsen, J. (2000). *Designing web usability*. Indianapolis: New Riders Publishing.

Nutbeam, D. (1998). Evaluating health promotion—progress, problems, and solutions. *Health Promotion International, 13*, 27–44.

Rinegold, D.J. (2002). Boomerang effects in response to public health interventions: Some unintended consequences in the alcoholic beverage market. *Journal of Consumer Policy, 25*, 27–63.

Rootman, I., Goodstadt, M., McQueen, D., Potvin, L., Springett, J., and Ziglio, E. (Eds.). (2001). *Evaluation in health promotion: Principles and perspectives*. WHO (EURO), Copenhagen.

US Department of Health and Human Services, Office of Disease Prevention and Health Promotion. (2010). *Quick Guide to Health Literacy*. Retrieved from http://www.health.gov/communication/literacy/quickguide/

Webb, E.J., Campbell, D.T., Schwartz, R.D., & Sechrist, L. (1972). *Unobtrusive Measures: Nonreactive Research in the Social Science*. New York: Rand McNally & Company.

Editors and Chapter Contributors

Do Kyun Kim, Ph.D., *Corresponding Editor*, is an Assistant Professor in the Department of Communication and the Richard D'Aquin / BORSF Endowed Professor at the University of Louisiana at Lafayette. He is also an affiliate researcher of the Center for Climate Change Communication at George Mason University, and president of Acadiana Community Education Center (ACE Center). He is an expert in the fields of diffusion of innovation, social network analysis, global media effects, and social empowerment. He earned his PhD in communication research from Ohio University where he received the first Everett M. Rogers Award and was named the Everett M. Rogers Scholar for the 2005–2006 academic year. He has additional degrees (BAs and MAs) in economics and political science and is particularly interested in examining the intersections between media, politics, economy, and social forces as they influence the diffusion of information and innovations that are of benefit to society. Currently, his interest is extended to issues of communication and social change. In addition to his work in the US, he has led and worked for several international projects in Africa and Asia.

Arvind Singhal, Ph.D. is the Samuel Shirley and Edna Holt Marston Endowed Professor of Communication and Director of the Social Justice Initiative at the University of Texas at El Paso, and has also been appointed, since 2009–2010, as the William J. Clinton Distinguished Fellow at the Clinton School of Public Service, Little Rock, Arkansas. Singhal teaches and conducts research in the diffusion of innovations, the positive deviance approach, organizing for social change, the entertainment-education strategy, and liberating interactional structures. His research and outreach spans sectors such as health, education, peace, human rights, poverty alleviation, sustainable development, civic participation, democracy and governance, and corporate citizenship. The Social Science Research Council & the International Communication Association recognized him as the winner of the Communication Research as Collaborative Practice Award in 2009, and the winner of the Communication Researcher as an Agent of Change Award in 2008. Singhal's research has been supported by many academic and governmental institutions. He has served as an advisor to the World Bank, UN-FAO, UNICEF, UNDP, UNAIDS, UNFPA, the BBC World Service Trust, and private corporations such as Procter & Gamble (U.S.A and Thailand), Telenor AS (Norway), SpareBank (Norway), and others.

Gary L. Kreps, Ph.D. is a University Distinguished Professor at George Mason University, where he serves as Chair of the Department of Communication and Directs the Center for Health and Risk Communication. He examines the ways strategic interpersonal and mediated communication can enhance health promotion, risk prevention, health advocacy, and quality of care, especially for vulnerable populations. He is a Fellow of the American Academy of Health Behavior and has received numerous scholarly awards. He serves as a scientific advisor to domestic and international health agencies, foundations, and corporations. Before joining the faculty at George Mason University, he was Chief of the Health Communication and Informatics Research Branch at the National Cancer Institute, Dean of the School of Communication at Hofstra University, Executive Director of the Greenspun School of Communication at UNLV, and a professor at Northern Illinois, Rutgers, Indiana, and Purdue Universities.

Editors and Chapter Contributors

Agaptus Anaele, M.A. is a Ford Foundation International Fellow from Nigeria, West Africa. At present, he is a doctoral student in the Brian Lamb School of Communication, Purdue University with concentration in Global Public Health Communication, Development, and Culture. His work is guided by the Culture Centered Approach (CCA), which promotes academic and community partnerships in problem identification and articulation of culturally situated solutions that lead to sustainable social changes. He has a Master's Degree in International Affairs (MIA) from Ohio University in Athens, Ohio, U.S.A, and a Bachelor's Degree in English Education (B.A.ED) from University of Port Harcourt, Nigeria.

Charles K. Atkin, Ph.D. chaired the Communication department at Michigan State University. He published 160 journal articles and chapters dealing with media effects on health, political, and social behavior, and six books. The Decade of Behavior consortium recognized his work with the 2006 "Award for Applied Social Science Research," and he received the 2008 "Outstanding Health Communication Scholar Award" from the ICA and NCA Health Communication Divisions and the "Distinguished Applied Communication Research Award" from NCA in 2010. Sadly, Chuck passed away in August 2012.

Wayne A. Beach, Ph.D. is Professor in the School of Communication at San Diego State University, Adjunct Professor, Department of Surgery, and Member of the Moores UCSD Cancer Center, University of California, San Diego. His research on health communication includes books on *Conversations about Illness*, *A Natural History of Family Cancer*, and *Handbook of Patient-Provider Interactions*. A wide variety of articles and chapters focus on issues ranging from medical interviews during clinical encounters, to how family members communicate throughout cancer journeys. External funding has been awarded from the National Institutes of Health (NIH)/National Cancer Institute (NCI), the American Cancer Society (ACS), and several philanthropic foundations in San Diego. Current work examines how patients make available and oncologists respond to hopes, fears, and uncertainties about cancer. He is also collaborating with theatre professionals in a production, funded by NCI and adapted from actual family phone calls, documenting how family members communicate about and manage cancer on the telephone.

Ellen Burke Beckjord, Ph.D. Ellen Beckjord is an Assistant Professor in the Department of Psychiatry at the University of Pittsburgh working in the Biobehavioral Medicine in Oncology Program at the University of Pittsburgh Medical Center Cancer Center. Her research is focused on cancer survivorship and the role of informatics in promoting health behavior. Dr. Beckjord was a Cancer Prevention Fellow at the National Cancer Institute (NCI), which is when she began her work with the Health Information National Trends Survey, including data analysis and survey development. She earned a doctorate in clinical psychology from the University of Vermont, her master's degree in public health with a focus on epidemiology and biostatistics from the Johns Hopkins Bloomberg School of Public Health, and a bachelor's degree in psychology from the Pennsylvania State University.

Kelly D. Blake, Sc.D. is a health scientist in the National Cancer Institute's (NCI) Health Communication and Informatics Research Branch. She serves on the management team for

NCI's Health Information National Trends Survey, and examines how media exposure and inequalities influence health behavior and attitudes toward public health policy. Dr. Blake was a cancer prevention fellow at the Dana-Farber Cancer Institute. Before that, she was a science writer in NCI's Division of Cancer Control and Population Sciences. Prior to that, she was a health educator for the West Virginia Rural Health Education Partnerships and a health communication research fellow at the Centers for Disease Control and Prevention, National Institute for Occupational Safety and Health. She earned a Doctor of Science degree in social epidemiology from the Harvard School of Public Health, a master's degree in community health education from West Virginia University and a bachelor's degree in journalism from Marshall University.

Jane Brown has over 20 years in development communication and production, with an emphasis on gender, adolescent reproductive health, HIV and AIDS as well as program management, and mass media. She has experience developing Social/Behavior Change Communication (S/BCC) strategies, messages and materials including radio distance learning programs and toolkits. Ms. Brown has worked extensively with government and non-government partners to build their capacity to produce high-quality, high-impact S/BCC programming. She has also worked with the private sector. She was one of the principal innovators of the evaluated *African Transformation* toolkit which enables women and men to explore the underlying gender barriers and facilitators to practicing positive health behaviors and develop realistic solutions, and *Go Girls!* a special Pepfar initiative to reduce girls' vulnerability to HIV. She provides leadership roles on many regional S/BCC projects and over a dozen country projects.

David B. Buller, Ph.D. is an expert in health communication, conducting research sponsored by the National Cancer Institute, the Robert Wood Johnson Foundation, and the U.S. Centers for Disease Control and Prevention since 1979. David was previously a Professor at the University of Arizona, a Senior Scientist at AMC Cancer Research Center, and the Harold Simmons Senior Scientist for Health Communication and Vice President of The Cooper Institute - Denver. Many of David's current projects are centered on educating targeted groups about relatively small changes they can make in their lives that can save them from years of chronic illnesses. Avoiding extreme sun exposure, developing healthier eating habits, and avoiding cigarette smoke are the focus of some of David's most recent and successful programs. His *Sunny Days Healthy Ways* program has been recognized as a national resource for complying with the CDC and American Cancer Society's recommendations for skin cancer education.

Mary K. Buller, M.A. has more than 20 years of experience leading research projects to develop skin cancer prevention and nutrition education programs for school children, college students and adults using print, interpersonal training and the Internet. Her research has been funded by grants and contracts from the National Institutes of Health and the U.S. Centers for Disease Control and Prevention. In 2006, Klein Buendel received the national Tibbetts Award for excellence and achievement in the Small Business Innovation Research program. Prior to co-founding Klein Buendel, Mary was president of Partners For Health Systems, Inc. (PHS), an affiliate of the AMC Cancer Research Center in Denver. Prior to PHS, Mary worked at the Arizona Cancer Center at the University of Arizona in Tucson for 11 years. From 1998 to

2001, she founded and directed the American Sun Protection Association (ASPA), a nonprofit trade association for the sun protection industry.

Wen-ying Sylvia Chou, Ph.D. is a Program Director in the Health Communication and Informatics Research Branch of the National Cancer Institute. Her recent publications have examined the role of Web 2.0/ social media in health, patient-provider communication, and end-of-life communication. Trained as a sociolinguist, she has extensive experience conducting mixed methods research on patient-provider interactions and illness narratives. As a Program Director, she supervises a portfolio of research on health literacy, patient-centered communication, health disparities, and the impact of technologies on clinical care and public health. Dr. Chou completed a fellowship through NCI's Cancer Prevention Fellowship Program; she holds an M.S. and Ph.D. in Linguistics from Georgetown University, and a Master of Public Health from the Interdisciplinary MPH program at UC Berkeley.

James W. Dearing, Ph.D. is Professor and Chairperson of the Department of Communication at Michigan State University. He has been Senior Scientist with Kaiser Permanente and on the faculties of several universities. He studies the strategic use of diffusion of innovation concepts to accelerate the spread of evidence-based practices, programs, and policies. He studied under and worked closely with Everett M. Rogers for 20 years. A recent book of his is *Communication of Innovations* (2006, co-edited with Arvind Singhal). Dearing served as a member of the National Academy of Science/Institute of Medicine framework committee for a five-year programmatic review of the National Institute for Occupational Safety and Health, and on a Centers for Disease Control and Prevention *Community Guide* health marketing and health communication review. Recently he has focused on the spread of approaches for improving healthcare delivery, and cancer care coordination and communication, lifestyle physical activity, pediatric care, university-community knowledge transfer, work-family balance in corporate settings, and innovations in the teaching and learning of chemistry, math, engineering, and physics.

David M. Dozier, Ph.D. is a professor in the School of Journalism and Media Studies at San Diego State University and heads the public relations emphasis in the school. He is the 2001 recipient of the Jackson, Jackson & Wagner Behavior Science Prize. In 2008, the Public Relations Society of America named him the Outstanding Educator, a national award. In 2009, the Institute for Public Relations named him a research fellow. The author or co-author of more than 50 books, book chapters, articles and scholarly papers, he is the 1990 recipient of the Pathfinder Award from the Institute for Public Relations Research and Education for his contribution to original scholarly research in the field. He is the second most cited scholar in the public relations discipline. A recognized expert on research applications to communication management, he has been an invited speaker throughout the United States, as well as in Canada, Europe, and the Middle East.

Lucía Durá, Ph.D. is Assistant Professor of Rhetoric and Composition in the Department of English at The University of Texas at El Paso (UTEP). Her work in the design, implementation, evaluation, and dissemination of system, culture, organization, and social change interventions focuses on how change happens rhetorically (how health, advocacy, intercultural, and change-related messages are designed, implemented, and evaluated). She has presented and published her work at multiple local, national, and international venues, including peer reviewed journals, book chapters, and international reports. Durá has been the recipient of numerous honors and awards such as the UT-Arlington Academy of Distinguished Scholars Public Interest Award and the Dodson Dissertation Fellowship.

Mohan J. Dutta, Ph.D. is Professor and Head of the Department of Communications and New Media at the National University of Singapore and Courtesy Professor of Communication at Purdue University. At NUS, he is the Founding Director of the Center for Culture-Centered Approach to Research and Evaluation (CARE), directing research on culturally-centered, community-based projects of social change. He teaches and conducts research in international health communication, critical cultural theory, poverty in healthcare, health activism in globalization politics, indigenous cosmologies of health, subaltern studies and dialogue, and public policy and social change. Currently, he serves as Editor of the "Global Health Communication Book Series" with Left Coast Press and sits on the editorial board of seven journals. Before arriving to NUS, he served as Associate Dean of Research in the College of Liberal Arts at Purdue University, a Service Learning Fellow, and a fellow of the Entrepreneurial Leadership Academy. Also at Purdue, he served as the Founding Director of the Center for Poverty and Health Inequities (COPHI).

Laurel J. Felt, M.A. is a doctoral candidate at the University of Southern California (USC)'s Annenberg School for Communication and Journalism. She is an Instructional Design Specialist with the USC Dornsife Joint Educational Project, and formerly was the Instructional Design Coordinator for the USC Shoah Foundation. From 2010–2012, Felt was lead Research Assistant for USC Annenberg Innovation Lab's project Participatory Learning And You! (PLAY!). Felt has designed research, curricula, and programs to nurture youths' social and emotional competence, new media literacies, and powerful play. Analyses of her original, theory-driven pedagogical interventions appear in *The Journal of Media Literacy Education* and in the edited volume *African Childhoods: Education, Development, Peacebuilding, and the Youngest Continent.*

Anat Gesser-Edelsburg, Ph.D. is a lecturer in the Department of Health Promotion, School of Public Health, University of Haifa and teaches in the Cheryl Spencer Department of Nursing, University of Haifa and at the Sammy Ofer School of Communications, the Interdisciplinary Center in Herzliya. She is also a senior researcher at the Participatory Social Marketing Program at Tel-Aviv University. Her research areas include entertainment-education, health and risk communication, social marketing, persuasive communication and health-promotion programs. Anat is a member of research teams that have received research grants from The Israel Anti-Drug Authority, Israeli Ministry of Immigrant Absorption, the Tami Steinmetz Center for Peace Research, Or Yarok, The Israel National Institute for Health Policy and Health Services Research, The Research Fund on Insurance Matters, affiliated with the Israel Insurance Association, The National Road Safety Authority, Maccabi Healthcare Services, Choices Israel Organization, European Union (FP7-Health), Pfizer Forum for Health Policy and Israel Ministry of Health. Her co-authored book *Talking Pupils* is used as a recommended textbook for criminology and sociology studies and by organizations such as the Association of Rape Crisis Centers in Israel. Her co-authored book *Peace and Tolerance Encouragement among Youth by Using Theatre: Are Educational Plays an Important and Effective Tool?* treats the multifaceted issue of peace through the prism of edutainment tools and theories of psychological health and wellbeing.

Dave Gustafson, Ph.D. is Research Professor of Industrial and Systems Engineering at the University of Wisconsin-Madison where he founded and directs the Center for Health Enhancement Systems Studies. The Center includes a Center of Excellence in Cancer Communication Research (National Cancer Institute), the national program office for the Network for the Improvement of Addiction Treatment (NIATx), and Center of Excellence on Active Aging Research (Agency for Healthcare Research and Quality). His individual change research develops and tests computer systems to help people deal with serious illness; organizational change research produces models to predict and explain implementation, sustainability and diffusion of innovations, as well as models to measure quality of care and understand customer needs. Dave is a member of the National Academy of Engineering, a Fellow of the Association for Health Services Research, the American Medical Informatics Association, the W K Kellogg Foundation, co-chaired the federal Science Panel on Interactive Communications in Health and helped found and is a Fellow and past vice-chair of the board of the Institute for Healthcare Improvement. He is a member of the NIH Healthcare Implementation and Dissemination Study Section.

Kyle Gutzmer, M.A. is a candidate in the Joint Doctoral Program in Public Heath at San Diego State University and the University of California, San Diego. Her research focuses on patient-doctor communication during oncology interviews and how families manage cancer.

Kari Hartwig, Ph.D. is an Adjunct Professor at Walden University teaching in the master's and doctoral public health program. She has more than 20 years' experience working and teaching in global public health including previous positions at Yale University, the University of Minnesota, and Family Health International.

Bradford W. Hesse, Ph.D. is Chief of the Health Communication and Informatics Research Branch at the National Cancer Institute (NCI). Trained as a psychologist, Dr. Hesse has spent most of his career working to improve the ways in which mediated communication environments can be used to improve decision making, enhance the user experience, influence group outcomes, and support adaptive and healthy behaviors. His work has taken him into the areas of human-computer interaction, medical informatics, health psychology, media psychology, interpersonal communication, health communication, and public health surveillance. Dr. Hesse currently serves as program director for the Health Information National Trends Survey (a national survey of adults' use of health information technologies), the Centers of Excellence in Cancer Communication Research, and has a rich portfolio of basic science communication projects and grants. He has authored or co-authored over 160 publications including peer-reviewed journal articles, technical reports, books, and book chapters.

Editors and Chapter Contributors

Andrew Isham, M.S. is a researcher at the Center for Health Enhancement Systems Studies, University of Wisconsin - Madison. His focus is on the innovative adaptation of information technologies to support behavioral change in people with chronic health conditions. Isham has a BS in mechanical engineering, a minor in psychology, and an M.S. in industrial engineering, with a specialization in health systems engineering. Isham is the director of development for three randomized clinical trials. The first involves the development and testing of a smartphone application designed to help underserved teens with asthma manage their disease (Mobile Comprehensive Health Enhancement Support System, or M-CHESS), the second involves the development and testing of a smartphone application designed to help patients leaving inpatient addiction treatment avoid relapse (Addiction-CHESS), and the development of web and mobile apps designed to help the elderly live independently (Elder—CHESS).

Caroline Jacoby, M.P.H. is an associate at the Johns Hopkins Bloomberg School of Public Health and teaches a graduate level Entertainment Education and Behavior Change Communication course. She has over 15 years experience in behavior and social change communication with an emphasis on Family Planning, Maternal and Child health (FP/MCH), Nutrition, Reproductive Health, Nutrition, Communication Strategy Development, Entertainment Education and Community Mobilization. A Senior Program Officer at Johns Hopkins Bloomberg School of Public Health/ Center for Communication Programs (JHU·CCP), she currently provides technical assistance to entertainment education programs in Nigeria and Nepal. Between 2006 and 2008 she was based in Nepal serving as the JHU·CCP Communication Advisor for a Safe Motherhood and Newborn Health Program. In Nepal she provided technical guidance to Nepali government and NGO partners in strategy development, program design, advocacy, implementation, monitoring, and evaluation. She has also worked on programs in Bangladesh, Ethiopia, Malawi, Botswana and Mozambique.

Matthew W. Kreuter, Ph.D. is founder and director of the Health Communication Laboratory at Washington University in St. Louis, one of five NCI-designated Centers of Excellence in Cancer Communication Research. His research explores strategies to increase the reach and effectiveness of health information in low-income and minority populations to help eliminate health disparities. He received his PhD and MPH in Health Behavior and Health Education from the School of Public Health at the University of North Carolina-Chapel Hill.

Uttara Bharath Kumar, M.P.H. has worked for JHU·CCP since 1997 based in Baltimore till 1999 and then in Zambia field office supporting Southern and East Africa programmes from 1999–2009. She is currently a Senior Technical Advisor for JHU·CCP based in Chennai, providing support to programmes in India and in Asia and Africa. In her global work she has led various health communication programmes and initiatives including ones that won awards (The Red Ribbon Award 2006, Silver Medal at the New York Film Festival 2007, Africommnet Award for Best Multimedia Campaign in Africa, 2009). She co-founded Nalamdana, a Chennai-based health communication NGO, in 1993 with a seed grant from the Echoing Green Foundation and was its executive director until 1996. She continues to actively serve on Nalamdana's Board of Trustees and provides technical guidance and fundraising support to Nalamdana's projects.

Editors and Chapter Contributors

Carolyn Lauckner, M.A. is a doctoral student at Michigan State University in the department of Telecommunication, Information Studies, and Media. Her research interests lie in the realms of health and social media, mHealth, and online health information. Previously, she has published research related to eHealth interventions for physical activity, the content of breast cancer websites, and mobile applications for diabetes.

Edward Maibach, Ph.D. is a University Distinguished Professor at George Mason University and director of the Center for Climate Change Communication. He has extensive experience as an academic researcher and as a communication and social marketing practitioner in government, business, and the non-profit sector. His research focuses on the broad question of how public engagement in climate change can be expanded and enhanced. Ed is currently a Principal Investigator on several climate change education grants funded by the National Science Foundation, NASA, Robert Wood Johnson Foundation, Grantham Foundation for the Protection of the Environment, and Town Creek Foundation. He also currently serves on the National Climate Assessment Development and Advisory Committee and advises a wide range of organizations on how to improve their climate change communication, education and outreach. Previously, Ed served as associate director of the National Cancer Institute, worldwide director of social marketing for Porter Novelli, co-chairman of the board for Kidsave International, and as a faculty member at Emory and George Washington universities. He has published over 100 peer-reviewed journal articles and book chapters.

Richard P. Moser, Ph.D. is a Research Psychologist within the Science of Research and Technology Branch, Behavioral Research Program, at the National Cancer Institute (NCI). He is the data coordinator for the Health Information National Trends Survey (HINTS) and directs the Grid-Enabled Measures (GEM) project, which is a web-based portal to promote the use of standardized health research measures and data sharing using technologically mediated social participation. He has particular interests in conducting and promoting integrative data analysis, which involves merging or linking independent data sets and analyzing them as a whole to help build a cumulative knowledge base. His research interests include statistical and survey methodology, health cognitions, and end-of-life issues. He is an author or co-author on more than 65 peer-reviewed journal articles and several book chapters spanning a range of topics including survey methodology, analytic procedures, health behaviors, and innovative uses of data.

David E. Nelson, M.D. is the Director of the Cancer Prevention Fellowship Program at the National Cancer Institute. Over his career, Dr. Nelson has conducted applied research on a wide range of topics, including alcohol, tobacco, and other risk factors; health services; communication; survey methodology; and injury prevention. He received his medical degree from the Oregon Health Sciences University, his master's degree in public health from the University of Michigan, and his master's degree in communication from the University of Delaware. He is an author on 90 articles in the peer-reviewed literature, and was the lead editor of the book "Communicating Public Health Information Effectively: A Guide for Practitioners," which was published by the American Public Health Association in 2002; he was the lead author of "Making Data Talk: Communicating Public Health Data to the Public, Policy Makers, and the Press" with co-authors Bradford Hesse and Robert Croyle.

Linda Neuhauser, Ph.D. is Clinical Professor of Community Health and Human Development at UC Berkeley and Co-Principal Investigator at Health Research for Action. Her research and teaching are focused on transdisciplinary, translational, and participatory approaches to improve health interventions. She has a special interest in collaborative design and evaluation of mass communication that meets people's literacy, language, cultural, disability, and other needs. In addition to her work at HRA, she serves on national task forces on translational research, communication, and Internet health. She has won numerous awards for her work in health promotion and communication. She formerly served as a health officer in the US State Department in West and Central Africa. She holds Ph.D. and M.P.H. degrees from the UC Berkeley School of Public Health.

Matthew Nisbet, Ph.D. is Associate Professor of Communication and Co-Director of the Center for Social Media at American University. His research investigates the role of communication in policymaking and public affairs, focusing on debates over science, sustainability, and public health. Nisbet is the author of more than fifty peer-reviewed studies, book chapters, and monographs. He has been a Health Policy Investigator at the Robert Wood Johnson Foundation, a Google Science Communication Fellow, and a Shorenstein Fellow in Press, Politics, and Policy at Harvard University's Kennedy School of Government. In 2011, the editors at the journal *Nature* recommended Nisbet's research as "essential reading for anyone with a passing interest in the climate change debate," and the *New Republic* highlighted his work as a "fascinating dissection of the shortcomings of climate activism." Since 2002, Nisbet's scholarship has been cited more than 850 times in the peer-reviewed literature and in more than 300 books.

Ronald E. Rice, Ph.D. is the Arthur N. Rupe Chair in the Social Effects of Mass Communication, Co-Director of the Carsey-Wolf Center, and former ICA President (2006–2007). He has published over 160 journal articles and book chapters, and 13 books, the two most recent of which are *Organizations and unusual routines*, and, with Atkin, *Public communication campaigns* (4th ed.).

Rajiv N. Rimal, Ph.D. is an Associate Professor in the Department of Health, Behavior, & Society and Senior Evaluation Officer at the Center for Communication Programs at the Johns Hopkins University Bloomberg School of Public Health. He is the former Chair of the Health Communication Division of both the International Communication Association and the National Communication Association. His work seeks to understand how individuals, across a variety of countries and cultures, process risk information, and how societal norms affect human behavior. His current work focuses on developing, implementing, and evaluating HIV-prevention interventions through the use of mass media, mobilization of community resources, and promotion of interpersonal communication in sub-Saharan Africa.

Editors and Chapter Contributors

Lila J. Rutten, Ph.D. is currently the Associate Scientific Director of Population Health Science in the Center for the Science of Healthcare Delivery at Mayo Clinic. Dr. Rutten's research is focused on population-level disease prevention and health promotion and the development, implementation, and evaluation of high-value, patient-centered health care to improve population health and health outcomes. Prior to her work with the Mayo Clinic, Dr. Rutten provided scientific and programmatic support to the National Cancer Institute's Health Communication and Informatics Research Branch as a Senior Behavioral Scientist with SAIC-Frederick, Inc., National Cancer Institute. Dr. Rutten also served the Health Communication and Informatics Research Branch as a Project Officer overseeing a multi-million dollar portfolio in health communication and informatics research, and serving as the Research Coordinator for HINTS. Dr. Rutten received her Ph.D. in Psychology from Miami University of Ohio and a Masters in Public Health from Harvard University.

Bret R. Shaw, Ph.D., is an Assistant Professor in the Department of Life Sciences Communication at the University of Wisconsin-Madison. His research focuses on how people with chronic health conditions benefit from online support and tailored information systems. He has published in a diverse range of journals, including *Health Education Research, Health Communication, the Journal of Health Communication, CIN: Computers, Informatics and Nursing, American Behavioral Scientist, Information Technology and Behaviour, the International Journal of Medical Informatics, PsychoOncology, the Journal of Computer-Mediated Communication,* and *Patient Education and Counseling*. Shaw also conducts research on developing and evaluating social marketing campaigns to encourage environmental behavior change.

S. Leonard Syme, Ph.D. is Professor of Epidemiology and Community Health (Emeritus) in the School of Public Health at UC Berkeley. During more than 20 years as Co-Principal Investigator at HRA, he has worked on developing community interventions to prevent disease and promote health. Pursuing his research interest on the relationship between health and such psychosocial factors as poverty, stress and social isolation, he has studied San Francisco bus drivers, civil servants in London, and Japanese living in Japan, Hawaii, and San Francisco. He has been elected to the Institute of Medicine of the National Academy of Science and won the J. D. Bruce Award for Distinguished Contributions in Preventive Medicine from the American College of Physicians, as well as the Wade Hampton Frost Award from the American Public Health Association for developing the field of Social Epidemiology. Len holds a Ph.D. in Medical Sociology from Yale University, following a B.A. and an M.A. in Anthropology and Sociology at UCLA.

Tess Thompson, M.P.H. received a master's degree in Victorian Literature from Oxford University and a master of Public Health at Washington University in St. Louis. She is currently a doctoral student in social work at Washington University in St. Louis, studying health behavior and the impact of family on health.

Sanjanthi Velu, Ph.D. has over 15 years of experience in developing and implementing integrated, strategic health communication programs in close collaboration with national programmatic goals and effective utilization of government resources, while engaging critical stakeholders, including end-audiences from conception to conclusion of programs. Sanjanthi's combined expertise in media, communications and public health have enabled her to assess capacity needs, strengthen capacities and provide technical assistance in public health communication. She has worked on issues ranging from HIV/AIDS prevention, stigma reduction, family planning, maternal and child health to water, sanitation and environmental conservation and has worked with many media formats, including electronic, print and traditional media, information communications technologies and offline strategies such as activations. As a journalist both in India and in the US, she has produced science, health, business and community news, documentary films and educational science videos. She currently serves as the country representative for JHU·CCP in India.

Hua Wang, Ph.D. is an Assistant Professor in the Department of Communication and Research Assistant Professor at the Department of Community Health and Health Behavior, University at Buffalo, The State University of New York. Her research interests include communication technologies, social networks, health promotion, and social change. She is particularly interested in the use of new media and communication networks to improve the well-being of individuals, communities, organizations, and societies at large. She has participated in interdisciplinary projects funded by the National Science Foundation, Robert Wood Johnson Foundation, Annenberg Foundation, and National Institutes of Health. Her work has been published in top journals such as *Communication Research*; *American Behavioral Scientist*; *Cyberpsychology, Behavior & Social Networking*; and *Journal of Medical Internet Research: Research Protocol*. Wang has presented her work in the United States, Canada, Germany, United Kingdom, Norway, Australia, Japan, Singapore, and Hong Kong.

Melinda R. Weathers, Ph.D. is an Assistant Professor in the Department of Communication Studies at Clemson University. Her scholarly interests include health communication, interpersonal communication, intercultural communication, new communication technologies/social media, gender communication, and qualitative research methods. Dr. Weathers' research has encompassed a range of topics addressing issues related to interpersonal and intercultural messages within relational, institutional, societal, and health contexts. Specifically, she has explored communication-related issues between doctors and patients, caregivers and older adults, and in heterosexual dating relationships. Ultimately, her research seeks to better understand how effective communication relates to the mental and physical health and well-being of persons and society. She has published in journals such as *Patient Education and Counseling, Journal of Participatory Medicine,* and *Communication Education.* Her research has been recognized through top paper awards from the National Communication Association and Central States Communication Association.

Pamela Whitten, Ph.D. enjoys an international reputation as a leading researcher in the field of telemedicine. Specifically, her research focuses on the use of technology in health care with a specific interest in telehealth and its impact on the delivery of health care services and education. Her intervention research projects range from telepsychiatry to telehospice and telehome care for COPD and CHF patients. In addition to her work assessing outcomes and impacts of telemedicine, she also conducts research that examines innovative uses of mediated communication to reach underserved populations, such as the creation of health websites for low literate adults. Her most recent work addresses the role of social media as a health communication intervention strategy.

Index

Accuracy 270, 275
Action research 338, 342, 348
Addiction 38
Aesthetic 137, 141, 145, 147
AIDS 244–245, 251, 253, 257–258
Asset-based approaches 177
Asthma 39
Audience segmentation 198

Behavior 319–320, 321, 323, 328
Biographic interview process 120, 123
Breast cancer 120–125, 128–130
Bridging individuals 157

Campaign case studies 28–30
Campaign design framework 13
Campaign effectiveness 28
Campaign limited effects 30
Campaign message framing 15
Campaign opportunities and barriers 13
Campaign resources 31
Cancer 320, 321, 326, 327, 328, 329
Catharsis 144 146–147
Change position 137
Civic education 203
Civic engagement 202
Climate change 191
Club risky business 83–96
Cognitive testing 324, 325, 326, 329
Collective narrative 124
Colon cancer 40
Communication 317, 319, 320, 321, 327, 328, 329
Communication in public health 103–106
Communication network analysis 153
Communication-persuasion matrix 14
Community 334, 336, 338, 339, 340, 344
Community-based prevention marketing 14
Composite stories 118
Comprehensivity 273, 275
Computer games messages 25
Conflict 138, 141–143, 146–147

Conversations About Cancer (CAC) 101–115
Critical mass 46
Crowdsourcing 69, 71, 72
Cultural & global adaptations 112–113
Cultural beacons 335, 336, 337, 338, 342, 344, 346
Cultural ecology 244–246, 255, 259
Cultural relevance 272, 275
Culturally embedded 335, 336, 339
Culture 265
Culture-centric approach 123, 126

Decision making 317
Demonstration 142, 146–147
Diffusion 154, 156, 187, 208, 210, 264
Digital games 67–76
Diverse 337, 344, 349
Drama 134–147

Eco, Umberto 271
Education 69, 73–74
Edutainment 102
EE development process 87–94
Entertainment Education 83–98
Environment 317, 318, 319, 320, 321, 329, 330
Epistemologies 336, 342
Ethics, of narratives 125
Evaluation 46
Exercise 69–70
Extended Elaboration Likelihood Model 119

Faith-based 244, 247, 250, 251, 256–259
False catharsis 144
Family communication 101–115
Firsthand experiential stories 118
Focus groups 43
Formative evaluation 15–17
Framing 195
Freire, Paulo 245, 249

Games for health 67
Gender analysis 244–245
Global Warming's Six Americas 198
Grassroots 335, 336, 338, 342, 347

Health communication 84
Health information 319, 320, 321, 328, 329
HIV 244–245, 251, 253, 257–258
HIV prevention 209, 214
Human health 191

Identification 119, 123, 126, 135, 138–141, 145–147
Informal opinion leaders 212
Informants' rating method 160
Innovation attributes 156
Interactivity, message 22
Internet 320, 321, 329
Internet messages 23
Intervention 334, 335, 337, 338, 347, 348
Invented stories 118

JHU-CCP 83–86, 98

Kato 75, 77

Lieberman 67–70, 73, 77
Local wisdom 335, 338, 342
Logo (health campaign) 262

McGonigal 68, 70, 72, 77
Media campaign length 27
Media campaign reach 26
Media dissemination factors 25–26
Media, mass and local 20–22
Media, online and digital applications 23
Media, online and digital attributes 22–23
Medical experts/Cancer professionals 113
Message testing 198
Messages, awareness 18
Messages, direct to goal audiences 17
Messages, five quality factors 19

Messages, indirect to interpersonal influencers 17
Messages, indirect to societal and organizational policymakers 18
Messages, instructional 18
Messages, persuasive 18
Messenger, source characteristics 20
·Mobile apps for health
  developing 60
  evaluating the use of 63
  examples of 54
  issues to address before using 64
MSM (men who have sex with men) 208
Mythical layer 138–139, 145, 147

Narrative (narrativity) 269, 274, 275
Narratives 118–127
Network centrality 166
Non-textocentric 337, 345

Observation method 162
Obstacles & solutions 114–115
Opinion Leaders 212
Opinion leadership 155
Overlooked indicators 335, 347

Participatory 336, 337, 338, 339, 342, 345
Participatory methods 245, 249, 250, 259
Persuasion 134, 135, 137, 155
Persuasive communication 135
Phase I Feasibility study 107–111
Phase II Dissemination and Effectiveness trial 111–112
Phone conversations 102
physical activity 69–70, 72
Platform Selection 41
Podcast messages 24
Popular opinion leaders 212
Population 318, 319, 320, 323, 326, 327, 328,
Positive deviance approach 174–189
  to combat malnutrition in Vietnam 177–180
  to reduce maternal and newborn mortality in Pakistan 181–186

as applied to formative research 174–176
and community participation 182
and self-discovery of PD practices 181, 184, 188
and acting One's Way 187
applications of 187
and differences with diffusion of innovations and social marketing 187
Precaution Adoption Process Model 120
Pre-production information gathering 16
Pretesting messages 16–17
Privacy 45
Process evaluation 27–28
Public awareness 194
Public engagement 195
Public health 317, 318, 319, 321, 327
Public health frame 196
Public health professionals 200
Public understanding of culture 265

Red-Ribbon 266
Rehearsal 69, 72
Research on 53
  steps for creating projects with 59
Research on 55
  steps for creating projects with 59
Rhetoric 135–137, 141, 145, 147
Rhetorical change model in drama 134, 144, 146–147

Self-designating method 162
Self-Determination Theory 40
Self-report 320, 323,
Semiotics 263, 267
Shannon & Weaver 271
Snowball method 161
Social Cognitive Theory 120
Social ecological framework 244, 246, 249, 259
Social influence 153, 287
Social marketing 208, 211, 214
Social marketing framework 14
Social media 45
Social media for health

developing 60
evaluating the use of 63
examples of initiatives in 56
issues to address before using 64
Social media messages 25
Social proof 176, 187
Social support 69–70
Sociometric method 160
Stakeholders 342, 344, 345
Storytelling 269
Strategic Integration 214
Summative evaluation 27–28
Survey 318, 319, 320, 322, 323, 324, 325, 326, 327, 329

Tailoring, message 22, 102–103, 107
Talkback sessions 107–108
Tanzania 251–253
Technical Brief 87–92
Texting messages 24
The Cancer Play 102, 110, 114, 115
The rhetoric of the aesthetic 145, 147
The spectator as ghostwriter 137, 145, 147
Theory 87–90
Theory of Reasoned Action 120
Transportation Imagery Model 119
Treatment 69, 74–75
Trends 319, 320, 324, 328,
TV drama 84, 85
Twitter messages 24

User-defined 335, 337

Validity 346 348

Web 2.0 messages 24
Website messages 23–24

Zambia 84, 89, 90, 92, 96

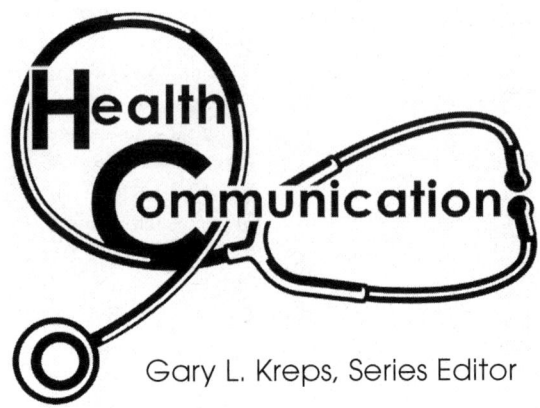

Gary L. Kreps, Series Editor

This series examines the powerful influences of human and mediated communication in delivering care and promoting health.

Books analyze the ways that strategic communication humanizes and increases access to quality care as well as examining the use of communication to encourage proactive health promotion. The books describe strategies for addressing major health issues, such as reducing health disparities, minimizing health risks, responding to health crises, encouraging early detection and care, facilitating informed health decisionmaking, promoting coordination within and across health teams, overcoming health literacy challenges, designing responsive health information technologies, and delivering sensitive end-of-life care.

All books in the series are grounded in broad evidence-based scholarship and are vivid, compelling, and accessible to broad audiences of scholars, students, professionals, and laypersons.

For additional information about this series or for the submission of manuscripts, please contact:

Gary L. Kreps
University Distinguished Professor and Chair, Department of Communication
Director, Center for Health and Risk Communication
George Mason University Science & Technology 2, Suite 230, MS 3D6
Fairfax, VA 22030-4444
gkreps@gmu.edu

To order other books in this series, please contact our Customer Service Department:

(800) 770-LANG (within the U.S.)
(212) 647-7706 (outside the U.S.)
(212) 647-7707 FAX

Or browse online by series:
www.peterlang.com